ADVANCES
IN SLEEP RESEARCH
Volume I

ADVANCES IN SLEEP RESEARCH

Volume I

Edited by Elliot D. Weitzman, M.D.

SP

SPECTRUM PUBLICATIONS, INC.
Flushing, New York

Distributed by Halsted Press
A Division of John Wiley & Sons
New York   Toronto   London   Sydney

Spectrum Publications, Inc.
75-31 192 Street, Flushing, New York 11366

Distributed solely by the Halsted Press Division of John Wiley & Sons, Inc., New York.

ISBN 0-470-93300-3

Library of Congress Catalog Card Number: 73-17440

Printed in the United States of America

Second Printing

Contributors

Edward O. Bixler, Ph.D.
Department of Psychiatry and Sleep
  Research and Treatment Facility,
Milton S. Hershey Medical Center
Pennsylvania State University
Hershey, Pennsylvania

Michael H. Chase, Ph.D.
Departments of Physiology and
  Anatomy and The Brain Research
  Institute,
University of California—
  Los Angeles
Los Angeles, California

William C. Dement, M.D., Ph.D
Department of Psychiatry and Sleep
  Disorders Clinic and Laboratory,
Stanford University School of Medi-
  cine
Stanford, California

Mary Fairbanks
Sepulveda Veterans Administration
  Hospital,
Los Angeles, California

Leonard Graziani, M.D.
Department of Pediatrics,
Jefferson Medical College
Philadelphia, Pennsylvania

Christian Guilleminault, M.D.
Department of Psychiatry and Sleep
  Disorders Clinic and Laboratory,
Stanford University School of Medi-
  cine
Stanford, California

Ronald M. Harper, Ph.D.
Sepulveda Veterans Administration
  Hospital and Department of Anat-
  omy,
University of California—
  Los Angeles
Los Angeles, California

J. Allan Hobson, M.D.
Department of Psychiatry,
Harvard Medical School
Boston, Masachusetts

Anthony Kales, M.D.
Department of Psychiatry and Sleep
  Research and Treatment Facility,
Milton S. Hershey Medical Center
Pennsylvania State University
Hershey, Pennsylvania

Joyce D. Kales, M.D.
Department of Psychiatry and Sleep
  Research and Treatment Facility,
Milton S. Hershey Medical Center
Pennsylvania State University
Hershey, Pennsylvania

Daniel F. Kripke, M.D.
Department of Psychiatry,
University of California—San Diego
  and Veterans Administration
  Hospital
San Diego, California

Dennis J. McGinty, Ph.D.
Sepulveda Veterans Administration
  Hospital and Department of Psy-
  chology,
University of California—
  Los Angeles
Los Angeles, California

Peter J. Morgane, Ph.D.
Laboratory of Neurophysiology,
Worcester Foundation for Experi-
  mental Biology
Shrewsbury, Massachusetts

Warren C. Stern, Ph.D.
Laboratory of Neurophysiology,
Worcester Foundation for Experi-
  mental Biology
Shrewsbury, Massachusetts

Edward S. Tauber, M.D.
Department of Psychology,
Yeshiva University, Departments of
  Psychiatry and Neurology, Mon-
  tefiore Hospital and Medical
  Center and Fellow of the William
  Alanson White Institute of Psy-
  chiatry
New York, N.Y.

Elliot D. Weitzman, M.D.
Department of Neurology,
Montefiore Hospital and Medical
  Center and Albert Einstein Col-
  lege of Medicine
Bronx, New York

Preface

The past 20 years have been extraordinarily productive ones in the area of sleep research. We have accumulated much observational and experimental data and have thereby elaborated many new insights and challenging concepts. However, with this explosive research effort, there is also a need for thoughtful, critical analysis. The introduction of this first volume of "Advances in Sleep Research" is an attempt to supply, in part, a forum for such critical reviews.

The field of sleep research has been a very fruitful and exciting one, to a large extent because of a multi-disciplinary approach. The meetings of the Sleep Society have provided a forum for direct intellectual communication and challenge across disciplines ranging from biochemistry, cellular neurophysiology, pharmacology and general physiology to biological rhythm research, ontogeny and phylogeny. In addition, psychological, neurologic, psychiatric and other clinical medical disciplines have been an active and important aspect of the field. In that same spirit, I have invited critical summaries and reviews across a broad spectrum of research areas from individuals directly involved in their areas of review. The papers in this first volume do not cover the full range of areas of sleep research, however, it is planned to include critical reviews of most of the important areas of sleep in subsequent volumes.

Elliot D. Weitzman, M.D.

November, 1973

Contents

CONTENTS

ADVANCES IN SLEEP RESEARCH
Volume I

Advances in Sleep Research, Vol. 1
© 1974, Spectrum Publications, Inc.

CHAPTER 1

Chemical Anatomy of Brain Circuits in Relation to Sleep and Wakefulness

PETER J. MORGANE
WARREN C. STERN

I. GENERAL INTRODUCTION

There is little doubt that the dramatic emergence of biochemical neuroanatomy has resulted in a significant merging of pharmacology, physiology, and biochemistry so that a new level of understanding of the organization of the nervous system is being achieved. The study of brain pathways, many of them previously unsuspected, based on the presence of specific chemical substances, presumably transmitters elaborated by these neurons, has opened up new vistas well beyond imagination just a few years ago.

Some questions we propose to discuss in this review, among others, are whether there is approximate congruity between histofluorescence and anatomical boundaries and how brain areas, coded as to their chemical anatomy, relate to nonfluorescing nuclear areas of the brainstem (previously identified by cytoarchitectonic analyses) and to various fiber systems. Terminological problems have been a major stumbling block in this area as many reticular structures go by eponymic names and purely topographical (e.g., latero-dorsal, medio-lateral, etc.) designations. Further, the correspondences, or homologies, of well known brain areas and fiber systems with fluorescing areas have not been worked out with any degree of precision. If chemical morphology is going to help unravel brain relations and functions then we must translate it into a more precise topographic reference, relate chemical systems to other non-chemically identified areas and, perhaps, place its formations into stereotaxic coordinates so that they can be manipulated by conventional physiological techniques.

Any attempt to study the various neural systems subserving the states of vigilance must take into account the architecture of morphological substrata, comprised of diverse neural subsystems, which overlap neural fields long related to the regulation of sleep-waking cycles. The elucidation of the anatomical underpinnings subserving sleep-waking states and other behaviors received its greatest impetus with the development of fluorescence histochemical techniques with which, for the first time, it has been possible to directly identify neural cellular assemblies and pathways on the basis of their transmitter chemistry, i.e., chemical neuroanatomy. This type of morphological analysis developed at a most opportune time since various attempts, using pharmacological and lesion approaches, were being made to correlate brain chemistry and behavior. Hence, direct visualization of transmitter substances within specific neuronal assemblies, i.e., direct visualization at a cellular level, was a significant advance. Application of histofluorescence methods allowed for the derivation of entirely new maps of the brain and identified neural pathways not previously seen by conventional anatomical studies. For example, the amine-containing neurons form systems of small diameter fibers with diffuse terminal distribution, and these do not often correspond to recognized ascending and descending pathways. Hence, there is some question whether most of these chemical pathways have ever really been seen at all by studies of normal anatomy or those using silver degeneration techniques. It is, thus, likely that the technique of fluorescence histochemistry has demonstrated neuronal cells and pathways that were previously unrecognized by all conventional methods of neuroanatomy. Nevertheless, using these techniques, various poorly understood areas of the brain, especially the reticular formation, have acquired histochemical specificity, whereas previously it had been a vast area defying orderly subdivision, and difficult to manipulate physiologically with any confidence of approaching exact structures in a repeatable fashion.

Of particular interest, of course, is that many of these neural areas, now identifiable by transmitter histochemical approaches, are composed of regions where manipulations had previously been shown to affect the vigilance states. Hence, a knowledge of the anatomical organization of chemically coded neurons is a prerequisite for any firm elucidation of the role of brain areas in the sleep-waking cycle, and, especially, for attempting to correlate chemical changes in the brain with the vigilance states. In this review, we will concentrate on the study of those chemical systems whose organization has been charted in some detail, i.e., the monoaminergic and cholinergic systems and relate these, as precisely as possible, to neural areas where physiological studies have indicated involvement of these regions in sleep-waking activity. It should be emphasized that concentration on monoaminergic and cholinergic systems should not be taken to indicate that other putative neurotransmitters do not also play important roles. However, at present, there is limited knowledge concerning the topography of neurons containing histamine, gamma-aminobutyric acid (GABA), glycine, glutamic acid, etc. No doubt, in time, when these systems are better known, they too can be worked into a general chemical schema of control of the arousal continuum. Since the anatomical organization of chemical circuits is of paramount importance for understanding the possible role of monoamines and acetylcholine in the regulation of sleep-waking behavior, the details of topography of these chemical systems will be discussed, especially in relation to known anatomical areas and fiber systems. It is well to point out that most of the histofluorescence tracing of chemical systems in the brain has been done in the rat, whereas the cat has been the animal most commonly used for studies of sleep-waking behavior. What is known about differences in chemical anatomy of the cat, and other species, especially the monkey, will be mentioned in the discussion below, where appropriate. This approach is obviously needed in considering the possible underlying causes of species differences in normal sleep-waking cycles and in following pharmacological and other manipulations.

II. CHEMICAL NEUROANATOMY

The important work of the Swedish group dealing with histofluorescence mapping of chemical pathways in the brain has been of inestimable value in developing correlations between morphology, physiology, brain chemistry, and behavior. This group has primarily confined themselves to studies of monoamine systems and have shown that there exist two distinctly different types of neurons which contain in their cell bodies and processes concentrations of primary catecholamine (dopamine or norepinephrine) and indoleamine (serotonin), respectively. Most importantly, they have traced axonal processes from these cell bodies and shown that these give rise to monoamine-containing synaptic terminals in which the catecholamines and serotonin are accumulated in very high concentrations. One of the most important aspects of the histofluorescence mapping technique is that it has allowed chemical neuronal systems to be traced continuously from the lower brainstem to forebrain areas, the many implications of which we will develop in detail below. Although the monoamine-containing nerve cells have a wide-spread distribution within the lower brainstem it has been difficult to systematize them on account of quite scanty knowledge as to what functional or anatomical systems they might belong. The fact that these chemical systems overlap morphological areas which, when lesioned or stimulated, affect the sleep states, has led to their direct implication in sleep-waking behavior, especially when it developed that these manipulations affecting sleep were correlated with specific changes in amine levels in brain areas to which these chemical neurons project. Obviously, there is a great necessity to precisely localize transmitter substances in the brain before endeavoring to understand such complex phenomena as sleep, arousal, sexual activity, etc., all of which are dependent on synaptic linkages whose transmitters can now be studied histochemically, physiologically, and pharmacologically. In this context, identification of the neurons responsible for the biosynthesis and storage of monoamines is clearly essential to any understanding of the functional role of these biologically active substances in the central nervous system.

As is well known, it is likely that several chemical substances are involved in synaptic transmission in the mammalian central nervous system. The Falck-Hillarp technique (1962) has demonstrated norepinephrine, dopamine, and serotonin within nerve cell bodies and terminals and the belief that these amines act as neurohumors is strengthened by observations that activation of nerve fibers leads to their release from the terminals. Since histochemical evidence suggests that discrete systems of neurons are identifiable by their content of particular amines, it seems likely that such neurohumorally homogeneous systems may well have a functional, as well as a chemical, identity. Chemical neuroanatomy makes use of the histochemical for-maldehyde fluorescence method of Falck et al. (1962). This method is based on the fact that certain monoamines like dopamine, norepinephrine, and serotonin, on reaction with formaldehyde vapor, are converted to fluorescent isoquinolines (derived from dopamine and norepinephrine) or beta-carbolines (from serotonin), which can be directly visualized in a fluorescence microscope (Corrodi and Jonsson, 1967). The method is considered highly specific and sensitive and it has been calculated that only about 4×10^{-16} g of norepinephrine is necessary to obtain a reaction product visible in the microscope provided the amount is concentrated in a small volume such as in a varicosity of a nerve terminal (Jonsson, 1971). With the help of such highly sensitive and specific histochemical fluorescence methods it has been possible to study the precise cellular localization of monoamines in the nervous system as well as plot the trajectory of their processes. In the mammalian brain norepinephrine and serotonin have been found to be accumulated in high concentrations within the fine, varicose, terminal parts of the nerve fibers, with lesser concentrations in the cell bodies and axons. The axons of neurons usually have concentrations of monoamines that are too low to be seen distinctly. However, these can usually be brought out either by axotomy, following which there is a buildup of transmitters in the proximal stump of the axon, or by use of monoamine oxidase inhibitors which prevent enzymatic destruction of monoamines.

Björklund, et al. (1971a) have emphasized that fluorescence histochemistry of biogenic monoamines is a very sensitive, precise, and versatile method which has proved extremely useful not only for mor-phological studies but also in pharmacological and physiological research. However, a critical point in all these studies is the actual identification of the fluorogenic compound, i.e., the compound that yields fluorescence after formaldahyde gas treatment. Thus, final identification of a fluorogenic compound requires a direct characterization of its fluorophore. For this reason microspectrofluorimetry is now considered indispensible for con-firmatory identifications in monoamine histochemistry. This is discussed in more detail with reference to several fluorescing systems of neurons identified by the Björkland group (1971a) and Aghajanian and Asher (1971) in the section immediately following the review of chemical circuits and areas.

III. THE CONCEPT OF THE RETICULAR CORE SYSTEM
(FORMATION) OF THE BRAINSTEM

To understand the immense significance currently attributed to the reticular formation in the total activity of the brain requires a precise description of its finer structural peculiarities and an exact as possible definition of this core complex as an anatomical and physiological concept. At present there is no overall agreement even on the criteria for determining which brain structures are to be considered as part of this system. However, in this section several of these possible criteria will be discussed and the concept of the reticular formation will be extended considerably beyond its classical confines.

As is well know, it has been customary to epitomize neuroanatomical data as a series of circuits that presumably represent those lines of communication, cell sequences, and synapses over which information is most likely to flow, i.e., in one sense the pathway becomes the message. It is necessary now to look at the profusion of neurochemically discrete subsystems that have recently been identified in the reticular core of the brainstem in relation to classical anatomical areas described and defined by older anatomical techniques. The Golgi method, as far as is known, is entirely silent on the chemical nature of the neural ground, but has been the method *par excellence* for unraveling many of the intricacies of the reticular fields. Degeneration methods, such as the classical Nauta procedure and its variations (Fink-Heimer method, etc.), and studies of normal material (myelin stains, cell stains, etc.), have all been of more limited, albeit complementary, value in this regard. Recently, radioautographic techniques have been applied to study the reticular areas since fibers of passage do not confound   the interpretations when this method is used. Naturally, combinations of all of these methods, each with its own unique advantages, offer the best opportunity for shedding light on the organization of the reticular formation. Thus, modern anatomical redefinition of the reticular formation,   in terms of Golgi analysis, dendritic pattern resolution, and, especially, the newer histofluorescence chemical codings and delineation of chemical systems, has provided a structural substrate within which an otherwise diverse mass of neurophysiological data may now be better assessed. The concept of the "isodendritic core" (see below) has led to an expansion of the older view of the reticular formation so that it now extends from the reticular core and spinal cord to the basal telencephalon and, perhaps, even into the cerebral cortex. Also, the work of the Scheibels (1970) has clearly indicated a bilaminar projection of reticular axons into the forebrain with the ventral lamella, or extrathalamic by-pass (via the zona incerta), terminating within the septal area and basal forebrain zones. This will be discussed further below.

The reticular formation of the lower brainstem is most logically the point of initial discussion of the neural substrata of the vigilance states. Classically, this area has been most associated with the arousal continuum dating from the experiments of Moruzzi and Magoun (1949), and before. Thus, in our discussion we will first define and delimit it and discuss its special characteristics before attempting to parcellate it into neurocytological elements whose processes we will trace into the basal forebrain and cerebral cortex. There is little question, then, that the beginnings of analysis of the multiple circuitries concerned with sleep-waking behavior should logically be the reticular formation. As Ramón-Moliner and Nauta (1966) have pointed out, one can accept neither the amalgamation of a number of physiological properties on the basis of an assumed unitary morphology nor, conversely, an assembling of anatomical regions on the basis of an assumed common physiological role. It has for some time been assumed that the generalized dendritic pattern is a cardinal identifying characteristic of the reticular formation. Of course, one can question whether dendritic peculiarities, alone or in combination with other histological properties, can be regarded as valid criteria in the conceptualization of the reticular formation. Ramón-Moliner and Nauta have proposed the term "isodendritic core" to define the vast region which extends throughout the brainstem and spinal cord, forming a matrix in which other cell groups, with more specialized dendritic features, lie embedded. The generalized dendritic patterns are usually found in cells having polygonal cell bodies, with irregularly dispersed Nissl bodies. In general, it appears to be that cytological polymorphism is one of the very striking features of the isodendritic core of the brainstem. Further, Mannen (1960) has stressed that a close commingling of passing fibers and dendrites can be considered a major feature of the core of the lower brainstem. Ramón-Moliner and Nauta have reiterated, however, that this is by no means a peculiar feature of that lower brainstem core, since the deeper layers of the cerebral cortex, reticular nucleus of the thalamus, subthalamus, zona incerta, and certain intralaminar nuclei of the thalamus are examples of the same type of histological configuration. Of course, if these areas are all considered as forebrain extensions of the reticular core, then Mannen's criterion can be accepted. In this same vein, Nauta and Haymaker (1969) have pointed out that the septal area, especially its medial, relatively magnocellular, component also exhibits a dendritic configuration and relationship of dendrites to passing fiber bundles entirely comparable to those found in the brainstem reticular formation and hypothalamus.

Leontovich and Zhukova (1963) include within the reticular formation the raphé nuclei, the central gray, the nucleus tegmenti pontis of Bechterew, nucleus of the solitary tract, vestibular nuclei, the entire substantia nigra, the parafascicular and reticular thalamic nuclei, the nucleus ventralis anterior, nucleus anteromedialis, nucleus paracentralis, nucleus centralis medialis, nucleus centralis lateralis, nuclear medialis dorsalis, nucleus medialis ventralis, the midline and commissural nuclei, the lateral habenular nucleus, the whole subthalamus or ventral thalamus (zona incerta), the ventral part of the lateral geniculate nucleus, the fields of Forel, parts of the hypothalamus and preoptic area as well as the pallidum, the area diagonalis with its anterior pole extending into the septal area (bed nucleus of anterior commissure), stria terminalis and substantia innominata. All are brain regions characterized by afferent connections of heterogeneous origin. Thus, according to this concept, the reticular formation stretches as an uninterrupted cell column throughout the brainstem and extends to the diencephalon and the basal regions of the telencephalon and, perhaps, beyond.

From classical anatomy it has long been known that the lateral zone of the hypothalamus is directly continuous with the ventral tegmental area of Tsai, an ill defined cell territory in turn laterally continuous with the so called deep tegmental nucleus (Gudden), which extends lateralward over the substantia nigra. Further, the medial and periventricular zones of the hypothalamus—in particular, the posterior hypothalamic nucleus—merge with the periaqueductal gray substance of the midbrain. Hence, the hypothalamus is considered as part of a neural continuum or extension of the reticular core from the midbrain forward. Whether or not one chooses to designate the forebrain continuum, along with the remainder of the brainstem tegmentum, as *reticular formation*, depends on the interpretation given to the latter term. From a histological point of view, it is justifiable to consider the hypothalamus as highly comparable to those mesencephalic and bulbar regions which are held to represent brainstem reticular formation. Thus, the hypothalamus shares with the major part of the bulbar and mesencephalic tegmentum the following characteristics: 1) neurons of the isodendritic type, i.e., having long, rectilinear and sparsely branching dendrites; 2) widely overlapping dendritic fields; and 3) a free mingling of dendrites with fascicles of axons in transit. If the reticular formation implies heterogeneity of afferent connections, then certainly the hypothalamus and its extensions into the forebrain would fall under this categorization. It might be well to emphasize that the medial forebrain bundle, the principal forebrain fiber system in this complex, is composed, in part, of relatively short neural links but the system is also pervaded with longer axonal conduction routes (Valverde, 1965).

In this review we would stress that the hypothalamus is directly continuous with the vast "nonspecific" neuronal apparatus of the brainstem reticular formation and should be considered a direct extension of it. Nauta and Haymaker (1969) point out that the hypothalamus could, in fact, be regarded as the ventro-medial part of a more generalized "nonspecific" diencephalic apparatus which extends the mesencephalic reticular formation rostralwards and encompasses, in addition, the so called nonspecific thalmic cell group and the subthalamic region. From this it can be seen that the subthalamus is also regarded as a direct rostral extension of the mesencephalic tegmentum.

Some examples of morphological specifics are of interest here relative to characteristics of the reticular formation, especially its relation to the raphé complex (see below) and other brainstem areas related to sleep-waking behavior. Thus, Ramón-Moliner and Nauta have shown that the average dendritic length found in the reticular continuum is well over 300 microns. For example, in their Golgi-stained material, they have seen neurons of the raphé nuclei which emit dendrites extending bilaterally as far as the magnocellular portion of the trigeminal nucleus. Further, some dendrites of the dorsal motor nucleus of the vagus overlap with those of the solitary tract and the latter nucleus has dendrites entering the area postrema (Morest, 1960). These are examples of special morphological characteristics that may relate to sleep-waking behavior since the solitary tract and the area postrema appear to be EEG synchronizing structures (Bronzino et al., 1972).

A wide variety of data makes it obvious that we are not dealing with a unitary concept of the reticular formation and this broader view then necessitates consideration of connectivity and nuclear specializations of relevance when one examines the necessity of accurately reporting the location of electrodes, lesions, fields of axonal distribution, etc. It should be stressed that there is not one single histological feature which can be attributed to the reticular formation which cannot also be found in other regions of the nervous system. This includes the consideration that the reticular formation consists largely of 'cells with axons that divide into ascending and descending branches and the concept that reticular axons are characterized by a richness of their collateralization. Thus, the heterogeneous nature of the afferent supply to its constituent cells might appear to be the most typical of all its attributes, but even that is shared with other neural territories as, for example, the superior colliculus. In the context of the present review, it is then to be noted that one of the ways of circumscribing specialized areas within the reticular formation is by use of histochemical techniques identifying amine-specific neurons on the basis of their presumed neurotransmitter agents. Therefore, as emphasized below, circumlineation along the entire trajectory of neurons lying in special fields in the reticular formation is now possible based on their chemical identification and profiling heretofore unseen systems against the dark background of neuropil of this complex area.

With the above in mind, the reticular formation may generally be defined as an extensive neural territory displaying, in Golgi-stained material, a relatively uniform histological appearence as follows: 1) generalized dendrites—these are long, radiating and relatively rectilinear processes arborizing in such a manner that the distal segments are generally longer than the proximal ones; 2) polymorphism of its cytological units—various sized neurons are found side by side and their dendritic trees show a wide diversity in overall profuseness of ramifications; 3) considerable degree of dendritic overlapping—as a result of the generally great length attained by the dendrites, and their rectilinear course, a continuum of overlapping dendritic fields is formed that extends throughout the length of the neuraxis; 4) apparent lack of distinctive regional dendritic characteristics; and 5) free intermingling of dendrites and passing myelinated and unmyelinated fiber bundles—in this latter regard, the dendrites of the reticular core (including its redefined extensions) differ markedly from those of most other cell regions.

Thus, from the above, even though the reticular formation is "diffuse" and its boundries quite "ill defined", it may still be looked at morphologically as a unitary concept, i.e., all of the above-mentioned attributes taken together describe a type of neural tissue that is present throughout the length of the core of the brainstem. Since similar coincidences of attributes have now been identified as extending forward into the diencephalon and basal forebrain areas , this simply means that these comparable neural formations represent extensions of the reticular formation further forward in the brain than was originally conceived. To extend this somewhat farther, it is noted that Bishop (1958) even regarded areas of the cortex as a variety of reticular formation.

In summary, the reticular core is made up of polysynaptic and even monosynaptic pathways from the bulbar, pontine, and mesencephalic reticular formations down to the cord or up to the thalamus, subthalamus, and hypothalamus, and, most importantly, some reticular fibers from the pontine and mesencephalic tegmentum project directly to the corpus striatum, septal area, basal forebrain area, and cortex. Golgi material conclusively indicates that the brainstem reticular core is not characterized simply by chains of short-axoned cells but rather contains numerous long axons of fine caliber and circuitous pathways are made by the innumerable collaterals of the long reticular fibers.

IV. THE NONSPECIFIC THALAMIC SYSTEM

As soon as the concept of a "reticular ascending activating system" was proposed by Moruzzi and Magoun (1949) it was hypothesized that the "diffuse" thalamo-cortical projections might also play a critical role in the generation of EEG arousal patterns. From many of these earlier studies Hunter and Jasper (1949) developed the term "thalamic reticular system" and many investigators thought of this as the cephalic end of the reticular activating or "waking" system.

It is well established that a reticulo-thalamo-cortical system plays a significant role in arousal, alerting, and attention. High-frequency stimulation of the mesencephalic reticular formation of the midline, so-called non-specific thalamic nuclei, will arouse a sleeping animal or alert a waking animal and cause desynchronization or activation of ongoing electrocortical activity. Conversely, low-frequency stimulation of the midline thalamic nuclei produces inattention, drowsiness, and sleep, and is associated with slow waves and spindle bursts in the EEG. Repetitive stimulation of midline and intralaminar nonspecific thalamic nuclei at a rate in the frequency range of spontaneous synchronized activity gives rise to recruiting responses, comprised of incrementing waves of synchronized activity.

It is essential in considering the neural circuits concerned with the states of vigilance, that the structural organization of the nonspecific thalamic nuclei and their projections to the neocortical formations be discussed in the context of this entire system, being an extension of the reticular formation. There is now good evidence that the anterior half of the medial thalamic fields projects indirectly to the cortex. The posterior third of the system, especially the centre median-parafascicular complex, appears to project no further than the caudate and putamen. Many electrophysiological studies have been instrumental in establishing the existence of a thalamo-cortical mechanism, based in the non-specific nuclear mass and characterized by the dispersion of incrementing amplitude, long latency negative waves upon the cortex following stimulation almost anywhere within the thalamic fields. Elicitation of this cortical recruitment phenomenon thus quite early became the paradigm of non-specific activity. The studies of Schlag and Chaillet (1963) and Weinberger et al. (1965) first showed that the pathway for transmission of thalamically induced cortical activation could be functionally dissected from that of cortical hypersynchrony. This is considered in more detail below.

The Scheibels (1967), in particular, using Golgi techniques, have attempted to develop morphological information about the thalamic non-specific system and to extract certain circuit paradigms which may be considered as substrate characteristic of intralaminar mechanisms. They have stressed general features of the field structure of the midline thalamic nuclear areas which seem common to the entire complex. It is well to note at the beginning that the terms "non-specific", "diffuse", and "intralaminar" are used interchangeably to denote the same thalamic field complex. These areas encompass that system of fields occupying the medial one-third of the dorsal thalamus and are characterized anatomically by radiative dendritic neuropil and heterogeneously converging (so called "nonpatterned") presynaptic afferents. As noted, these fields truly represent extensions of the lower brainstem reticular formation.

As to architecture, neurons of most of this thalamic nonspecific system resemble those of the reticular formation of the brainstem in that they are multipolar, variable in size and shape, and characterized by some variation of the dendrite pattern which can be described as radiating, poorly ramified, and spine-bearing. Afferents to this system from more caudal brainstem levels are largely, though not completely, represented by 1) the spinothalamic, and 2) the system of ascending reticular axons. The spinothalamic tract innervates a large portion of the posterior pole of the diencephalon including the posterior nucleus, parts of the ventro-basal complex of the thalamus and large portions of the posterior lateral intralaminar system, as well as the entire substance of the brainstem reticular core. Also, masses of fine collaterals leave the spinothalamic tract at or near the diencephalic border and strongly infiltrate the entire posterior half of the non-specific thalamic field.

The concept that the nonspecific nuclei of the thalamus play an important role in development of high amplitude, low-frequency, "synchronized" activity on the cortex, in the form of spindles, recruiting, or augmenting responses, has received a great deal of experimental support since the original observations of Morison and Dempsey (1943). Currently this concept states that a group of thalamic nuclei, termed "non-specific" nuclei, act as a unified whole in synchronizing activity over widespread cortical areas through their diffuse cortical projections. How these cortical projections are affected will be discussed below. The non-specific nuclei to which we refer include those of the midline (centralis medialis nucleus, rhomboidalis nucleus, reuniens nucleus), intralaminar (centralis lateralis nucleus, paracentralis nucleus, centrum medianum-parafascicularis nucleus) and remaining paramedian nuclei (ventralis anterior nucleus, reticular nucleus, ventralis medialis nucleus, submedius nucleus). Various workers consider other subdivisions of the midline thalamic areas as part of these three groups but a detailed discussion of this is beyond the scope of the present review. With regard to the organization in both specific and non-specific thalamic fields from the comparative morphological point of view, the jump in circuit complexity from the rat to the most usually utilized recording subjects—cats and monkeys—seems to involve several orders of magnitude. The comparison problem of species differences must always be entertained. For example, there is virtual absence of the centre median component of the centre median-parafascicular complex in mice and rats which undergoes rapid development from cat to monkey to man.

The relationship of ascending reticular fibers to the thalamus has been described in some detail by the Scheibels (1958, 1966, 1967, 1970). Examination of sagitally sectioned Golgi material at the mesodiencephalic level shows a splitting of the main current of fibers from the brainstem reticular core just posterior to the centre median-parafascicular complex. The long ascending fibers of the brainstem reticular formation that bifurcate (see Figs. 1 and 2) send a powerful ventral division through the zona incerta to the anterior thalamus, septum, and basal forebrain areas. This more ventral branch of the reticular bifurcation proceeds through the subthalamus with one or more branches continuing rostrad in the zona incerta. Many of these axons continue in the subthalamus and finally enter the septum and basal olfactory area. The dorsal division of this bifurcating reticular stream projects through the intralaminar system as far rostral as the dorsomedial nucleus, the reticular nucleus, and the striatum. The dorsal contingent of axons can be followed into the intralaminar fields as well as the posterior-ventral portion of the dorsomedial nucleus, the fibers from this system collateralizing widely throughout these areas. Via this system synaptic drive of reticular origin is spread broadly over an extensive thalamic field including both the specific thalamic nuclei and the intralaminar groups. It should also be noted that even so-called specific thalamic nuclei, such as those of the ventro-basal complex, receive synaptic contributions from ascending reticular components. The centre median-parafascicular complex signifies that fiber-cell field which is the most posterior component of the thalamic intralaminar system and which centers about the descending fibers of the habenulo-interpeduncular tract. The neurons of the centre median-parafascicular complex are characterized by a multipolar "reticular" configuration, lack of obvious dendritic orientation, and a range of cell body sizes from moderately large to small. Very little dendritic specialization is seen. There is a powerful axon system from the intralaminar fields that plays back upon the posterior thalamus and midbrain reticular formation and the Scheibels, using Golgi analysis, have clearly shown that a very large number of intralaminar thalamic cells project caudally in this recurrent path (Figs. 1 and 2).

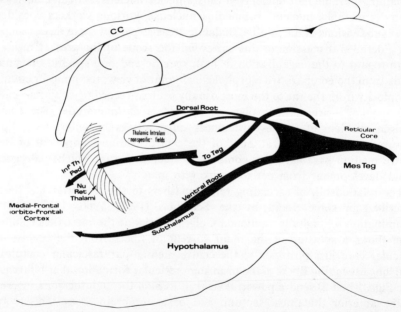

Fig. 1. Diagram of projection pathways of the brainstem reticular core. From the reticular core system, ascending through the mesencephalic tegmentum (Mes Teg), two major non-specific pathways diverge, forming a dorsal root and ventral root. The dorsal root projects primarily to the thalamic intralaminar ("nonspecific") and dorso-medial fields and regathers into pathways that pierce the reticular nucleus of the thalamus (Nu Ret Thalami) to form the inferior thalamic peduncle (Inf Th Ped), in turn, projecting to the basal forebrain/orbito-frontal area. From the dorsal nonspecific system a recurrent bundle projects back into the mesencephalic reticular core. The ventral root projects ventral and lateral through the sub-thalamus and hypothalamus, eventually entering the basal forebrain area including the or-bito-frontal fields. Other Abbreviation: CC = .corpus callosum (adapted from the Scheibels, 1967).

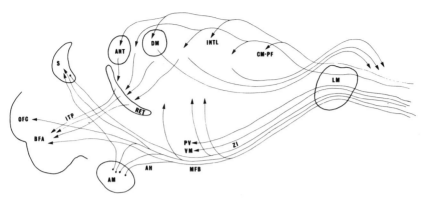

Fig. 2. Schematic representation of ascending reticular system projecting, in part, through and near the limbic midbrain area (LM) and then bifurcating, just posterior to the centre median-parafascicular thalamic nuclear complex (CM-PF), into a dorsal leaf (which is shown entering the CM-PF complex), intralaminar nuclei (INTL), dorso-medial thalamic nuclei (DM), and anterior thalamic area (ANT), and a ventral leaf projecting rostrally via the zona incerta (ZI) and medial forebrain bundle system (MFB). Note that from the dorsal leaf dispersions of fibers regather to pass through the reticular thalamic nucleus (RET) and, from there, form the inferior thalamic peduncle (ITP) passing into the basal forebrain area (BFA). Components of the ventral leaf leave the MFB in a dorso-lateral trajectory to enter many of the midline thalamic fields while others enter the periventricular (PV) and ventro-medial (VM) hypothalamic areas. Also shown in this figure are projections from the amygdaloid complex (AM) which join the MFB, via the direct amygdalo-hypothalamic projections (AH), and which also pass to the septal area (S). Note also projections from the MFB to the orbito-frontal cortex (OFC).

There are also descending afferents from more rostral brain centers approaching the non-specific thalamic fields primarily via two routes: 1) from the region of the basal forebrain area via the inferior thalamic radiation; and 2) from the hypothalamus via an extensive collateral system from the medial forebrain bundle complex (Figs. 2 and 3). There is little doubt that the fibers which enter the anterior pole of the thalamus via the inferior thalamic radiation are largely derived from orbito-frontal cortex. The collateral system, which ascends from fibers coursing caudally in the medial forebrain bundle, originates in large part from the basal forebrain area as well as the region anterior and ventral to the anterior commissure, and from the olfactory bulb and tract, orbital cortex, hippocampal formation and amygdaloid complex.

As noted, the most obvious feature of axons of the thalamic non-specific system is multiple branching and collateralization, an organizational pattern similar to that of axons of the neurons of the lower brainstem reticular core. In general, non-specific conductors appear organized to achieve maximal divergence of information within and outside of the intralaminar system. Characteristically, axons from many intralaminar cells quickly divide into long rostral and caudally coursing components, the former generally running rostro-laterad and either dorsad or ventrad, depending on the orientation of the field. The majority of such fibers appear to join the internal capsule and project at least as far as the basal ganglia. The caudally coursing components of intralaminar cells typically run posteriorly and medially, either reentering a more posterior thalamic non-specific area, or continuing back into the the mesencephalic tegmentum (Fig. 2). The axons from the anterior non-specific fields continue rostrally in the inferior thalamic peduncle. These bundles can be followed through the medial part of the caudate nucleus close to the

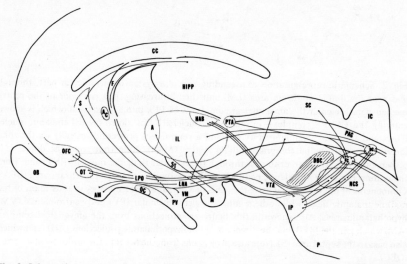

Fig. 3. Schematic representation of reciprocity of connection between basal forebrain/limbic forebrain fields and limbic midbrain area. This reciprocity of connections is mediated largely via the medial forebrain bundle passing through the lateral preoptic area (LPO) and lateral hypothalamic area (LHA). Rostrally the dispersions of the medial forebrain bundle systems enter the septal area (S), orbit-frontal cortex (OFC), olfactory tubercle (OT) and components of the amygdaloid complex (AM). Both caudally and rostrally directed components of the medial forebrain bundle pass somewhat dorso-laterally in its diencephalic trajectory to enter the intralaminar thalamic fields (IL). Offshoots from the medial forebrain bundle enter the subthalamus (ST) and some components of the bundle pass in the ventral subthalamic area. Medial forebrain bundle components also enter the preiventricular (PV) and ventro-medial (VM) zones of the hypothalamus. This figure shows the well-developed fibers entering and leaving the limbic midbrain zone which comprises, in part, the dorsal (DG) and ventral (VG) nuclei of Gudden and the nucleus centralis superior of Bechterew (NCS). Note the numerous fibers from this area entering and passing in close proximity to the interpeduncular nucleus (IP), mainly via the ventral tegmental area of Tsai (VTA). Many of these fibers run in the narrow space between the mammillary body (M) and the substantia nigra (not shown on this figure). Other pathways shown in this figure run in the periaqueductal gray (PAG) to the posterior thalamic area (PTA), between the habenular nuclear complex (HAB) to the interpeduncular nucleus and nucleus centralis superior of Bechterew; also note fornix (F) projections to the hypothalamus, and projections from the mammillary body (M) to the anterior thalamic nuclei (A). Other Abbreviations: IC = inferior colliculus; SC = superior colliculus; DBC = decussation of the brachium conjunctivum; HIPP = hippocampus; CC = corpus callosum; AC = anterior commissure; OB = olfactory bulb; OC = optic chiasm; P = pons.

lateral ventricle and appear to occupy, in the cat, the most antero-medial portion of the internal capsule. These axons of the inferior thalamic peduncle can be traced to the deepest layers of the orbito-frontal cortex (Fig. 2).

The Scheibels (1958, 1966) have stressed structural similarities between axons of the thalamic non-specific neurons and those of the brainstem reticular core. However, they have also noted one outstanding difference between the rostral projections of these two axonal groups, i.e., all of these thalamically derived fibers pass through the nucleus reticularis thalami while brainstem reticular axons, swinging ventrally through zona incerta and hypothalamus (ventral limb of reticular bifurcation), avoid this field entirely (Figs. 1 and 2). They have observed that the nucleus reticularis thalami (Fig. 1) is a sheet-like nuclear complex surrounding the lateral and anterior borders of the thalamus and has, until recently, been considered a final common pathway on the route from non-specific systems in the thalamus to the cortex. However, Golgi preparations clearly show that the vast majority of reticularis-cell axons project caudally upon the thalamus and upper brainstem rather than rostrally upon the neocortex. As noted by the Scheibels, virtually all specific and non-specific thalamo-cortical systems perforate the nucleus reticularis on their rostral path. With regard to their chemical anatomy, the thalamic systems and nuclei are discussed in the cholinergic section (below). Suffice it to note here that the uneven distribution of cholinesterase can now be used as a criterion to delineate more precisely anatomical subdivisions within the thalamus.

Thalamic Physiology

With the above morphological orientation, we will now present a brief description of manipulative procedures bearing on organization of the midline thalamus and its projections, especially as these relate to cortical desynchronization and synchronization.

Moruzzi and Magoun (1949) first showed that high-frequency stimulation of the reticular formation of the brainstem is capable of desynchronizing the cortical EEG, producing the familiar low-voltage, fast pattern of arousal. Although similar stimuli applied to thalamic intralaminar fields produced the same results, the studies of Schlag and Chaillet (1963) and Weinberger et al. (1965) have shown that the pathway for the thalamically-induced effect initially passes back to the mesencephalon since tegmental lesions behind the point of thalamic stimulation abolish the cortical response. Thalamic intralaminar stimulation at low frequencies (6-12/sec) produces typical incrementing negative waves on the cortex independent of tegmental lesions. Lesions involving the mesial sectors of the antero-ventral and nucleus reticularis, or the inferior thalamic peduncle just anterior and ventral to these areas, effectively block the development of cortical recruitment waves, leaving thalamically-induced cortical desynchronization uneffected. Clearly then, separate paths are involved in the production of cortical desynchronization and cortical recruitment phenomena. Continuing studies along similar lines, Villablanca and Schlag (1968) found that placing lesions in the region of the inferior thalamic peduncle in an intact hemisphere abolished both thalamic and cortical spindles. This effect persisted after complete mesencephalic transection, but the spindles reappeared after complete decortication. They postulated that EEG spindles are basically thalamic in origin and their occurrence is shomehow controlled by antagonistic cortico-thalamic influences which operate independently from influences of the caudal brainstem. Additional data suggesting the same dichotomy between pathways involved in cortical desynchronization and cortical recruitment phenomena was presented by Jouvet and Jouvet (1963). They showed that ventrally placed lesions throughout the septum, hypothalamus, subthalamus, and interpenduncular regions suppress, partially or totally, fast cortical activity associated with the REM sleep phase. On the other hand, dorsal lesions involving the posterior thalamus and/or the tegmento-thalamic junction, did not eliminate high-frequency cortical activity. Both bodies of data may be interpreted as indicating that the ventral route alone may be effective as a pathway for cortical desynchronization while the dorsal thalamic route projecting rostrally produces only slow, high voltage potentials on the cortex, i.e., spindles, recruitment waves, etc.

In analysis of thousands of Golgi impregnated sections the Schiebels (1958, 1966) noted that the most likely system mediating *all forms* of low voltage, fast cortical activity is the ventral leaf of the ascending axonal projections of the brainstem reticular formation. Convincing data have been assembled pointing to the medial sectors of ventral anterior and nucleus reticularis as the route via which recruiting effects are directed rostrally. This pathway, as noted, has been traced forward by Skinner and Lindsley (1967), via the inferior thalamic peduncle, through the basal forebrain to the orbito-frontal cortex. From their studies they suggested that the orbito-frontal cortex may, in fact, function as the principal cortical distribution center for recruitment phenomena and spindle bursts. Their findings suggest that the anterior path, through the inferior thalamic peduncle, is the major means of cortical access for incrementing negative potentials. All of these data are in essential agreement with those of Schlag and Chaillet (1963) who believe that lateral and posterior portions of the thalamic non-specific system project augmenting-recruiting complexes directly to the superior-lateral portions of the hemisphere without mediation by the orbital-frontal cortex. One of the main implications of the work of Schlag and Chaillet (1963) was that it also demonstrated that the thalamo-cortical systems of conduction responsible for EEG desynchronization and synchronization were different. They have tended to emphasize that the thalamic reticular system and the actual lower brainstem reticular formation are not quite the same functional continuum. It was further shown that the thalamic mechanisms responsible for cortical synchronization can be activated by high-frequency as well as by low-frequency shocks. Careful mapping of the medial thalamus further revealed that the recruiting and desynchronizing areas, although overlapping, do not coincide entirely. It might be emphasized that the Golgi impregnations by the Schiebels have left little doubt that a well-defined fiber complex can be followed rostrally to the orbito-frontal cortex, along the path of the inferior thalamic peduncle. The data of Skinner and Lindsley (see below) imply that the intralaminar projection through the inferior thalamic peduncle to the orbital-frontal cortex may, in fact, constitute the only significant pathway in the development of cortical synchronous wave activity. If so, the elucidation of the pathway of secondary dispersion to other cortical areas becomes a critical problem. Golgi impregnations confirm the results of degeneration studies (see below) in revealing the presence of massive projections from orbital-frontal cortex back upon the thalamus and a complex of pathways utilizing intracortical and subgriseal routes from one cortical area to the other.

Weinberger et al. (1965) had shown that thalamo-cortical pathways for recruiting responses appear to course rostrally to the frontal pole of the thalamus, via the nucleus ventralis anterior and nucleus reticularis, before entering the internal capsule since lesions in these nuclei were shown to prevent or attenuate cortical recruiting responses. Skinner and Lindsley (1967) have attempted to delimit the thalamo-cortical system anatomically and functionally and, to accomplish this, have produced lesions in the thalamo-cortical system, namely, the rostral thalamus, the anterior thalamic radiations (inferior thalamic peduncle), and the orbital cortex. They have noted that the exact source and destination of the non-specific thalamo-cortical system is not known, but that it appears that the dorsomedial nucleus, and other portions of the midline thalamic nuclear group, project, via the inferior thalamic peduncle, to the latero-ventral and orbital surface of the frontal lobe. In these studies they showed that blockade of the non-specific thalamo-cortical synchronization system i.e., the orbital cortex, anterior thalamic radiations, and rostral thalamus, abolish both spindle bursts and recruiting responses. Specifically, they showed that blockade of the non-specific thalamo-cortical system in any one of three regions: the rostral thalamus (nucleus ventralis anterior), the forebrain (inferior thalamic peduncle), or the orbito-frontal cortex (granular cortex) has three significant effects: (1) reduction or abolition of recruiting responses and spontaneous spindle bursts; (2) enhancement of sensory evoked cortical responses; and (3) interference with the performance of certain learned, operant, behavioral tasks. They noted that the non-specific thalamo-cortical system, although influenced by projections from the ascending reticular formation, appeared to be anchored in the non-specific nuclei of the thalamic midline nuclear group. From this work they concluded that the orbital-frontal cortex, which receives projections from the midline thalamic group via the inferior thalamic peduncle, is the principal link in this system for synchronizing and regulating electrocortical activity. Their studies also showed that another functional role of the midline nuclear group of the thalamus, when driven by a high-frequency, direct electrical stimulation, or a high-frequency discharge from the reticular formation, is to exert, through the non-specific thalamo-cortical projections, an activation manifested by a desynchronizing effect. This effect may also be one of tonic nature, but it is usually slightly overridden by the dominant inhibitory effect characterized by EEG syn-chronization, in both waking (alpha) and sleeping states (spindle bursts and slow waves). They further showed that there are separate projection path-ways for incrementing responses induced by low-frequency stimulation in non-specific and specific thalamic relay nuclei.

In summary, thalamo-cortical desynchronization is achieved by stimulation of the medial thalamic nuclear complex at relatively high frequencies. As noted, when the mesencephalic tegmentum directly behind the thalamus is destroyed, cortical desynchronization can no longer be obtained after high-frequency stimulation of the medial thalamus. Schlag and Chaillet (1963), among others, have thus concluded that "activation" of the cortex apparently depends exclusively on the mediation of the ascending reticular formation of the brainstem. As indicated, there is a crucial bran-ching point in the reticular formation which occurs just caudal to the centre median-parafascicular thalamic complex, with the shorter dorsal branch being lost in a group of posterior and medial thalamic nuclei. The ventral component ascends through the zona incerta and hypothalamus and con-tinues forward into the fields of the preoptic and basal forebrain regions. The Scheibels have clearly shown that the axons of a single cell in the anterior third of the thalamic non-specific system may project major branches an-teriorly upon orbito-frontal cortex and posteriorly upon the mesencephalic tegmentum. The influences of these cells are, therefore, extremely widespread. Finally, with regard to the ascending reticular system and wakefulness, Nauta (1954) has observed that it would seem that the region of the lateral hypothalamus is, in part, involved in the transmission of ascending impulses from the midbrain reticular system. He has conjectured that it is possible that this fiber system contains ascending elements that will, directly or indirectly, lead to the basal and medial parts of the telencephalon in-cluding the septal region and hippocampal area. He has observed, and this has been confirmed by Golgi studies, that there is a very powerful bilateral offset from this system into the intralaminar nuclei of the thalamus (see Figs. 2 and 4). A variety of studies indicate that some fibers from the medial forebrain bundle send collaterals ascending at right angles into specific thalamic fields. Others ascend to the thalamic midline and medial nuclei along the trajectory of the medial forebrain bundle. Some of these appear to first pass medially into the periventricular areas before ascending to the thalamic fields. On the other hand, Magoun (1954) has pointed out that the most efficacious area in EEG arousal includes the dorsal hypothalamus and subthalamus, the region of the ventro-medial thalamic nucleus and at least the ventral portions of the centre median, intralaminar nuclei, and ventralis anterior. Thus, quite early, the medial forebrain bundle system, including both its ventral and dorsal components, became a prime candidate for mediating activating influences on the cerebral cortex.

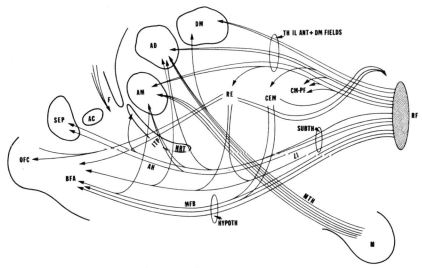

Fig. 4. Rostral projections from the reticular formation (RF) are shown dividing into dorsal and ventral limbs. The dorsal limb enters the centre median-parafascicular nuclei of thalamus (CM-PF), central medial (CEM) nucleus, reunions (RE), as well as the dorso-medial (DM), antero-dorsal (AD) and antero-medial (AM) nuclei. From these systems fibers gather to penetrate the nucleus reticularis thalami (NRT) and form the inferior thalamic peduncle (ITP) and pass to basal forebrain area (BFA) and orbito-frontal cortex (OFA). The ventral limb of the reticular division projects through the subthalamus (SUBTH) and zona incerta (ZI) and forms a major component of the medial forebrain bundle (MFB). This system receives and sends fibers into the midline thalamic area (RE and CEM). Components pass through the anterior hypothalamic area (AH) to the septal area (SEP). Also shown in this diagram are the projections from the mammillary body (M) to the anterior thalamic fields via the mam-millothalamic tract (MTH). Other abbreviations: F = fornix; AC = anterior commissure; TH IL ANT + DM Fields = thalamic intra-laminar, anterior and dorso-medial fields; HYPOTH = hypothalamus.

V. THE MONOAMINE SYSTEMS

A. Organization

1. *General Orientation*

The topology of amine systems as seen at different levels within the brain are helping provide us with a framework for thinking about their metabolism and possible functions in neural regulations. It is important to point out at the beginning that the localization of the serotonin type fluorescing neurons is entirely different from that of the catecholamine neurons. Their cell bodies are found predominantly in the raphé (medial) region throughout the medulla, pons, and mesencephalon, while the catecholamine cell bodies occupy a more lateral position except in the rostral part of the midbrain where they converge toward the midline at the interpeduncular level. No serotonin-containing cell bodies are found in the spinal cord, diencephalon, or telencephalon. First we will define the major fluorescing cell assemblies and present the general features of their fiber trajectories. In later sections, dealing with the raphé complex and locus coeruleus, we will present the more detailed picture of the fiber projections.

2. The Serotonergic Cell Groups and Pathways

(a) Organization. Most of the cell bodies containing serotonin are located in the nuclei of the raphé complex (groups B1 to B9 coding system of Dahlström and Fuxe, 1964), and in other nuclear formations not coded by the Swedish workers. These serotonin-containing cell bodies extend from the nucleus raphé pallidus (group B1) in the caudal medulla to the linearis group of nuclei in the anterior mesencephalon. They will be discussed individually from caudally to rostrally as to their topography and relations to other brain structures (Fig. 5).

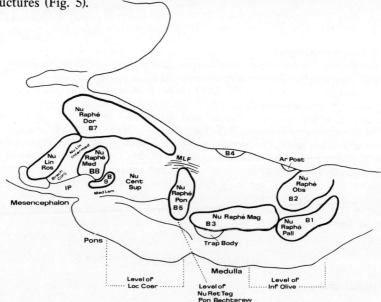

Fig. 5. Profiles of the raphé nuclei indicating their approximate relations in the brainstem. Their anatomical and B-code names are given. B6 is omitted since it is not a designated nuclear formation (is in midline just beneath ventricle). Abbreviations other than raphé nuclei: Trap Body = trapezoid body; Ar Post = area postrema; MLF = medial longitudinal fasciculus; Med. Lem. = medial lemniscus; Nu Lin Intermed. = nucleus linearis intermedius; Brach Conj. = brachium conjunctivum; IP = interpeduncular nucleus.

The nucleus raphé pallidus (B1) is comprised of cells surrounding the medial and ventral surfaces of the pyramidal tract from the level of the pyramidal decussation up to the level of the facial nucleus. Most of the fibers of the raphé pallidus pass to the spinal cord gray matter along with those of the adjacent nucleus raphé obscurus (B2). Topographywise, the fibers of the two groups join and lie close to the ventral surface of the brain just lateral to the pyramidal tract. The nucleus raphé magnus (B3) is comprised of cells surrounding the pyramidal tract at different levels of the facial nucleus. Its cells are interspersed among the fibers of the medial lemniscus just dorsal to the pyramidal tract and also lie within an area just lateral to the pyramidal tract corresponding to the nucleus paragigantocellularis lateralis in the cat. It sends fibers to the spinal cord mainly lying just lateral to the pyramidal tract. The cells of nucleus B4 (not comprising an architecturally defined nucleus) lie just under the fourth ventricle dorsal to the vestibular nuclei and the abducens nerve nucleus. Also in the medulla, though not originally coded by Dahlström and Fuxe (1964), is the area postrema which contains some serotonin (as well as catecholamine) cells. Fuxe and Owman (1965) have shown that there are large amounts of norepinephrine and serotonin in the area postrema in the rat, guinea pig, rabbit, cat, dog, and monkey and that the monoamines are localized to nerve cells and not to glial cells in this organ. The catecholamine-type cells are present in the dorsal part of this structure while the serotonin cells appear to be concentrated in the ventral part (see further discussion of area postrema below).

Cell groups B5 and B6 are in the pons. Group B5 is entirely a pontine nucleus lying at the level of the motor nucleus of the trigeminal and the cells are concentrated in the nucleus raphé pontis. Nucleus B6, also a pontine nucleus, is in the midline just under the ventricle, though not within a named anatomical nuclear formation.

At the mesencephalic level are cell groups B7, B8, and B9. Cell group B7 is situated in the central gray substance with the majority of cells concentrated in the nucleus raphé dorsalis, especially in the part just above and medial to the medial longitudinal fasciculus. Group B8 is situated from the caudal end of the inferior colliculus to the caudal third of the interpeduncular nucleus, being largely found within the nucleus raphé medianus. Some cells of B8 extend into the caudal portion of the nucleus linearis. In fact, cell group B8 largely comprises the so-called nucleus linearis caudalis (see further below). Cell group B9 is in and around the medial lemniscus from the caudal end of the inferior colliculus to the caudal third of interpeduncular nucleus. Some cells of this group lie just dorsal to the medial lemniscus within the mesencephalic reticular formation. At the junction of the mesencephalon and diencephalon some cells are concentrated in a tract just dorso-medial to the habenulo-interpeduncular tract and pass just dorso-lateral to the mammillary body where some terminate. The rostrally directed fibers are in the medial forebrain bundle and lie medial and parallel to noradrenergic fiber systems in the same bundle.

Since there has been lengthy debate as to the coincidence or correspondence of fluorescing elements to known nuclear formations in the brainstem, it might be pointed out that B3 has been taken by Baumgarten and Lachenmayer (1972) as equivalent to the nucleus paragigantocellularis basalis, while B6 and B7 have been referred to as the nucleus raphé dorsalis by these same workers. Shute and Lewis (1963) have referred to B7 and B8 as the nucleus centralis superior of Bechterew. Since Bechterew's nucleus was not mentioned in the original studies of Dahlström and Fuxe (1964), it might be emphasized that its nearest equivalent appears to be nucleus B8. On the other hand, Björklund et al. (1971) refer to nucleus B8 and B7 as the nucleus linearis caudalis. The nucleus centralis superior of Bechterew has also been variously termed the raphé nucleus of Bechterew and nucleus centralis tegmenti superior. Baumgarten and Lachenmayer refer to B8 as nucleus raphé medius. In the Swedish studies B8 was the cell code for the nucleus medianus raphé and was also described as having some cells present in the caudal portion of the nucleus linearis. Cell group B9 has been referred to as the nucleus linearis caudalis by Baumgarten and Lachenmayer (1972). In the original studies of Dahlström and Fuxe (1964), B9 was described as being in and around the medial lemniscus within the mesencephalic reticular formation.

In general, the serotonergic fibers assemble in dense bundles just dorso-lateral to the interpeduncular nucleus and ascend in the ventral part of medial forebrain bundle in medial and lateral components, passing through the septum and cingulum, and some appear to leave the hypothalamus in a lateral direction. A large proportion of the ascending fibers entering the medial forebrain bundle, especially from the anterior raphé system (nucleus raphé dorsalis and medianus), maintain a rather specific trajectory within this bundle (Figs. 6 and 7). It is noteworthy that the cells of B7 (nucleus raphé dorsalis), the most prominent of the "anterior" raphé group related to slow-wave sleep (see below), send axons ventrally toward the interpeduncular nucleus which then make a sharp bend and run parallel to the ventral surface of the brain just dorsal to this nucleus. At the junction between the mesencephalon and diencephalon some of them are concentrated in a tract just dorso-medial to the habenulo-interpeduncular tract. This tract then bends around the habenulo-interpeduncular tract on its medial side and passes through the dorso-lateral part of the mammillary body where many of its fibers appear to terminate. Further rostrally, the fibers appear to lie mainly within the medial forebrain bundle (see below), medial and parallel to the catecholamine fibers, which are also situated mainly within this bundle. Serotonergic terminals have been found in many of the nuclei of the surrounding brainstem areas throughout the ponto-mesencephalic reticular formation, and in the lateral hypothalamic and lateral preoptic areas, hippocampal formation, amygdaloid complex, lateral geniculate nucleus, and extending into the neocortex. On the whole, the distribution of the serotonin nerve terminals is not known to the same degree as are catecholamine nerve terminals owing to technical difficulties, but findings to date are reviewed in more detail below.

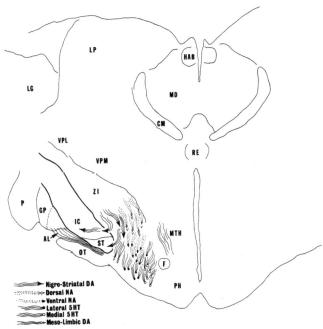

Fig. 6. Topography of chemical systems in the medial forebrain bundle as seen in frontal section. This schematic shows the relative positions of the serotonergic (5-HT), noradrenergic (NA) and dopaminergic (DA) fibers in the medial forebrain bundle (lateral hypothalamic area). Note the more medial position of serotonergic fibers and dorso-lateral position of the noradrenergic systems, some of the components of the dorsal noradrenergic system passing in the zona incerta (ZI) and subthalamic zones. The nigrostriatal dopamine system is seen entering the internal capsule (IC) and subthalamic nucleus (ST) on its passage to the striatum. Other abbreviations: HAB = habenular complex; MD = medio-dorsal nucleus of thalamus; CM = central medial nucleus; RE = reuniens nucleus; LP = lateral posterior nucleus; VPM = postero-medial ventral nucleus; VPL = postero-lateral ventral nucleus; LG = lateral geniculate nucleus; OT = optic tract; AL = ansa lenticularis; GP = globus pallidus; P = putamen; PH = posterior hypothalamic area; F = fornix; MTH = mammillo-thalamic tract.

Although most of the anatomical plotting of the organization of the serotonergic systems. have been done in the rat some limited work has also been done in the cat. In general, the two species exhibit many similarities in this system (Sladek, 1971a, b). Basically in both species the primary axons, especially from the nuclei raphé dorsalis and medialis, largely enter the medial forebrain bundle and have terminals throughout the lateral hypothalamic and lateral preoptic areas, septal areas, amygdaloid complex, basal forebrain area, and neocortical formations.

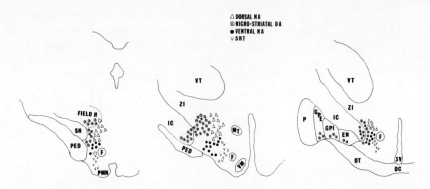

Fig. 7. Frontal views of three brain levels extending (left to right) from the premammillary nuclear area (PMN) to the ventro-medial hypothalamic nuclear level (VM) to the level of the optic chiasm (OC). Topography of the dorsal and ventral noradrenergic (NA) pathways, serotonin (5-HT) pathway, and nigro-striatal dopamine (DA) pathway are shown. In the first schematic note the clustering of the nigro-striatal dopamine fibers in the prerubral field (Field H of Forel) and their gathering medio-dorsal to the substantia nigra (SN) and cerebral peduncle (PED). In the second drawing they are shown passing through the zona incerta (ZI) and penetrating the internal capsule (IC), and in the third drawing they are shown passing through (or near) the entopeduncular nucleus (EN) and into the internal (GPI) and external (GPE) parts of the globus pallidus on their way to the putamen (P). In the left-hand drawing the dorsal noradrenergic pathway forms the dorsal part of the medial forebrain bundle with ventral noradrenergic fibers immediately below. At the level of the middle of the hypothalamus (middle drawing) the clearly lateral position of the noradrenergic pathways in the medial forebrain bundle is shown. These relative positions are maintained as these fiber systems ascend to the anterior hypothalamic area (right-hand drawing) at the level of the optic chiasm. In all three drawings the serotonin fibers form the more ventro-medial components of the medial forebrain bundle. Other abbreviations: F = fornix; MT = mammillo-thalamic tract; VT = ventral thalamic nuclear complex; 3V = third ventricle; OT = optic tract.

In both species the serotonin fibers ascend medially in the mesencephalon just lateral to the midline and enter the medial forebrain bundle by turning somewhat laterally when reaching the border between the mesencephalon and the diencephalon. At this point most of the serotonin fibers are densely aggregated, lying ventral and immediately medial to the habenulo-interpeduncular tract. In the medial forebrain bundle the serotonin fibers, in both rat and cat, appear to be spread out in numerous bundles, some of which lie immediately lateral to the fornix and some of which occupy a more ventro-lateral position along the dorsal surface of the optic tract (Figs. 6 and 7). Some also lie immediately ventral to the ventral part of the cerebral peduncle and the retrolenticular part of the internal capsule. Further details of species differences in organization of amine systems in rat, cat, and monkey are given in a later section.

(b) *The Raphé Complex.* The raphé nuclei are present and well organized in birds and other lower vertebrates indicating that this nuclear complex is probably a primitive part of the brainstem which shows relatively little differentiation during the phylogenetic ascent of vertebrates. Correspondingly, one might be inclined to ascribe to it rather fundamental and important tasks in the function of the brain. We would emphasize that certain anatomical similarities between the raphé complex and the reticular formation are sufficiently close to suggest functional relationships and, in fact, the raphé nuclear assemblies meet the various morphological criteria of "reticular" organization. It is, of course, possible that the raphé nuclear complex may even comprise part of the structural bases of the "ascending activating system" of Moruzzi and Magoun. Thus, high-frequency stimulation of the medial reticular formation may well have activated components of this nuclear complex since most of the positive regions are usually shown as extending to the midline. However, their established relation to slow-wave sleep and serotonin systems has tended to relate them more to sleep than to arousal mechanisms (see below).

Several general characteristics of the raphé system should be emphasized at the onset. It is important to keep in mind that most of the nuclei of the raphé are traversed by large numbers of fibers which makes the identification of terminal degeneration extremely difficult. Therefore, establishing connectivities of this area by conventional degeneration techniques has so far been relatively unrewarding. Also, considering the wealth of axonal branching and of collaterals of the cells of the reticular formation and their diverse and widespread distribution, it appears likely that many cells of the reticular formation may have synaptic contact with cells of the raphé nuclei. It should be emphasized that there are long neural pathways passing immediately lateral to the raphé nuclear groups, such as the medial longitudinal fasciculus, the tectospinal tract, and the medial lemniscus. Thus, manipulations such as lesioning procedures that extend slightly beyond the confines of the raphé nuclei may be interrupting these various fibers of passage. This proximity to long pathways lying immediately lateral to the raphé also has made it difficult to trace degeneration from these nuclei. Since most of the nuclei are thin in the latero-lateral dimension and platelike in shape it is extremely difficult to limit a lesion to the raphé itself without involving these laterally placed fiber systems.

Because of the inconsistencies in the literature with regard to the nomenclature and delimitations of the raphé nuclei, it was deemed necessary to discuss the normal topography and cytoarchitecture of these nuclei, especially in the cat. At the onset it should be pointed out that Valverde (1962) found no important differences in the raphé nuclei in the rat from the raphé map of the cat as made by Taber et al. (1960). This is discussed more in detail under species variations below. The cat is the experimental animal most widely used in sleep research and considerable confusion exists with regard to the subdivisions and nomenclature of the nuclei of the raphé. At some levels in the brainstem these nuclear masses are situated along the midsagittal plane and are separated on either side from other cellular aggregations by fiber masses, thus permitting their unequivocal delimitation in most instances. However, at some sites in the sagittal plane these elements fuse more laterally with groups of cells making delimitation quite arbitrary. For example, the lateral borders of the nucleus centralis superior, in particular, are poorly defined against the reticular formation. The cells of the nucleus raphé magnus especially resemble in cytoarchitecture the laterally adjoining reticular formation but in most places it is separated from this formation by longitudinally running fiber bundles. Some of the raphé nuclei fuse rather imperceptably with each other, and, while some are clearly characterized by their cytoarchitecture as being different from neighboring cell groups, this is not always the case. Thus, in most places the transition from one raphé cell group to its neighbors is diffuse and the cytoarchitectonic pattern changes gradually as one passes from one nucleus of the raphé to the adjoining ones. Most important in this regard, it is generally thought that many cells of the reticular formation may have synaptical contact with the cells of the raphé nuclei.

The raphé complex in the cat forms a continuous mass of cells along the midline of the brain but there are cytoarchitectonic differences between them. As noted, the anatomical similarities between the raphé complex and the reticular formation are sufficiently close to suggest strong functional relationships. Some of the earlier literature has indicated that this nuclear complex may be part of the structural basis of the "ascending activating system" of Moruzzi and Magoun (1949). It has long been known that activating effects are obtained on high-frequency stimulation of the *medial* reticular formation, the positive regions usually being shown in published works as extending to the midline, and have been obtained from the mesencephalon, pons, and medulla.

The similarities between the reticular formation and the raphé nuclei are especially marked with regard to the nucleus raphé magnus and, to a lesser extent, from the nucleus raphé pallidus. The fiber connections, as well as the architecture of the nucleus raphé magnus, and to a lesser extent the nucleus raphé pallidus, in addition to suggesting a close functional similarity to the reticular formation, furnish evidence that these particular nuclei differ functionally, more or less, from the other cell groups of the raphé. This has, of course, been borne out in physiological experiments (below).

Taber et al. (1960), in a study of the raphé nuclei of the cat by cytoarchitectonic methods, distinguished 8 nuclear formations (Fig. 5): the nucleus raphé dorsalis, nucleus centralis superior of Bechterew, nucleus linearis intermedius, nucleus linearis rostralis, nucleus raphé magnus, nucleus raphé pontis, nucleus raphé obscurus, and the nucleus raphé pallidus. It can immediately be seen that this grouping does not precisely correspond to the histochemical fluorescence classification of specific serotonin fluorescing areas of the brainstem. With regard to the "linear" group of nuclei, these are in the mid-regions of the midbrain tegmentum, except where interrupted by decussating fibers such as those of the superior cerebellar peduncles. They form rows of dorso-laterally extending cells on either side of the midline. Rostral, intermediate, and caudal portions of these nuclei have been recognized in various mammals.

The nucleus raphé dorsalis is approximately 2.8 mm in length in the cat and extends from the level just caudal to the caudal pole of the dorsal tegmental nucleus of Gudden to the level of the caudal pole of the oculomotor complex. It is located predominantly in the ventral periaqueductal gray matter, especially in the part above and medial to the medial longitudinal fasciculus. Rostral to the level of the ventral tegmental nucleus of Gudden the nucleus fans out laterally and, at the level of the trochlear nucleus, it is composed of one midline concentrated group of cells with somewhat dispersed, bilateral wings. The nucleus merges for a short distance with both the nucleus centralis superior or Bechterew and the nucleus linearis intermedius.

The nucleus centralis superior of Bechterew or raphé nucleus of Bechterew, not mentioned in histofluorescence mapping studies, has been termed the nucleus linearis caudalis by Brown (1943). Winkler and Potter (1914), in their atlas of the cat, described a formation they termed nucleus ventralis raphé which seems to be coextensive to a part of the nucleus centralis superior. It is important to point out that fluorescence coded cells B-8, the so called nucleus raphé medianus, corresponds, in large part, to the nucleus centralis superior of Bechterew. This nucleus has also been variously termed in the literature the central reticular nucleus and nucleus reticularis superior. The nucleus centralis superior of Bechterew extends from the level of the rostral portion of the nucleus reticularis tegmenti pontis of Bechterew (a pontine nucleus) to the caudal portion of the decussation of the brachium conjunctivum (approximately 2.2 mm in the cat). It is a midline, ovoid-shaped, loosely structured concentration of cells which, caudally, at the level of the ventral tegmental nucleus of Gudden, extends dorsally between the medial longitudinal fasciculi and merges with the nucleus raphé dorsalis. The rostral pole of the nucleus lies just dorsal to the caudal pole of the interpeduncular nucleus. The nucleus centralis superior of Bechterew may be said to continue the nucleus raphé pontis in a rostral direction. Decussating fibers of the brachium conjunctivum pass across the dorso-rostral aspect of the nucleus centralis superior and separate it from the rostral or major part of the nucleus raphe dorsalis. The decussation also separates the nucleus from the nucleus linearis intermedius. As noted, the lateral boarders of the nucleus centralis superior are poorly defined against the reticular formation.

The nucleus linearis intermedius is a raphé nucleus that extends from approximately the mid-level of the decussation of the brachium conjunctivum to the level of the caudal pole of the red nucleus (approximately 1.2 mm). It is an unpaired nucleus, which extends rostrally dorsal to the decussating fibers of the brachium conjunctivum. Caudally, the nucleus merges with both the nucleus centralis superior of Bechterew and the nucleus

raphé dorsalis. The rostral pole of the nucleus lies dorsal to the interpeduncular nucleus and merges with the nucleus linearis rostralis. The
nucleus linearis rostralis extends from about the level of the mid-
caudorostral extent of the red nucleus to the level of the junction of the mid-
and forebrain. This is a bilateral nucleus and forms a band of cells that lies
medial to and follows the contour of the root fibers of the oculomotor nerve.
Caudally, the nucleus merges with the nucleus linearis intermedius.

Detailed discussion of the nuclei raphé obscurus, pallidus magnus, and
pontis are beyond the scope of this review, since they bear less directly on
problems related to morphological substrata of sleep-waking activity. The
very close relationship between the nucleus raphé pontis and cerebellum
should, perhaps, be noted. Also, the interpeduncular nucleus, although
largely a midline structure, is not considered part of the raphé group.

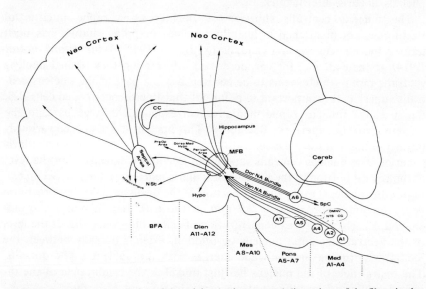

Fig. 8. Schematic representation of the origins, trajectory, and dispersions of the fibers in the
dorsal (Dor NA) and ventral (Ven NA) noradrenergic bundles. Note that the ventral bundle
arises from most of the A coded noradrenergic cell groups in the medullary and pontine
regions and projects into many parts of the hypothalamus, including the periventricular zone
(Periven Area) and dorso-medial hypothalamic area (Dorso-Med Hypo). Also, strong
projections from this bundle enter the preoptic area (PreOp Area), septal area, and nucleus of
the stria terminalis (N St). The dorsal noradrenergic system is shown arising largely from the
locus coeruleus area (A 6) and projecting rostrally in the dorsal components of the medial
forebrain bundle (MFB) to the hippocampus and neocortex. Details given in text. Other
abbreviations: Med=medulla; Mes=mesencephalon; Dien= diencephalon; BFA = basal
forebrain area; Cereb = cerebellum; CC = corpus callosum; SpC = spinal cord; DMNV =
dorsal motor nucleus of vagus; NTS = nucleus of the tractus solitarius; CG = central gray.
The numbers below the brain areas Med, Pons, Mes, and Dien represent the noradrenergic
coded cell groupings described by Dahlström and Fuxe (see text). A3 and A13 not shown in
figure.

However, due to its intimate topographic relations to many chemical fiber systems, we will briefly define its position. This nucleus extends throughout the length of the mesencephalon as an unpaired, midline nucleus located in the floor of the interpeduncular fossa between the two cerebral peduncles. The caudal pole is oval-shaped with its long axis directed dorso-ventrally, and lies ventral to the rostral portion of the nucleus centralis superior.

3. *The Catecholaminergic Cell Groups and Pathways*

(a) *General Orientation.* The catecholamine-type cellular formations have been classified according to the Swedish group from A1 through A13 (Fig. 8). These are organized into two major systems: the dopamine and the noradrenergic cell groups.

(1) Dopamine. Most of the dopamine-containing cell bodies are located in the pars compacta of the substantia nigra (group A9) and in an area (A10) dorsal to the interpeduncular nucleus. Another group of dopamine cells (A8) lie in the reticular formation just behind the red nucleus dorsal to the lateral part of the medial lemniscus, i.e., in the lateral mesencephalic reticular formation. Cell groups A8 and A9 contribute primarily to the nigro-striatal system while A10 sends fibers, via the meso-limbic system, to the olfactory tubercle region, amygdaloid complex, and nucleus accumbens. Although the locus coeruleus (A6) is not within this topographic area, it is noteworthy that Gerardy et al. (1969), using biochemical methods, have reported dopamine (as well as norepinephrine) in the locus coeruleus of the rabbit, cow and rat.

(2) Norepinephrine. Most of the norepinephrine-containing cell bodies are in the lateral part of the brainstem tegmentum, with cell groups A1 through A4 situated in the medulla (Fig. 8). They lie in close relation to the inferior olivary complex, the motor nucleus of the vagus, the accessory olivary nucleus, and the facial nerve nucleus. This group of cells primarily send descending fibers to the spinal cord. Jouvet (1972c) has described ascending fibers which run medially from this group to the locus coeruleus (A6) in the reticular formation of the pons. The medullary A1-A4 groups constitute the beginnings of the ventral noradrenergic pathway (Fig. 8) which runs in the anterior mesencephalon dorso-lateral to the interpeduncular nucleus. These fiber bundles, joining other noradrenergic systems rostrally, enter the medial forebrain bundle and innervate the lateral hypothalamic and lateral preoptic areas and portions of the limbic forebrain area.

Group A1 is comprised of cells extending from the pyramidal decussation up to the rostral half of the inferior olive lateral to the nucleus reticularis lateralis. In a transverse section most of these cells are seen at the mid-olivary level. They stand out in comparison to the very large, nonfluorescing multipolar cells of the nucleus reticularis lateralis. Most cells of A1 have axons that appear to form descending fibers to the spinal cord. The cells of group A2 are in the medulla near the nucleus of the tractus solitarius and dorsal motor nucleus of the vagus nerve and some extend rostrally into the rostral components of the nucleus of the tractus solitarius. Cell group A3, best observed in transverse sections, lies in the dorsal accessory olivary nucleus. Group A4 lie in the lateral part of the roof of the fourth ventricle with maximum development at the level of the facial nerve nucleus. They are just under the ependyma ventral to the cerebellar nuclei.

At the level of the pons lie cell groups A5, A6, and A7 of the catecholamine type. In the cat the organization of noradrenergic cell bodies in the pontine area is much more diffuse than in the rat and is divisible into the main nucleus of the locus coeruleus proper (A6), the subcoeruleus (A7), the nucleus parabrachialis medialis, and lateralis (the nucleus parabrachialis is synonymous with the nucleus parapeduncularis cerebellaris superior or nucleus brachii conjunctivi), and group K (A5). Cell groups A5 are present among the fibers of the rubro-spinal tract mainly at the level of the middle and caudal third of the superior olivary nucleus medial to the emerging fibers of the facial nerve and lateral to the superior olivary nucleus. Some of the processes appear to run in the general direction of the motor nucleus of the trigeminal nerve.

Also lying within the pons is cell group A6 which is identical to the locus coeruleus or nucleus dorso-lateralis tegmenti. It is of particular importance because of the many experiments that have related this area to sleep and detailed discussions of this formation will be given in the sections below dealing with physiological experiments. Some of the cells of group A6 that are in the lateral part of the nucleus stream medially toward the raphé area (Fig. 9) while others run ventrally to the trigeminal motor nucleus. The locus coeruleus also contributes strong innervation to the cerebellum and to the surrounding reticular formation of the pons. At the level of the caudal third of the pontine gray, the locus coeruleus fairly well fades out. The fluorescing cells of the locus coeruleus stand in sharp contrast to the nonfluorescing, but immediately adjacent, mesencephalic nucleus of the trigeminal nerve. In general, the locus coeruleus contributes ascending projections through the dorsal noradrenergic bundle (Figs. 8 and 9) which lies just lateral to the central gray substance (Olson and Fuxe, 1971; Ungerstedt, 1971a, b). Some ventral components of the locus coeruleus may also project rostrally through a so-called intermediate pathway (Maeda and Shimizu, 1972). These fiber groups, once joined, abruptly turn ventrally at the border between the mesencephalon (Fig. 9) and diencephalon and, after coursing through the subthalamic region, pass rostrally in the dorso-lateral hypothalamic area. The dorsal noradrenergic bundle appears to innervate the cerebral neocortex and the hippocampal formation. Additional fibers from the locus coeruleus terminate in the lateral geniculate bodies but their exact route is undetermined. This is discussed in considerable detail in the section on ponto-geniculo-occipital spikes and lateral geniculate innervation (below). Olson and Fuxe (1971, 1972) and co-workers have observed a strongly flurorescent medium-sized group of multipolar cells with the same general appearance as the locus coeruleus cells passing from the ventral part of the rostral portion of the locus coeruleus in an arch medial to the motor nucleus of the trigeminal nerve down to the cells within group A5. This constitutes the "subcoeruleus" complex and is discussed more in detail further on. Cell group A7 lies at the level of the caudal third of the pontine gray and is seen in the reticular formation ventral to the ventral portion of the dorsal cerebellar peduncle and dorsal to the rubro-spinal tract.

At the level of the mesencephalon are cell groups A8, A9 and A10, with the localization of catecholaminergic neurons being generally similar in the rat and cat. These cell groups can be topographically divided as follows: (1) Cells in the lateral mesencephalic reticular formation just behind the red nucleus and dorsal to the lateral part of the medial lemniscus comprise A8; (2) cells mostly in the pars compacta of the substantia nigra comprise A9; and (3) cells in the baso-medial area dorsal to the interpeduncular nucleus comprise group A10. There are indistinct boundaries between A8 ventro-medially against A10 and ventro-laterally against A9. Cell group A9 is not clearly separated from A10 medially and, laterally, separation between A9 and A8 is also not clear. Fibers of cell group A8 form one major system of the nigro-striatal pathway projecting, mostly via the ventral part of the cerebral peduncle, through the far-lateral hypothalamus and internal capsule, to the putamen and caudate nucleus. Cell group A9 is located mostly in the pars compacta of the substantia nigra. In the rostral part of this group many cells lie in the ventral tegmental area of Tsai and surround the non-fluorescent nucleus of the basal optic tract. There appears to be no distinct borderline between the pars compacta of the substantia nigra and the ventral tegmental area of Tsai. Fibers of A9 run in Forel's field H_2 (fasciculus lenticularis) and the ventral portion of the cerebral peduncle, these latter passing, via the lateral hypothalamus into the internal capsule to the caudate nucleus and putamen. Many fibers in field H_2 enter the lateral part of the hypothalamus via the medial forebrain bundle and terminate in the hypothalamus. Cells of group A10 form the largest group in the midbrain and lie primarily dorsal to the interpeduncular nucleus and somewhat lateral to it. Most of the fibers run cranially in Forel's field H_2 in the medial forebrain bundle and many terminate in the hypothalamus while others project to the limbic forebrain areas.

In summary, cell groups A9 and A10 appear to give rise to fiber bundles which run cranially mainly within Forel's field H_2 and within the ventral portion of the cerebral peduncle. Most of the fiber bundles within Forel's field H_2 pass into the lateral part of the hypothalamus as components of the medial forebrain bundle and some of these probably terminate in the hypothalamus. Cell group A10 is the largest fluorescent group in the mesencephalon and is situated mainly in the area dorsal to the interpeduncular nucleus and extends caudally to the intermediate and caudal parts of the nucleus linearis groups. Some cells of group A10 extend forward between the fascicles of the habenulo-interpeduncular tract. Fluorescing cells just lateral to the interpeduncular nucleus are probably part of this same group. It appears that the fibers from group A10 run forward within Forel's field H_2 in the medial forebrain bundle with some of them terminating in the hypothalamus. In broadly summarizing all of these complex projections it appears that cell group A10 is the primary source of origin for the meso-limbic dopamine system while groups A8 and A9 form cells of origin primarily of the nigro-striatal dopamine system.

In the diencephalon, there are three groups of catecholaminergic neuronal systems: A11, A12, and A13. These are norepinephrine -containing cell bodies lying close to the third ventricle and around the habenulo-interpeduncular tract and in the periventricular gray. Some of the cell bodies are scattered in the posterior hypothalamic and supramammillary area. At the level of the diencephalon, cell group A11 is close to the third ventricle medial, dorsal and ventral to the habenulo-interpeduncular tract mainly within the periventricular gray. Some of the cells of this group are in the posterior hypothalamic region and supramammillary area. Cells of A12 are primarily in the arcuate nucleus and in the ventral part of the anterior periventricular area, with fibers ending in the hypophyseal-portal area. Cells of A13 are dorso-lateral to the dorso-medial nucleus. Jonsson et al. (1972) have shown that these latter cells contain dopamine and thus may be part of a dopamine system.

(b) The Locus Coeruleus and Other Noradrenergic Systems

(1) Orientation. The nucleus locus coeruleus or dorso-lateral tegmental nucleus is approximately 3 mm in length in the cat and extends from the mid-level of the motor nuclues of the trigeminal nerve to a level slightly rostral to the dorsal tegmental nucleus of Gudden. The caudal portion lies medial to the mesencephalic route of the trigeminal nerve, within the periaqueductal gray and the underlying tegmentum. The mid-portion extends ventrally deep within the tegmentum, medial to the brachium conjunctivum, while the rostral portion is located only within the periaqueductal gray and extends rostro-medially toward the nucleus raphé dorsalis.

Very few degeneration studies, using more conventional anatomical methods, have been carried out relative to connections of the locus coeruleus. In one such study following lesions in the hypothalamus of rabbits Mizuno and Nakamura (1970) demonstrated electron dense synaptic bags ipsilaterally in the locus coeruleus following lesions in the supramammillary area of the posterior hypothalamus. Some degenerated fine fibers were traced into the central gray substance close to the rostral pole of the locus coeruleus by the Nauta technique but no confirmatory light microscopic evidence of termination of hypothalamic efferents within the locus coeruleus proper was obtained.

The locus coeruleus, from the standpoint of cytoarchitecture and connections, has been extensively studied by Russell (1955) in several species. Throughout its extent the locus coeruleus is located in the angle of the periventricular gray substance and the underlying tegmental reticular formation. In the dog and cat the locus coeruleus extends from the level of the dorsal tegmental nucleus caudad (approximately the caudal level of the trochlear nucleus) to the middle of the masticator nucleus and, in both the cat and the dog, the cells are of two types. Embryologically the nucleus locus coeruleus is derived from the superior reticular nucleus. Crosby and Woodburne (1943) homologized the posterior portion of the latero-dorsal tegmental nucleus (nucleus dorso-lateralis tegmenti) of subprimate species with the locus coeruleus of primates, including man. Russell has presumed, on the basis of comparative morphological studies, that the locus coeruleus is not a part of the central somesthetic mechanism for the head and is not a part of the trigeminal complex. He cites a wealth of evidence supporting the hypothesis that the locus coeruleus is a subdivision of the reticular nuclei of the pontine tegmentum.

(2) Projection Pathways. Loizou (1969a), using histochemical fluorescence techniques, has studied the projections of the locus coeruleus in the rat. He has shown that the locus area has diffuse fiber dispersions, lending further support to the view that this nucleus is a reticular one. He outlined one projection of the locus coeruleus to the dorsal motor nucleus of the vagus and to the tractus solitarius. In addition, following lesions of the locus coeruleus, degenerative changes in norepinephrine-containing terminal systems, assessed by histofluorescence techniques (changes in pattern of distribution, density, intensity, and size of fluorescent variscosities in lesioned and normal rats), were seen in the central gray, the nucleus raphé dorsalis, in the premammillary and mammillary nuclei, posterior hypothalamus, and periventricular areas, as well as the arcuate nuclei. In some animals degeneration was seen in the nucleus raphé pallidus, raphé obscurus, reticular formation of the midbrain, perifornical area of the hypothalamus, preoptic area, septal area, hippocampus, and amygdaloid complex, among others. From these studies it is clear that the projections of the locus coeruleus are extremely widespread.

Loizou (1969b) also showed that projections from norepinephrine-containing cell bodies of the brainstem traversed the dorsal part of the reticular formation of the medulla and pons and entered the mesencephalic tegmentum dorsal and ventral to the superior cerebellar peduncle. He noted that the fibers shift dorso-medially in their ascent through the mesencephalon and enter the diencephalon dorsal to field H_1 of Forel (thalamic fasciculus) at the level of the infra-mammillary recess. From here some of the fibers course ventro-medially to terminate in medial hypothalamic nuclei and some pass ventro-laterally to join the medial forebrain bundle and terminate in the lateral hypothalamic area and amygdaloid complex. Arbuthnott et al. (1970), also using fluorescence histochemical mapping techniques, observed that the dorsal noradrenergic bundle ascends just lateral to the central gray substance and arises primarily from noradrenergic cell bodies in the locus coeruleus. They noted that this bundle innervates primarily the cerebral cortex and hippocampal formation and that the pathway turns abruptly ventrally at the border between the mesencephalon and diencephalon, and approaches the dorso-lateral hypothalamic area after passing through the subthalamus. On the other hand, the ventral noradrenergic pathway was shown to arise from noradrenergic cell groups other than those in the locus coeruleus which are present mainly in the medulla and pons and ascends in the lateral reticular formation of the medulla, pons and mesencephalon. This pathway lies ventro-lateral to the dorsal bundle at the level of the caudal portion of the interpenduncular nucleus. It gives rise to noradrenergic terminals which are primarily in the hypothalamus, the preoptic area, ventral parts of the limbic forebrain area, and septum. The ventral noradrenergic pathway passes through the lateral A10 area after having turned medially along the dorsal surface of the medial lemniscus. It is important to note that a large number of serotonergic fibers pass through the A10 area but lie closer to the midline. These topographic orientations are critical in interpreting the effects of amine-specific lesions in the brain (see below).

Olson and Fuxe (1971) studied the projections from the locus coeruleus noradrenergic neurons to the cerebellum and showed that cerebellar noradrenergic innervation originates mainly from the principal locus coeruleus. From these studies they suggested that a single locus coeruleus nor-adrenergic nerve is capable of innervating all cortices of the brain. They found that nor-adrenergic cell bodies of the locus coeruleus project in a distinct bundle in the dorsal tegmentum just ventro-lateral to the medial longitudinal fasciculus with the individual fibers lying aggregated in bundles. This rostral projection was described as originating mainly from the rostral part of the locus coeruleus, particularly the dorso-lateral or principal nucleus. In addition, a medial fiber system was shown in horizontal sections to project to the raphé and these probably represent partly crossing fibers. The medial fiber projection from the locus coeruleus to the raphé appears to constitute a partially crossed fiber system, responsible for part of the cortical innervation and at least some of the innervation of the vagal area, raphé area, and the hypothalamus, especially in view of Loizou's (1969a) findings of a disappearance of noradrenergic nerve terminals in the latter areas following bilateral lesions of the locus coeruleus. This medially oriented fiber projection originates from the most ventro-medial part of the locus coeruleus which contains the largest cell bodies and exhibits the strongest fluorescence intensity. No bundle formation was observed in this fiber system. Following cerebellectomy in rats noradrenergic fibers have been traced all the way to the dorso-lateral locus coeruleus cell bodies as well as to nuclear group A4 in the roof of the fourth ventricle which, as shown by retrograde fluorescence changes after lesions, represents the caudal extension of the dorso-lateral part of the locus coeruleus. These studies showed that a major part of the cerebellar noradrenergic innervation originated from the dorso-lateral part of the locus coeruleus, including cell area A4.

Ungerstedt (1971a, b) and Olson and Fuxe (1971) favor the view that one single noradrenergic neuron in the dorso-lateral locus coeruleus area can monosynaptically innervate both the cerebral cortex and cerebellum and that such a pattern would enable these neurons to immediately and simultaneously influence the neural activity in practically all cortical areas of the brain. They further noted that the ascending noradrenergic pathways on their course from the locus coeruleus to the cerebral cortex give collaterals to the colliculi, the geniculate bodies and parts of the thalamus. Olson and Fuxe (1971) have postulated that since the locus coeruleus system also innervates the geniculate bodies this system may be involved in regulation of ponto-geniculo-occipital discharges of REM sleep. They have suggested that noradrenergic neurons from the locus coeruleus may be involved, not only in REM sleep, but also in the maintenance of cortical EEG activation. Some evidence for this is that DOPA causes an increase in waking whereas destruction of the noradrenergic neurons are known to increase cortical synchronization (Jones et al., 1969). In summarising their work, Olson and Fuxe (1971) have speculated that it seems a distinct possibility that the "activating" effects of the locus coeruleus noradrenergic neurons on all cortices form an important component of the reticular activating system.

Maeda and Shimizu (1972), in a comprehensive study, mapped the ascending projections of the locus coeruleus and other pontine aminergic neurons at the level of the forebrain of the rat. From one system (coerulo-cortical pathways), these workers identified very small noradrenergic varicosities at the level of the neocortex as well as in the meso-, archi-, and paleo-cortices, such as the cingular area, hippocampus, dentate gyrus, en-torhinal area, and pyriform lobe. The complete destruction of the locus coeruleus in their experiments brought about the total disappearence of fluorescing variscosities on the side which was manipulated, in all areas about a week following surgery. The same disappearance was observed when the lesions of the locus coeruleus left intact the antero-ventral part of the locus coeruleus ("anterior" locus coeruleus) as well as the subcoeruleus nuclei (which they term group A7). They concluded that there exists two major subdivisions of the locus coeruleus in the rat, at least in regard to the projections of the ascending fibers. The anterior or antero-ventral locus coeruleus was also distinguished from the posterior or principal locus coeruleus according to its fluorescence aspects. They observed that the anterior part of the locus coeruleus was found to be composed of large cells with stronger fluorescence than that seen in the caudal part, these cells being dispersed at the level of the pontine reticular formation to constitute what they termed the nucleus subcoeruleus. It is noteworthy that Olson and Fuxe (1971) pointed out that the ventro-medial part of the locus coeruleus has the largest and stronger fluorescing units and this may well correspond to the antero-ventral group of Maeda and Shimizu.

Maeda and Shimizu observed that large lesions of the principal (posterior) part of the locus coeruleus bring about a decrease of the catecholamine varicosities at the level of cortical areas. After the lesions, which resulted in a decrease of the fine varicosities of the cortex, they also observed a decrease of the fluorescence at the level of the thalamus. The thalamic varicosities which were decreased by the lesions were very small and similar to those found in the cortex and were distributed in a diffuse fashion at the level of the thalamus, including the dorsal part of the lateral geniculate nucleus. These were shown, however, to be different from the very small varicosities which are concentrated in the antero-ventral nucleus of the thalamus and which were not diminished by lesions of the locus coeruleus. The thick varicosities at the level of the hypothalamus (ponto-hypothalamic system) were not altered by lesions of the principal part of the locus coeruleus which suppressed the very small varicosities. Lesions involving the total locus coeruleus and the subcoeruleus resulted in major reductions of the thick varicosities, especially at the level of the periventricular part of the third ventricle, including the paraventricular nuclei.

The most abundant decrease of the thick varicosities at the level of the forebrain areas such as the septal area, hypothalamus, and subthalamus was observed by Maeda and Shimizu after deep destruction of the reticular formation located just medial to the caudal area of the motor nucleus of the trigeminal nerve. By destroying the reticular formation 2 mm posterior to the locus coeruleus they observed a decrease of thick varicosities in the dorsomedial hypothalamic nucleus, the basal part of the hypothalamus, and the lateral hypothalamic area. Some of these varicosities in the lateral preoptic area and the nucleus accumbens of the septum extended from this latter structure to form varicosities below the anterior commissure. This latter area was described as the interstitial nucleus of the stria terminalis (ventral part) by Fuxe and Lundgren (1965). These experiments indicated that ascending aminergic fibers exist which begin at the level of catecholaminergic nuclei of the pons, that is, the anterior part of the locus coeruleus, the subcoeruleus (which Maeda and Shimizu term A7) and the cell group K (A5). These nuclei were shown to innervate, via the ponto-hypothalamic system, especially the periventricular zone of the hypothalamus, and were distinguishable from ascending fibers coming from the medulla (which form the ventral noradrenergic pathway).

With lesions of the mesencephalic gray matter and a small part of the adjacent tegmentum at the level of the oculomotor nucleus retrograde fluorescence was observed posterior to the lesion just below the gray matter laterally and dorsally in regard to the medial longitudinal fasciculus. Such retrograde fluorescence changes were traced back as far as the locus coeruleus, thus indicating that the aminergic fibers which derive from the principal (posterior) part of the locus coeruleus pass through the dorso-medial part of the mesencephalic reticular formation in their ascending pathway to the thalamus and cerebral cortex. This bundle is probably identical to the dorsal noradrenergic bundle previously described. Maeda and Shimizu have pointed out that it is interesting that the accumulation of fluorescence in these bundles is not as marked as that provoked by lesions of the ventral part of the mesencephalic tegmentum. With destruction of the medio-dorsal part of the mesencephalic tegmentum, they observed an accumulation of fluorescence just ventral in regard to the bundles (dorsal noradrenergic pathways) arising from the principal part of the locus coeruleus. They pointed out that axons whose catecholamines acccumulate following these lesions are much thicker than those which originate from the principal part of the locus coeruleus and which extend as far as the cerebral cortex. These thicker fibers were traced back as far as the rostral (antero-ventral) part of the locus coeruleus and were separable into two bundles: 1) more dorsal fibers which are mixed with the fine fibers from the principal part of the locus coeruleus; and 2) more ventral fibers which were traced as far as the level of the disseminated neurons of the subcoeruleus (A7) and of the group K (A5). They observed that the more dorsal fibers probably have their route in the anterior part of the locus coeruleus and in the dorsal part of the subcoeruleus.

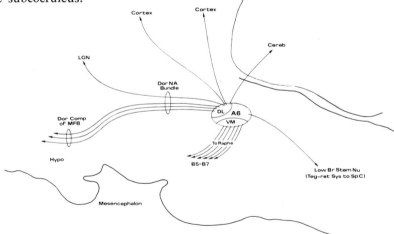

Fig. 9. Drawing of some projections of the locus coeruleus (A6) complex. The dorso-lateral (DL) portion of the locus coeruleus (principal locus coeruleus of Olson and Fuxe (1970); posterior locus coeruleus according to Jouvet (1972 c)) sends projections to the cerebellum (Cereb) and contributes mainly to the dorsal noradrenergic pathway with components projecting to the lateral geniculate nucleus (LGN) and, after turning ventrally at the anterior mesencephalic level, the dorsal component of the medial forebrain bundle system (Dor Comp of MFB) passes to the hippocampus and neocortical formations. The·posterior part of the locus coeruleus projects primarily to the medullary (Low Br Stem Nu) and spinal cord areas via the tegmento-reticular fiber systems (Teg-ret Sys to SpC). Powerful components from the more ventro-medial parts (VM) of the locus coeruleus pass into the raphé complex, especially nuclei B5, B6 and B7 (see text for details). Other abbreviation: Hypo = hypothalamus.

Thus, according to Maeda and Shimizu (1972), the catecholaminergic ascending fibers of the anterior part of the locus coeruleus, of the sub-coeruleus (A7), and of group K (A5) pass rostrally through a bundle (ponto-hypothalamic bundle) which is located in the dorso-medial part of the mesencephalon (just ventral to the dorsal noradrenergic pathway) and terminates especially at the level of the periventricular part of the ipsilateral hypothalamus. These neurons have relatively thicker axons terminating with thick varicosities. From these disseminated nuclei an independent bundle ascends from the pons and passes rostrad at the inside of the dorsal longitudinal fasciculus to innervate the hypothalamus. Maeda and Shimizu (1972) have termed this an intermediary bundle (intermediate noradrenergic pathway) which would thus be in addition to the so-called dorsal and ventral noradrenergic systems of the Swedish school. They also point out that the "real" ventral noradrenergic pathway seems to be composed of aminergic fibers which start almost exclusively at the level of the medulla (medullo-forebrain systems) and which ascend ventrally in the reticular formation of the pons and mesencephalon.

They have observed that some of the fibers of the two components of the intermediate fiber system which come up from the brainstem can be traced, via the zona incerta, to the periventricular hypothalamic zone. In accord with this finding, a significant decrease of the varicosities was observed at the level of the periventricular area when a lesion was placed in this intermediate bundle just laterally in regard to the periventricular nucleus.

Thus, from the careful analyses of Maeda and Shimizu (1972), it was concluded that at the level of the mesencephalon there are three major catecholaminergic bundles: (1) the dorsal pathway lying just ventro-lateral to the central gray substance; 2) the intermediate pathway lying just ventral to this; and 3) the so-called ventral noradrenergic pathways which lie ventro-laterally to the intermediate bundle. When viewed in sagittal section the dorsal noradrenergic bundle is seen emanating from the principal portion of the locus coeruleus. The intermediate bundle derives primarily from the pontine disseminated group of Maeda and Shimizu, i.e., the locus sub-coeruleus, the anterior portion of the locus coeruleus and from the K cell group immediately below. The true ventral noradrenergic pathway projects primarily from the medulla through the pons and lies ventro-lateral to the above pathways at the level of the mesencephalon finally passing into the diencephalon and comprising, with other fibers, the more ventral components of the medial forebrain bundle. In summary, the studies of Maeda and Shimizu (1972) indicate that there thus exist two ascending amine fiber systems from the pontine amine neurons to the forebrain, namely the coerulo-cortical and ponto-hypothalamic neuron systems. The coerulo-cortical systems would appear to be identical with the dorsal noradrenergic pathways described by the Swedish workers. The ponto-hypothalamic pathway, termed by Maeda and Shimizu as an intermediate noradrenergic pathway, has not previously been defined by the Swedish School. The ventral noradrenergic pathways, according to Maeda and Shimizu, are derived from cell groups A1 to A4 in the medulla. The axons of the coerulo-cortical neuron system originate from the principal portion of the locus coeruleus and ascend just beneath the central gray substance to innervate, with very fine varicosities, the neo-, meso-, archi-, and paleo-cortices, i.e., the entire cortical region. On their ascent they appear to give rise to axon collaterals to the diencephalon. Maeda and Shimizu could derive no topographical subdivision of the principal portion of the locus coeruleus from the studies of the fiber projections, but emphasized that single neurons of this division appear to innervate the whole cortical region and thalamus.

Olson and Fuxe (1972), using knife cut lesioning procedures and histofluorescence mapping techniques, further charted the so-called sub-coeruleus area. They found that the dorsal noradrenergic pathway mainly originates from the dorso lateral part (principal nucleus) of the locus coeruleus while the origin of the ventral noradrenergic pathway is more heterogeneous, with cell bodies both in the pons and in the medulla oblongata. In these studies they have proposed that the pontine noradrenergic cell bodies, of which the ventral part of cell group A6 as well as A7 is comprised, and the noradrenergic nerve cells connecting these two groups, constitute the "subcoeruleus area." This area lies ventral to the principal locus coeruleus and gives rise mainly to thick periventricular plexa of fibers along the third ventricle in the hypothalamus and the preoptic areas. Fuxe and Olson observed that the noradrenergic cell bodies in the medulla (A1 to A4) mainly innervate the basal and lateral parts of the hypothalamus, the preoptic area, and the ventral part of the interstital nucleus of the stria terminalis. They have noted the existence of descending noradrenergic pathways from the subcoeruleus area.

The nucleus subcoeruleus extends from the caudal level of the nucleus locus coeruleus to approximately the mid-level of the latter (approximately 1 mm). The caudal portion lies medial to the brachium conjunctivum and latero-ventral to the nucleus of the locus coeruleus with which it is directly continuous. The cells of the rostral portion are dispersed among fibers of the brachium conjunctivum. These workers also traced the fibers of the ventral noradrenergic bundle caudally to the area of group A5 and into the nucleus reticularis pontis oralis and caudalis. Olson and Fuxe interpret their results as giving rather clear-cut evidence that the ascending ventral noradrenergic pathway can be divided into two components: 1) the subcoeruleus and 2) the medulla oblongata components, respectively. They feel that the latter also contain fibers from the pontine cell group A5. In these studies the sub-coeruleus projection was shown to originate from the ventral part of A6, A7, and the noradrenergic cell bodies connecting these groups and to innervate mainly the periventricular areas of the hypothalamus and preoptic area. Olson and Fuxe have emphasized that this subcoeruleus projection rapidly joins the ascending medulla oblongata projection (they say primarily from A1 and A2 cell groups) to form the ventral noradrenergic pathway and does not itself constitute a distinct intermediate pathway. This interpretation thus differs from that of Maeda and Shimizu (1972) which indicated that the subcoeruleus projection forms a distinct intermediate pathway between the dorsal noradrenergic projection and the ventral noradrenergic path.

Olson and Fuxe (1972) feel that the principal locus coeruleus, i.e., the dorso-lateral part, is mainly concerned with coordinating cortical activities and with the regulation of vigilance states via its diffuse and widespread cortical innervation. On the other hand, they put forward the view that the noradrenergic cell bodies of the subcoeruleus area may be concerned with control of visceral and neuroendocrine functions via their hypothalamic, preoptic, and medullary projections. In their speculative functional interpretations, the large subcoeruleus noradrenergic neurons may also play a role as coordinators of activity in the visceral centers of the hypothalamus, medulla, and pons.

Fuxe et. al. (1968) have carried out a systematic description of the distribution of catecholamine nerve terminals in the cerebral cortex. They showed that the vast majority of these terminals represent norepinephrine nerve terminals since the norepinephrine concentrations are around 0.35 $\mu g/g$, whereas the dopamine concentrations are very low to insignificant. They pointed out that in spite of the relatively high concentrations of norepinephrine it has been difficult to visualize noradrenergic nerve terminals due to the fact that most of them appear to be very fine and that the varicosities contain only small amounts of norepinephrine as compared to those of the hypothalamic noradrenergic nerve terminals. These workers observed that there exists diffusely spread out noradrenergic nerve terminals in practically all parts of the cortex of the rat and that this pattern of distribution is also observed in the hippocampal region. In the neocortex there was no marked difference among the various regions. They showed that the high density of noradrenergic nerve terminals exists in the cingular region which forms a component of the limbic lobe and that the noradrenergic terminals arise from fine axons, which run in the cingulum. It was observed that these axons originate from cell bodies in the brainstem which reach the cingulum via the medial forebrain bundle after by-passing the septal area. It was also shown that the terminals seem to make axodendritic contacts, with close relations to nerve cells being in the minority. In several cortical areas the highest density was present in the molecular layer, indicating that close contacts are made with the terminal branches of the apical dendrites of the pyramidal cells. Thus, this distribution pattern is somewhat similar to the so called "unspecific afferents" (Scheibel and Scheibel, 1967), with the highest density of terminals being in the four outer layers. The well known specific thalamic projection systems, on the other hand, seem to distribute mainly to the inner granular layer. Thus, this study demonstrated the existence of a diffuse network of fine, varicose noradrenergic nerve terminals in practically all parts of the cerebral cortex of the rat. Recently Nystrom et al. (1972) have shown that both the cerebral and cerebellar cortices of man are richly provided with noradrenergic nerve terminals with a density equalling that of the rat.

It is of interest to note that Dahlström and Fuxe (1964, 1965) pointed out that cell groups of the "limbic midbrain area", with the exception of the ventral and dorsal nuclei of Gudden, contain numerous catecholamine and serotonin cells. There would appear to be somewhat of a misinterpretation as to the extent of the limbic midbrain zone as originally defined by Nauta (1958), since this region would appear more to overlap the raphé complex and the nucleus centralis superior of Bechterew rather than whose in which catecholamine cells have been described. This is a rather important point since the limbic midbrain zone has extensive reciprocal connections with the limbic forebrain zone. Terminals from cell groups A10, B7 and B8, in particular, seem to play an important role as part of the limbic forebrain limbic midbrain integration system since terminals from these regions are profusely distributed to the amygdaloid complex and the hippocampal gyrus. It is particularly important to note that serotonergic cell groups B7 and B8 send fibers to the neostriatum which has a relatively high content of serotonin.

In considering the projection systems from the limbic midbrain area, a few notes about this region are helpful, especially when discussed in relation to histochemical mapping studies (Figs. 3, 10). In this regard, Briggs and Kaelber (1971) placed lesions in the dorsal and deep tegmental nuclei of Gudden and showed degeneration coursing through the mammillary peduncle and dorso-lateral to the mammillary body. These degenerating fibers continued rostrally along the course of the medial forebrain bundle and terminate in the lateral hypothalamic and preoptic areas ipsilateral to the lesion. Degeneration was noted to be diffuse in the preoptic area but could not be traced further rostrally. It was observed that fibers from the dorsal and ventral tegmental nuclei of Gudden follow different paths in reaching the tegmento-peduncular tract (Figs. 10, 11). Those from the dorsal nucleus pass dorsal to the medial longitudinal fasciculus before entering the anterior raphé nuclei including the nucleus centralis superior of Bechterew, while those emanating from the deep or ventral nucleus of Gudden run ventrally to this bundle. Many fibers originating in both nuclei terminate throughout the nucleus centralis superior of Bechterew, while others continue ventrally to enter the interpeduncular nucleus. Some fibers run rostrally in the ventro-lateral tegmentum, ventro-lateral to the medial longitudinal fasciculus, and were shown to end in the nuclei centre median, parafasciculus, centralis medialis, and centralis lateralis of the thalamus, all in the thalamic intralaminar group. The work of Briggs and Kaelber showed that the dorsal and deep tegmental nuclei contribute fibers which terminate in the nucleus centralis superior of Bechterew and the interpeduncular nucleus via a tegmento-peduncular tract (Figs. 10, 11). In brains in which the lesions involved the pontine tegmentum the degeneration seen in the intralaminar nuclei of the thalamus could have been due to interruption of fibers of passage. These are important morphological considerations because of the powerful reciprocity of connections between the limbic midbrain area and the limbic forebrain zones, via the medial forebrain bundle in the lateral hypothalamus. Also, these limbic midbrain fields overlap to a considerable extent the anterior raphé complex. Lesions in restricted zones in this area (Morgane and Stern, 1972) have a selective depleting effect on basal forebrain serotonin (see below).

Andén et al. (1966c), using combined histochemical and biochemical approaches, have attempted to more precisely localize the noradrenergic cell bodies in the lower brainstem. In rats lesions were placed in the lateral reticular formation between pons and midbrain. Histofluorescence mapping showed a marked decrease in the number of noradrenergic terminals in the

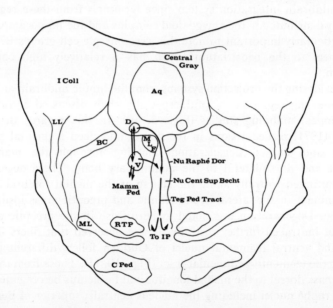

Fig. 10. Frontal schematic drawing of rostral projections from the limbic midbrain and anterior raphé zones. Note that the dorsal nucleus of Gudden projects into the nucleus raphé dorsalis (Nu Raphé Dor) and, via this, to the nucleus centralis superior of Bechterew (Nu Cent Sup Becht) forming the tegmento-peduncular tract (Teg Ped Tract) to the interpeduncular nucleus (IP). The ventral nucleus of Gudden (V) projects rostrally via the mammillary peduncle (Mamm Ped) and also sends components into the nucleus raphé dorsalis and nucleus centralis superior of Bechterew, joining with the fibers from the dorsal nucleus of Gudden (D). Other abbreviations: I Coll = inferior colliculus; Aq = aqueduct; MLF = medial longitudinal fasciculus; LL = lateral lemniscus; BC = brachium conjunctivum; ML = medial lemniscus; RTP = nucleus reticularis tegmenti pontis of Bechterew; C Ped = cerebral peduncle.

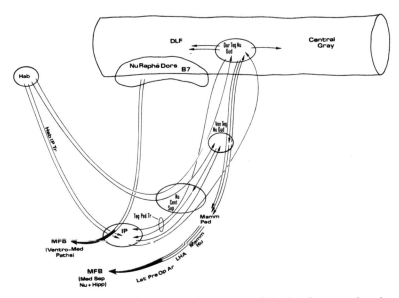

Fig. 11. Schematic representation of projection systems of the dorsal tegmental nucleus of Gudden (Dor Teg Nu Gud) and nucleus raphé dorsalis (Nu Raphé Dors, B7). Note projection from dorsal tegmental nucleus to interpeduncular nucleus (IP) via tegmento-peduncular tract (Teg Ped Tr). Some of these projections run through and possibly relay in the nucleus centralis superior of Bechterew (Nu Cent Sup). The heaviest projection from the dorsal nucleus of Gudden runs in the mammillary peduncle (Mamm Ped), through the lateral hypothalamic area (LHA), lateral preoptic area (Lat Pre Op Ar) in medial forebrain bundle (MFB) to the medial septal nucleus (Med Sep Nu) and hippocampus (Hipp). The raphé projections (serotonergic) are indicated as passing near (but not through) the interpeduncular nucleus and form the ventro-medial path (Ventro-Med Paths) in the medial forebrain bundle. Other abbreviations: DLF = dorsal longitudinal fasciculus; Hab = habenula; Ven Teg Nu Gud = ventral tegmental nucleus of Gudden; Hab IP Tr = habenulo-interpeduncular tract.

ipsilateral neocortex, limbic forebrain area, and hypothalamus while dopamine terminals were not affected. Biochemical data were in complete agreement with the histochemical findings. They concluded that two-thirds of the noradrenergic terminals in the telencephalon and diencephalon belong to neurons with cell bodies caudal to the mesencephalon, whereas practically all the dopamine cell bodies are present mainly in the mesencephalon and partly in the diencephalon. Since monoamine terminals in the pons, medulla, and cord were intact these terminals must derive from fibers originating from cell bodies in the pons and medulla. A marked increase in fluorescence intensity was seen in swollen catecholamine cell bodies in the lateral reticular formation of the medulla, especially cell group A1, and in catecholamine cell bodies of groups A5 to A7 in the pons. Most of the retrograde cell changes were seen on the side ipsilateral to the lesion indicating that the majority of the noradrenergic neurons appeared uncrossed. The fibers from the medulla were described as reaching the mesencephalon via the dorsal part of the reticular formation in the medulla, and from the reticular formation of the pons just medial to fibers of the facial nerve. They join the fibers from the noradrenergic cell bodies in the pons at the level of the motor nucleus of the trigeminal nerve where all the fibers appear to lie immediately medial and dorso-medial to this nucleus.

Andén et al. (1966b) mapped out a number of ascending monoamine neuron systems from the lower brainstem by studying the anterograde and retrograde fluorescence changes that occur in these neurons after various types of brain lesions. In this way they demonstrated: 1) ascending norepinephrine neuron systems with cell bodies situated mainly in the medulla and pons (locus coeruleus, reticular formation), and axons running uncrossed mainly in the medial forebrain bundle innervating the limbic forebrain structures, the neocortex, and the hypothalamus; 2) a dopamine neuron system, arising from cell bodies in the mesencephalon, ascending uncrossed in the medial forebrain bundle close to the nigro-neostriatal dopamine fibers, and innervating the tuberculum olfactorium and the nucleus accumbens; and 3) a large, uncrossed nigro-neostriatal dopamine neuron system. These workers have noted that there are ascending monoamine fibers in the medial forebrain bundle to the neocortex and that the neocortex does not seem to contain any monoamine nerve cell bodies. They further observed that these axons are very thin (1 to 2 microns) and appear to be unmyelinated. This latter fact may explain why various workers have failed to detect fiber degeneration in the neocortex following brainstem lesions using classical anatomical methods.

4. *Amine-Specific Pathways as Determined by Lesions*

In addition to tracing chemical systems by histofluorescence mapping (histochemical methods), it has also been shown that following discrete lesions, biogenic amine measures in terminal regions to which fibers systems project may indicate the type of amine pathway, thus complementing the histochemical findings. A large series of experiments using this approach has been carried out since the Heller et al. report (1962) of decreases in serotonin following medial forebrain bundle lesions in the rat. This was the first study in which there were attempts to assess the chemical identity of neurons using the lesion method and determine whether fiber systems can be delineated which show selective specificity for the various biogenic amines. In later studies Harvey et al. (1963) showed that the fall in cortical serotonin was related specifically to sectioning the medial forebrain bundle and the consequent degeneration of its fibers; i.e., the fall in serotonin began 2 to 3 days after the lesion and was complete by day 12. They showed the decreases in serotonin levels were restricted to areas innervated by the tract. Moore et al. (1965) also found that after lateral hypothalamic lesions there were significant decreases in serotonin levels in all regions of the telencephalon. In this same study they demonstrated that fractional lesions in the lateral hypothalamus involved various numbers of serotonergic fibers and observed that the lesion diminished not only serotonin but also the enzyme necessary for its synthesis (tryptophan hydroxylase). Thus, the selected lesions altered the levels of either serotonin and norepinephrine, in part, by affecting the synthesis of these amines. In this study they noted that with no known direct projections to the neocortex some type of transynaptic effect must be involved. They concluded that *distant* neurochemical effects must be of importance in determining the physiological and behavioral sequelae of brain lesions. Heller and Moore (1965) conclusively demonstrated the selective nature of chemical changes following restricted lesions in the trajectory of various pathways entering the hypothalamus, including the medial forebrain bundle and concluded that the medial forebrain bundle is involved with the maintenance of both serotonin and norepinephrine in the brain. They further showed that the lateral tegmentum is concerned only with norepinephrine. Lesions in the central gray at the level of dorsal nucleus of Gudden lowered only serotonin while dorso-medial tegmental lesions reduced both amines. Only those lesions sectioning the medial forebrain bundle or ablating areas contributing fibers to that tract led to decreases in amines. The appearance of degenerating fibers in the medial forebrain bundle coincided with onset of decreases in amines after lesions. Heller et al. (1966) showed that select lesions of the medial forebrain bundle produce significant decreases of norepinephrine content throughout the telencephalon on the half of the brain ipsilateral to the lesion. Medial hypothalamic lesions did not affect the norepinephrine content of any brain region.

Heller and Moore (1968), in an attempt to delineate the role of specific fiber groups in maintenance of amines in their terminal areas, placed lesions in a series of mesencephalic, diencephalic, and telencephalic areas and determined serotonin levels in whole brain of rats. Lesions in the septal area, dorso-medial tegmentum, and ventral midbrain tegmentum reduced brain serotonin by 12-15%. Lateral hypothalamic area lesions reduced serotonin by 36% while lesions in other areas produced insignificant changes. It appears that the integrity of the lateral hypothalamic-medial forebrain bundle system is necessary for the maintenance of serotonin in the brain. Thus, each lesion which significantly affected serotonin either transected the medial forebrain bundle or involved fiber systems contributing to it. Lesions in the medial forebrain bundle or the dorso-medial tegmentum produced a reduction in brain norepinephrine. Therefore, the concept that selective destruction of restricted brain areas could produce amine-specific effects was shown. Medial forebrain bundle and dorso-medial tegmental lesions both produced significant decreases in both serotonin and norepinephrine. The two tegmental lesions demonstrated lesion selectivity. Ventro-lateral tegmental destruction reduced norepinephrine in telencephalic areas and diencephalon without affecting serotonin whereas central gray lesions lowered only serotonin. It was concluded that lateral tegmental nuclei are necessary for maintenance of brain norepinephrine whereas normal serotonin levels appear dependent on the integrity of more dorsal and medial tegmental nuclei. These workers also showed that levels of norepinephrine and serotonin were decreased throughout the telencephalon following medial forebrain bundle lesions in both rat and cat, although by anatomical degeneration techniques only the septal area and amygdala were found to be directly innervated by this bundle. The dorso-medial tegmental lesion was shown to have a regional distribution of degenerating axons identical to that of the ventro-lateral tegmental lesions. A dorsal fiber group was shown to traverse the central reticular formation to enter the subthalamus and intralaminar thalamic nuclei. Degeneration in this group predominated following the ventro-lateral tegmental lesions. A second, ventral group of axons, was also demonstrated after each lesion and these fibers traversed the ventral tegmental area of Tsai to enter the medial forebrain bundle. Degeneration in this group predominated following the dorso-medial tegmental lesion. It was emphasized that both of these lesions destroy axons which contribute to the medial forebrain bundle.

Morgane and Stern (1972) carried out an extensive series of lesions in the medial forebrain bundle system extending from the limbic midbrain area, through the lateral hypothalamus, and into the preoptic areas in order to more precisely define the topography of amine-specific neurons in this system. Special attention was given to latero-lateral lesions in the lateral hypothalamus and it was found that mid-lateral hypothalamic lesions (Fig. 12) selectively reduced serotonin in the basal forebrain area with insignificant effects or norepinephrine, while upper far-lateral hypothalamic lesions (Fig. 13) selectively reduced norepinephrine with insignificant effects on serotonin. These findings confirmed the more lateral and dorsal trajectory of noradrenergic pathways in the medial forebrain bundle, with serotonergic elements being the more medial components in this heterogeneous bundle. Lesions in the ventral half of the central gray at the level of the dorsal nucleus of Gudden or in dorso-medial or ventro-medial tegmental areas selectively lowered basal forebrain serotonin with almost no effects on norepinephrine (Fig. 14). These studies indicate that the paramedial midbrain areas (limbic midbrain zone) overlap the serotonin cell groups of the anterior raphé and that the serotonergic fibers emanating from this zone pass more medially in the medial forebrain bundle. The implications of this are that the anterior raphé area is strongly related reciprocally with the limbic forebrain area and thus comes under possible regulation from many limbic forebrain structures.

There is some question whether the Nauta method is sufficiently reliable and sensitive to demonstrate all of the connections of the medial forebrain bundle. However, there is nothing to suggest that it is not. Heller and Moore (1968) pointed out that they have routinely resolved degenerating axons which have been measured to be 0.5 microns in diameter. This is well within

the size range which should include most, if not all, central axons and terminals, and, taking into account the well recognized swelling which occurs
during the process of axonal degeneration, they may well have been

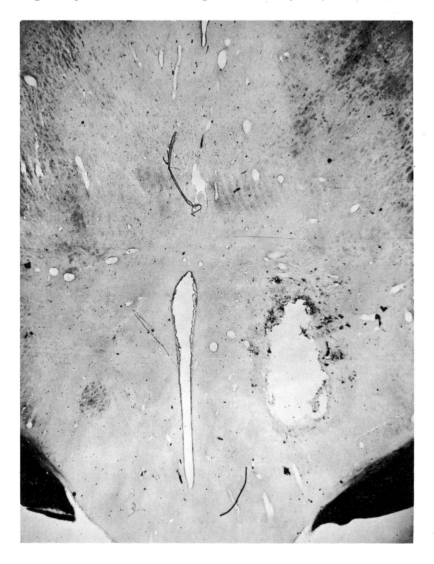

Fig. 12. Photograph of mid-lateral hypothalamic lesion in the cat that specifically lowers
serotonin levels in the ipsilateral basal forebrain area with insignificant effects on
norepinephrine. Note by comparing the lesioned side with opposite side that this lesion involves the part of the lateral hypothalamus immediately lateral to the descending column of
the fornix (mid lateral hypothalamic area). Klüver stain, approx. 20 X.

demonstrating axons whose normal diameter was in the range of 0.2 microns. In this regard, Moore and Heller (1967) carried out studies of the cross-sectional diameter of more than 100 axons measured by electron micrographs from the rat medial forebrain bundle. The vast majority of the axons in the tract were unmyelinated and ranged from 0.2 microns to 0.7 microns in diameter. The myelinated axons, which were relatively few in number, varied from 0.6 microns to 3.0 microns in diameter.

Heller (1972) has pointed out that with the use of degeneration studies it has been possible to follow fibers in the medial forebrain bundle to the medial hypothalamus, lateral hypothalamus, anterior hypothalamus and a moderate number to the anterior amygdaloid nuclei and medial septal nucleus, with a few degenerating fibers also seen in the lateral septal nucleus and nucleus accumbens. He noted that no fibers from the medial forebrain bundle terminate in the striatum, in other limbic or rhinencephalic areas, or in the neocortex. He has argued that the neurochemical effects of the lesions on norepinephrine and serotonin levels cannot be explained simply on the basis of section and degeneration of monoamine-producing neurons but that

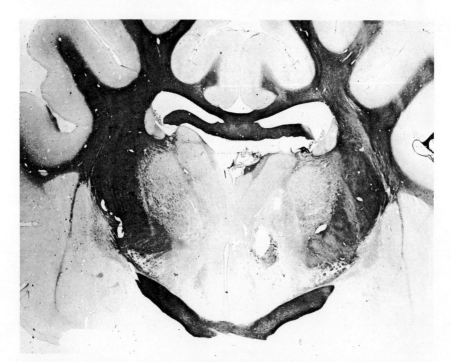

Fig. 13. Photograph of far-lateral hypothalamic lesion in the cat that specifically lowers ipsilateral basal forebrain levels of norepinephrine with insignificant effects on serotonin. This lesion extends about 0.5 mm laterally and 1 mm dorsally to that shown in Figure 10 and does not impinge on the lateral hypothalamic area just lateral to the fornix. Klüver stain, approx. 10 X.

the mechanism is more complex and represents, at least in part, a disruption of normal neuronal control of monoamine biosynthesis in the brain mediated across a polyneuronal system. He has observed that since transneuronal degeneration is an uncommon event in the central nervous system, outside of the sensory projections, the neurochemical changes are presumably occurring in intact cells. He feels that the reduction in biogenic amine-enzymatic activities results from an altered afferent input to monoamine-producing neurons rostral to the cells destroyed by the particular lesion. This explanation of lesion effects implies that under normal circumstances the level of enzymes essential for the biosynthesis of serotonin and norepinephrine is a function of afferent input to monoamine-producing cells and that the lesion removes the primary fiber tract over which such influences are transmitted rostrally in the brain. The loss of medial forebrain bundle axons and the afferent influences they transmit thus result in a reduction in enzyme content and, secondarily, in cellular content of the biogenic amines.

There is considerable controversy regarding the synaptic nature of the ascending monoaminergic pathways. Thus, the Heller, Harvey and Moore

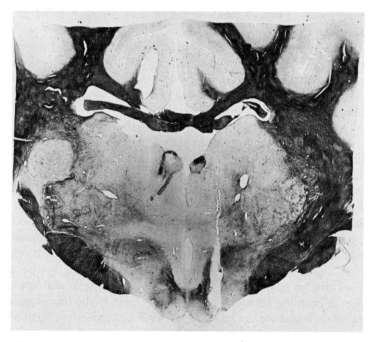

Fig. 14. Photograph of cat brain at posterior hypothalamic level (level of mammillary bodies) showing a highly amine-specific lesion occupying the narrow space between the mammillary body and substantia nigra. This lesion specifically lowers serotonin levels in the basal forebrain area on the ipsilateral side with insignificant effects on norepinephrine. Klüver stain, approx. 10 X.

group feel that they are mainly polysynaptic systems and that amine decreases following lesions of the medial forebrain bundle result from transynaptic metabolic changes in anatomically intact neuronal systems. On the other hand, the histochemical fluorescence technique has not identified monoamine cell bodies between the hypothalamus and the telencephalon and, thus, the Swedish group has direct evidence preponderantly supporting the view of direct monosynaptic fiber systems passing from the brainstem to the cerebral neocortex. In view of the organization of the medial forebrain bundle into both long (monosynaptic) as well as polysynaptic elements, both types of systems may project to the neocortex.

In other studies, Benetato et al. (1967a, b) have reported a fall of hypothalamic serotonin following bilateral lesions of the medial forebrain bundle at the level of the hypothalamus in the rat. Parent and Poirier (1969), and Parent et al. (1969) confirmed these findings following bilateral ventro-medial tegmental lesions in the cat. The interruption of the medial forebrain bundle rostral to the hypothalamus did not result in any decrease of hypothalamic serotonin, indicating that serotonergic fibers to the hypothalamus are exclusively ascending. These workers showed that interrupting many pathways to and from the hypothalamus does not modify the concentration of hypothalamic serotonin. For example, bilateral lesions of the fornix, the dorsal longitudinal fasciculus, the amygdalo-hypothalamic fibers, or the periventricular system did not interfere with the normal concentration of serotonin in the hypothalamus. All of this work confirms the view that ascending serotonergic fibers have their origin in medially located upper brainstem nuclei which have been shown to be rich in serotonin by histofluorescence mapping techniques.

Parent et al. (1969), using biochemical methods following lesions, showed that catecholaminergic neurons of the substantia nigra give rise to important ascending dopaminergic pathways which terminate in the ipsilateral striatum. In one study they found that interruption of a group of fibers different from those concerned with serotonin in the ventro-medial tegmental area of the midbrain resulted in retrograde degeneration of the cells of the substantia nigra as well as a marked decrease of dopamine in the ipsilateral striatum in the monkey and the cat. Most importantly, they showed that these nigro-striatal dopaminergic neurons may be under the direct control of the striato-nigral pathways which show an intense cholinesterasic activity that fades after striatal lesions. Their studies also suggest that specific intracerebrally coursing nervous pathways contribute to the biosynthesis, at a distance, of various chemical mediators, including serotonin, dopamine, and acetylcholine. Their results further indicate that, in contrast, hypothalamic norepinephrine appears to be elaborated independently of any centrally coursing pathways ending in the hypothalamus. In this latter regard both the work of Benetato's group and their own showed that there was no change in norepinephrine concentration of the hypothalamus following bilateral in-

terruption of the medial forebrain bundle in the rat. This latter finding does
not agree with the earlier work of Moore and Heller (1967), Heller and Moore
(1968), Heller (1972), and others who have shown that specific lesions in the
medial forebrain bundle may decrease hypothalamic norepinephrine. On the
other hand, Morgane and Stern (1972) showed that with medial forebrain
bundle lesions in the lateral (but not the medial) preoptic area there were
significant decreases in hypothalamic norepinephrine with insignificant
effects on hypothalamic serotonin.

In further studies to delimit chemical fiber systems in the medial forebrain
bundle, Parent and Poirier (1969) showed that unilateral lesions of the caudal
hypothalamus, the ventral tegmental area of the Tsai and ventro-medial
tegmental area resulted in a decrease in concentration of both dopamine and
serotonin in the ipsilateral striatum. Lesions of the rostro-medial
hypothalamus medial to the fornix and of the subthalamus did not interfere
with the concentration of either amine in the corresponding striatum.
Significantly, lesions of the rostro-lateral hypothalamus involving the medial
forebrain bundle were associated with an almost complete depletion of
dopamine without any change of the serotonin concentration in the
corresponding striatum. Caudal and latero-rostral hypothalamic lesions were
associated with a cell loss in the ipsilateral substantia nigra and nucleus
linearis area. These workers conclude that these results confirm previous
findings suggesting that the dopamine and serotonin ascending pathways
course in the ventro-medial tegmental area of the brainstem from the level of
the upper pons to that of the caudal hypothalamus. Moreover, they indicate
that at the level of the rostro-lateral hypothalamus, the medial forebrain
bundle contains the dopamine but not the serotonin fibers ending in the
striatum. Serotonin fibers deriving from the nucleus linearis and raphé
complex end in the baso-medial telencephalic structures after apparently
traveling within the more medial components of medial forebrain bundle.
Summarizing these results, Parent and Poirier showed that bilateral lesions
of the dorsal tegmentum, the dorsal or lateral hypothalamus, or the subthalamus do not interfere with a normal concentration of serotonin in the
striatum. Caudo-ventral hypothalamic lesions, however, resulted in a lower
serotonin concentration in the striatum. In the light of these and other
negative data, they concluded that the serotonin fibers terminating in the
striatum reach the latter structure through the rostral part of the cerebral
peduncle and the internal capsule. They summarized their data as follows: it
appears that the nigro-striatal dopamine pathway and serotonin fibers
ending in various areas of the diencephalon and telencephalon are
topographically related in the area of Tsai at the midbrain and caudal
hypothalamic level. More rostrally, the dopamine striatal afferents course in
the medial forebrain bundle, whereas the serotonin striatal afferents apparently travel in the cerebral peduncle (Fig. 15). On the other hand,
norepinephrine, which is mainly concentrated in the hypothalamus, appears

to be synthesized independently of the central nervous pathways to and from the hypothalamus. They noted that this peculiar arrangement of the above-mentioned monoaminergic mechanisms may, to some extent, explain certain behavioral and visceral disturbances associated with differently placed lesions at the hypothalamic level.

The data of Parent and Poirier (1969) appear to indicate that the ascending monoaminergic pathways ending in the striatum have a somewhat different course than that proposed by the Heller and Moore groups concerning the serotonin fibers and by Andén et al. (1966a, b) concerning the serotonin and

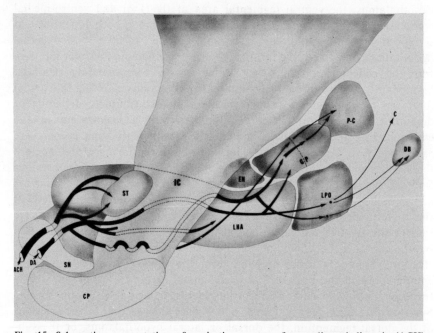

Fig. 15. Schematic representation of projection routes of ascending cholinergic (ACH) reticular fibers and dopamine (DA) fiber systems in their diencephalic trajectory as viewed from the right side seen from behind. As noted by Shute (1970), cholinergic axons from the dorsal hypothalamic neurons run rostrally by a more medial route to the reticular nucleus and globus pallidus (GP) and thence on to the caudate-putamen (P-C). Some of these fibers may terminate in the entopeduncular nucleus (EN). Other components of this system project forward in the medial forebrain bundle through the lateral hypothalamic (LHA) and lateral preoptic areas (LPO) to relay in the diagonal band area (DB), and some pass directly to the cerebral cortex (C). Fibers from cells of the subthalamic nucleus (ST) take a more lateral route across the cerebral peduncle (CP) to the entopeduncular nucleus and globus pallidus. The dopamine fiber systems, especially emanating from the substantia nigra (SN), pass rostrally in groups of fibers, one forming the nigro-striatal system that winds its way through the cerebral peduncle and projects to the globus pallidus and putamen-caudate. Another component of the dopamine system (meso-limbic component) passes rostrally in the medial forebrain bundle through the lateral hypothalamic area and the lateral preoptic region toward limbic forebrain terminal sites. Other abbreviations: IC = internal capsule.

dopamine fibers. Bedard et al. (1969) carried out a correlative study of the nigro-striatal pathway based on neuroanatomical and neurochemical criteria in the cat and the monkey. They noted that the striato-nigral fibers are distributed to the substantia nigra according to a topographical relationship which is strikingly similar to that of the nigro-striatal fibers. They postulated that the striato-nigral pathway, which is highly cholinergic (see below), may represent a feedback mechanism in a striato-nigro-striatal loop by which the corpus striatum controls its own levels of dopamine.

Many studies involving the tracing of degenerating terminals in the material prepared by the Nauta technique following lesions in the substantia nigra have failed to disclose any important group of nigro-striatal fibers. It is likely that such fibers are extremely small, a fact which could explain the failure to demonstrate them in material prepared for the study of terminal degeneration. Electron microscopic studies have disclosed numerous axons of very fine caliber, 0.6 microns or less, terminating in the caudate nucleus. Electrophysiological studies involving the recording of evoked potentials in single neurons of the caudate nucleus in response to stimulation of the substantia nigra have revealed the existence of long latency (15 to 20 msec) unit discharges, suggesting the presence of direct nigro-striatal fibers of very fine caliber. It is clear, however, that in the cat the nigro-striatal fibers do course in the lateral hypothalamus within the medial forebrain bundle as indicated by the studies of Moore et al. (1971). They have emphasized that it has not been possible to demonstrate a nigro-neostriatal projection by conventional anatomical techniques and that electrophysiological studies have also not yielded definitive data for a direct pathway. By combined anatomical and chemical studies they have shown that, following lesions in the pars compacta of the substantia nigra, degenerating axons can be traced rostrally in the ventral midbrain tegmentum to reach the ventral and lateral parts of Forel's field H (pre-rubral field). More rostrally in the diencephalon, the projection forms a compact tract which lies partly in the medial internal capsule and partly in the adjacent lateral hypothalamus where its fibers mingle with the more lateral components of the medial forebrain bundle (far-lateral hypothalamus). The demonstration of nigro-neostriatal projections in this study was made possible by application of the technique of Fink and Heimer which allows the selective silver impregnation of degenerating axons and terminals. They also found that when lesions are large and involve both the medial internal capsule and the lateral hypothalamic area, the fall in caudate nucleus dopamine content is as great as 90% and that there is extensive retrograde degeneration which involves both the pars compacta of the substantia nigra and the adjacent ventral tegmental nuclei, both of which have been designated (above) as the brainstem sites of dopamine-containing cell bodies.

Although the cholinergic systems will be discussed in a separate section (below), it is important to mention one cholinergic system at this point since it relates to the nigro-striatal pathways and may interrelate with the monoamine systems. Olivier et al. (1970b) studied the cholinesterasic striato-pallidal and striato-nigral efferents in the cat and the monkey. These workers showed that a considerable number of cholinesterasic fibers continue downward from the striatum, through the pallidum, and reach the substantia nigra. The existence of a relationship between these cholinesterasic fibers and those demonstrated by silver impregnation techniques was further supported by the fact that in this study lesions of the caudate nucleus led, after several weeks, to the disappearance of the cholinesterasic reaction in groups of fibers ending in the ipsilateral pallidum and substantia nigra in the cat. They further observed that the striatum is the richest cholinergic structure in the brain and that the presence of important cholinergic striatal efferents suggests that the outflow from the striatum to the pallidum and substantia nigra is mainly, if not exclusively, cholinergic. The pallido-fugal fibers, however, were shown to be devoid of cholinesterase. The matter is rather complicated, however, because of the work of Smelik and Ernst (1966) who reported some evidence in favor of cholinergic synapses ending on dopaminergic cells of the substantia nigra. Olivier et al. (1970b) feel that the cholinergic pathway represented by the striato-nigral system may regulate the rate of striatal dopamine formation by influencing enzymatic mechanisms involved in the synthesis of dopamine.

5. *Unidentified Fluorescing Systems* (*Monoamine-Like Systems*)

With the above elucidation of the chemical systems in the brain it is now pertinent to discuss the nature of some unidentified chemical systems using microspectrofluorometric and pharmacological methods. Using these techniques Björklund et al. (1971a) have shown that a yellow fluorescing compound exists in the brainstem which is similar, but not identical, to serotonin. The fluorogenic compound that gives rise to this new fluorophore has an intraneuronal localization, with major storage being in cell bodies and terminals. Since, after axotomy, the fluorophore is accumulated in the proximal end of the axon this suggests that the compound is transported from cell bodies to terminals along axons. Further, its depletion by reserpine is compatible with a granular storage mechanism for the compound in the neuron. However, the intraneuronal fluorogenic compound has not yet been chemically isolated or identified. Along the same lines, Aghajanian and Asher (1971) have pointed out that the histochemical fluorescence of those neurons in the raphé, which are presumed to contain serotonin, is selectively and stereo-specifically enhanced by L-tryptophan at doses that also produce an elevation in the concentration of serotonin. However, they showed that this increase in raphé fluorescence is not prevented by PCPA, an inhibitor of serotonin synthesis. They concluded that, under some conditions, derivatives of tryptophan other than, or in addition to, serotonin may be of significance in raphé neurons. They note that under such conditions the term serotonin-containing or "serotonergic" can be applied only tentatively to raphé neurons pending the acquisition of further data concerning the exact chemical identity of the fluorescent substance or substances in raphé cells. Björklund et al. (1971b) have now described three fluorescing systems, a serotonin system, a catecholaminergic system, and another system which contains a monoamine-like substance, possibly an indoleethylamine derivative not identical to serotonin. The catecholamine-containing neurons (A-type, fluoresce green) were depleted by reserpine and not notably affected by either PCPA or nialamide. The B-type neurons were depleted by reserpine and not affected by PCPA or nialamide, but fluoresced at the yellow wavelength, like that of serotonin. The C-type neurons (serotonin-containing) were depleted by reserpine and PCPA and fluorescence was increased by nialamide. These B-type neurons were described as found primarily in the nucleus linearis caudalis, the nucelus medianus raphé and the nucleus raphé dorsalis. They were also found lateral to the nucleus medianus raphé and ventrally and ventro-laterally within the reticular formation of the mesencephalon. It was observed that these cell bodies belong to the yellow fluorescent cell groups B7, B8 and B9 according to the nomenclature of Dahlström and Fuxe (1964). It is interesting that the C-type, or serotonin-containing neurons, have a similar distribution as the B-type cell bodies. The serotonin cell bodies occur intermingled with the B-type cell bodies in the anterior raphé nuclei, but their relative distributions are somewhat different. Most of the B-type cell bodies occur within the nucleus linearis caudalis, nucleus medianus raphé (B8), and winglike structures situated somewhat lateral to this latter nucleus. The serotonin cell bodies were identified mainly in the nucleus raphé dorsalis (B7) and in the B9 group around the medial lemniscus in the mesencephalic reticular formation.

At the level of the most anterior part of the interpeduncular nucleus fibers all three fluorescing cell types merge in a fairly well-defined bundle situated just latero-dorsal to the interpeduncular nucleus. The B-type fibers form a bundle that could be traced back to the nucleus linearis caudalis of the mesencephalon which is B8, according to Björkland et al. (1971b), or nucleus medianus raphé according to Dahlström and Fuxe (1964). These fibers project rostrally through the ventral tegmental decussation into the medial part of the ventro-medial tegmental area and run medially and laterally past the habenulo-interpeduncular tract into a position fairly well separated from the catecholamine and serotonin tracts. No fibers were seen to cross the midline. Rostrally the bundle of B-type fibers were shown to run in the medial part of the medial forebrain bundle. The serotonin-type fibers intermingle with the B-type fibers and the catecholamine-type (A-type) fibers at the level of the anterior part of the interpeduncular nucleus. In the posterior mammillary region the serotonin fibers (C-type) showed a rather scattered distribution. Thus, they were found both medial to the medial forebrain bundle, where they intermingle with the B-type fibers, and in the medial forebrain bundle and field H$_2$ or Forel (fascicularis lenticularis), where they are partially intermingled with the catecholamine fibers. As reviewed earlier, more rostrally the serotonin fibers run in the medial and ventral parts of the medial forebrain bundle (see Figs. 6 and 7).

The catecholamine fibers are mainly confined to both a ventral and a dorsal fiber system. The ventral fibers could partly be traced back to the catecholamine-containing cell bodies situated in the substantia nigra and to those found in the region anterior, dorsal and lateral to the anterior part of the interpeduncular nucleus, mainly situated within the ventral tegmental area of Tsai and the linear complex of nuclei. These cell groups are primarily the A9 and A10 groups. Some of the fibers of the ventral catecholamine tract could be traced further caudally, past these catecholamine cell groups, but their origin has not been clearly identified. No doubt these derive from the A1-A5 noradrenergic system of the medulla and pons, discussed above. The ventral system of catecholamine fibers from these different sources converge into a bundle in the ventro-medial tegmentum at the level of the interpeduncular fossa, and become intermingled with both the serotonin (C-type) and B-type fibers. Rostrally they run in the medial forebrain bundle mainly lying lateral and dorsal to the B-type and to the serotonin fibers. As previously discussed, the more dorsally situated catecholamine fibers form a tract that can be traced from a position just dorso-lateral to the medial longitudinal fasciculus, rostrally along the ventricle up to the level of the caudal median eminence where the fibers then turn ventrally to join the catecholamine fibers in the medial forebrain bundle. Along its course in the caudal hypothalamus, a substantial portion of the fibers leave the dorsal tract in a ventral and ventro-lateral direction to join the ventrally situated fiber systems.

Although two types of cell bodies are intermingled in the raphé nuclei, the bulk of the B-type cell bodies are found in the nucleus linearis caudalis and the nucleus medianus raphé and scattered just lateral to these areas. In the caudal hypothalamus the B-type fibers are almost exclusively confined to a well-defined bundle situated close to the midline. In contrast, the serotonin fibers are much more widespread, running in a poorly defined tract in the ventro-medial tegmentum. It is thus clear from this work that the B-type neurons form a well defined ascending neuronal system morphologically distinguishable from the system of serotonin neurons. Björklund and colleagues (1971a, b) have emphasized that the recognition of these B-type neurons as a special and separate entity should be considered in future functional studies. They have stressed that the B-type fluorophore is derived from a hitherto unknown intraneuronal monoamine-like substance.

6. Species Variations

Most of the neurophysiological experiments on sleep have been carried out in cats while much of the biochemistry and practically all the histofluorescence mapping of chemical circuits have been done in the rat. However, there are a few studies, summarized below, that have begun to compare chemical circuits in these two species and in monkeys.

Pin et al. (1968) and Jones (1969) have attempted to work out the topography of monoaminergic neurons in the cat. They have noted that the serotonin neurons are situated at the level of all of the raphé nuclei, with the exception of the linearis nuclei. Further, they have observed an important group of serotonin cells at the level of the mesencephalon in the magnocellular part of the red nucleus. These workers have stressed that in the cat the organization of monoaminergic neurons is comparable to the one described in the rat. Some significant differences, however, were noted. For example, in the cat there exists an important group of neurons containing serotonin at the level of the magnocellular part of the red nucleus and in the nuclei of the third and fourth cranial nerves, which were not seen in the rat. Regarding the catecholamine neurons, they observed that there exists no cellular groups at the level of the medulla which, of course, is contrary to the findings of the Swedish group in the rat. They also noted that in the pons of the cat the catecholamine-containing neurons were located mostly in the dorso-lateral part of the pontine tegmentum regions of the locus coeruleus, subcoeruleus, nuclei parabrachialis medialis and lateralis, and were very closely related with the localization of monoamine oxidase. In the cat catecholamine cells were located in the mesencephalic reticular formation in regions corresponding to group A8 in the rat. They observed that, corresponding to group A9 of the rat, were cells in the pars compacta of the substantia nigra and in the medial lemniscus.

Sladek (1971a, b) has also emphasized the differences in the distribution of catecholamine varicosities in cat and rat reticular formation. In the kitten, he noted a continuous pattern of varicosities in the reticular formation that were not present in the rat. In the mesencephalon these appeared in the sub-cuneiform nuclear area, while in the rostral pons they appeared within the nucleus reticularis pontis oralis. At mid-pontine levels, these patterns appeared within the nucleus reticularis pontis caudalis. In the caudal medulla these patterns were seen near the dorsal motor nucleus of the vagus and solitary nucleus extending ventrally into the remainder of the nucleus reticularis ventralis, and medially into the raphé. Sladek also observed that, with these few exceptions, the distribution of catecholamine varicosities in the remainder of the brainstem reticular formation of the cat corresponds closely to that of the rat.

Battista et al. (1972) have carried out a mapping of central monoamine neurons in the monkey using histochemical fluorescence techniques. The animals used were *Macaca-Irus* (cynomolgus) and the African Green Monkey (*Cercopeithecus sabaeus*). They observed that the distribution of both the catecholamine and serotonin cell bodies in the lower brainstem of the monkey was generally similar to that of the rat. The catecholamine cell bodies were localized in the lateral reticular formation of the medulla and the pons within the locus coeruleus, subcoeruleus area, substantia nigra, ventro-medial part of the rostral mesencephalon, and the nucleus arcuatus. They found that the number of catecholamine cell bodies in the subcoeruleus area of the monkey constituted a larger part of the catecholamine cell population than in the rat. The serotonin cell bodies were distributed in the raphé nuclei in a manner similar to that described in the rat. No serotonin cell bodies, however, were found in the red nucleus, which, as noted, Pin et al. (1968) and Jones (1969) have claimed to contain serotonin cell bodies in the cat. Battista et al. (1972) observed in the monkey three different kinds of catecholamine nerve terminals including very fine terminals which were scattered in practically all parts of the cerebral cortex in all cortical layers. They also found very fine densely packed catecholamine terminals in the neostriatum similar to those observed in the rat by Andén et al. (1964). Dense networks of these terminals were also found in the preoptic region and subcortical parts of the limbic system and are similiar to those seen in the same areas in the rat. The third type consisted of nerve terminals with strong fluorescence and varicosities and are found scattered in many brain areas, e.g., the cerebral cortex, the thalamus, and the globus pallidus. Battista et al., pointed out that these terminals had not been previously observed in the rat. They think that these types of terminals may belong to phylogenetically older neuronal systems rather than the other monoamine terminal systems described. Battista et al. noted that the serotonon nerve terminals were mainly observed in certain brainstem areas also found previously in the rat. For example, a high density of serotonin nerve terminals was observed in the suprachiasmatic nucleus. In sagittal series they showed that catecholamine fibers could be seen traversing the ventral reticular nucleus in the medulla, the parvo-cellular reticular nucleus of the pons, the caudal and oral reticular nuclei of the pons, the area medial to the motor nucleus of the trigeminal nerve, and the nucleus subcuneiformis of the mesencephalon. They noted that the course of these fibers is very similar to that of the ascending norepinephrine tracts in the rat. It was concluded that in the monkey the principal architecture of the central monoamine neurons is similar to that in the rat and other mammals such as the rabbit and the cat. Thus, the catecholamine and serotonin neurons of the lower brainstem in the monkey are reticular in type with long ascending monosynaptic connections with the telencephalon and diencephalon.

The most up-to-date consideration of species differences in monoamine systems is that Hubbard and DiCarlo (1973), who analyzed monoamine-containing cell bodies in the locus coeruleus of the squirrel monkey. They found that in most respects this area in the squirrel monkey resembles that in the rat with two major exceptions. One was the striking proximity of the fluorescing cell bodies to the mesencephalic tract of the trigeminal nerve. They found that in the squirrel monkey these fluorescing cell bodies are closely associated with the tract from its most caudal levels to the levels at which, rostrally, it takes a position lateral to the cerebral aqueduct. A second feature in the squirrel monkey, not described in the rat, was the preferential distribution of the larger cell bodies in the more dorsal portion of the locus coeruleus (where the cells are more compact) and of the smaller cell bodies in the ventral portion of the nucleus. It is especially interesting that Hubbard and Dicarlo consider cell groups A4, A6, and A7 (of Dahlström and Fuxe, 1964, 1965) as the locus coeruleus. This grouping was done on the basis that this cell complex has similar fluorescence intensity, similar Nissl staining characteristics, and are found in relative close proximity to each other. They consider that both in the rat and squirrel monkey these three groups (on anatomical and histochemical bases) should all be considered portions of the locus coeruleus. They observed similar retrograde fluorescence changes in A4 and A6 after cerebellar lesions and lesions rostral to the locus area. However, A7 did not show these changes and, thus, on these grounds, it is questionable if A7 should be grouped as part of locus complex. Especially since it contributes fibers to the ventral noradrenergic pathway while most of the locus sends fibers through the dorsal noradrenergic pathway. Hubbard and DiCarlo emphasize that, since they see fluorescence in the mesencephalic tract of the trigeminal nerve, this, too, may be considered a part of the locus complex. They correctly point out that brain atlases label this fluorescing zone as the nucleus of the mesencephalic tract of the trigeminal nerve. Hubbard and DiCarlo note that fiber systems of the locus coeruleus in the squirrel monkey are directed in a ventro-lateral as well as a dorso-medial direction which agrees somewhat with these trajectories in the rat. One puzzling aspect of this study was the notation that they found almost no nonfluorescing locus cells (what few there were appeared in the dorso-lateral portion). Thus, no accounting was given in this study for the presumed large number of cholinergic cells that are thought to contribute to the makeup of this nucleus (see below).

B. Physiological Manipulation of Monoamine Systems

1. *General Orientation*

Electrophysiological studies suggest that separate neuronal systems are involved in the mediation of states of wakefulness and attention, and it is possible that there may be neurochemical bases for such differences. The main portion of the noradrenergic pathway lies within what would usually be considered the lateral reticular formation of the brainstem, regions usually included in those portions whose activation is responsible for arousal and which produce the classical effects of the reticular activating system with desynchronization of the cortical electrical activity. One main problem which exists, however, is the relationship between noradrenergic systems and activated or REM sleep and the classical arousal response of waking.

It was originally shown by Dell (1963) and Rothballer (1956, 1959) that electrocortical activation, as well as behavioral awakening or arousal, can be produced by intracarotid injections of small amounts of norepinephrine. It was thought that this form of activation was due to excitation of the reticular activating system, which possessed adrenergic receptors in the brainstem, and that it was not due to a direct action on the cerebral cortex itself. The evidence for this was provided by experiments in which sections of the brainstem at the superior collicular level prevented arousal following injection of noradrenaline. Such experiments led to the conclusion that adrenergic cortical activation was, therefore, not direct, but that it was mediated by the brainstem activating system. Some questions about the nature of the direct action of norepinephrine have been raised by later experiments showing the failure of norepinephrine injected into the blood to be taken up by brain tissue. However, the existence of norepinephrine-containing neurons throughout a significant portion of the reticular activating system certainly suggests that norepinephrine is an important candidate for a part of the arousal mechanism. There is not sufficient evidence, however, that it is *the* cortical mediator of desynchronized activation accompanying behavioral arousal.

As reviewed, Olson and Fuxe (1971) have demonstrated that the cerebellar norepinephrine innervation originates mainly from the locus coeruleus in the same way as the cerebral cortical norepinephrine nerve terminals. They suggested that a single locus coeruleus noradrenergic nerve cell is capable of diffusely innervating all cortices of the brain. As noted earlier, they observed that the rostral projections from the locus coeruleus originate mainly from the cranial part, particularly the dorso-lateral or principal nucleus of the locus coeruleus. Most importantly, a medial fiber projection to the raphé (Fig. 9) was observed in horizontal sections which probably represents, in part, crossing fibers. These latter fiber projections partly originate from the most ventro-medial part of the locus coeruleus which, in the rat, contains the largest cell bodies and exhibits the strongest fluorescence intensity. These morphological points are reiterated especially because of the possibility that the locus coeruleus/raphé relations may play a key role in regulation of the sleep-waking cycle.

Following cerebellectomy the norepinephrine fibers can be traced all the way to the dorso-lateral locus coeruleus noradrenergic cell bodies. The same is true for the noradrenergic cell bodies in the roof of the fourth ventricle (cell group A4), which represents the caudal extension of the dorso-lateral part of the locus coeruleus. Similarly, knife cuts in front of the locus coeruleus, damaging primarily the dorsal noradrenergic bundle, are associated with retrograde cell body changes, especially in the dorso-lateral part of the locus coeruleus, and include cell group A4 in the roof of the fourth ventricle. Furthermore, a considerable disappearance of fluorescing noradrenergic nerve terminals is observed in the colliculi, the geniculate bodies, and in the thalamus on the lesioned side. Arbuthnott et al. (1970) have confirmed the fact that a single noradrenergic neuron in the dorso-lateral locus coeruleus area can monosynaptically innervate both the cerebral cortex and cerebellum. This, then, enables these neurons to immediately and simultaneously influence the neural activity in practically all cortical areas of the brain. They also confirmed that the ascending dorsal noradrenergic pathway gives collaterals to the superior and inferior colliculi, the geniculate bodies and parts of the thalamus. It is possible that this dorsal noradrenergic system is important for the induction of REM sleep since some evidence indicated an increase in norepinephrine turnover during the rebound phase following REM sleep deprivation (Pujol et al., 1968), and since DOPA induces a normal REM sleep in reserpine-pretreated rats. On the other hand, this latter finding has not been confirmed by Stern and Morgane (1973a). Pujol et al. also showed that the noradrenergic receptor blocking agent, phenoxybenzamine, diminishes REM sleep as does destruction of the locus coeruleus. The locus coeruleus system projecting to the cerebral cortex (dorsal noradrenergic pathways) also innervates the geniculate bodies and it is, therefore, possible (see below) that this system may be involved in the regulation of ponto-geniculo-occipital (PGO) discharges found in REM sleep. It is also important to remember that these discharges are particularly frequent after reserpine treatment (or destruction of the raphé area), an effect which may be due to disruption of serotonergic neurons.

Not only PGO spikes, but also the maintenance of cortical activation, may be dependent on the locus coeruleus noradrenergic neurons. Thus, it has been found that DOPA causes an increase of the waking state, and destruction of the noradrenergic neurons increases cortical synchronization (Jones et al., 1969). The importance of the locus coeruleus noradrenergic system for cortical "arousal" is also indicated by the marked inhibition of the activity of this system occurring after treatment with minor tranquilizers and barbiturates and by the high sensitivity of this system to the releasing action of amphetamine. Thus, it seems a distinct possibility that the activating effects of the locus coeruleus noradrenergic neurons on all cortices forms an important component of the reticular activating system.

In a recent study, Chu and Bloom (1973) recorded the activity of the noradrenergic neurons of the locus coeruleus of the unrestrained cat during sleeping and waking. The recorded neurons were subsequently identified by combined fluorescence histochemistry of catecholamines and identification of micro-lesions at recording sites. They found that these pontine units show homogeneous changes in discharge patterns with respect to sleep stages, firing slowly during drowsy periods and slow-wave sleep and firing in rapid bursts during REM sleep. They felt that these results provided a direct correlation between the activity of defined catecholamine-containing neurons and spontaneous occurrence of sleep stages. Thus, from this work it would appear that norepinephrine-containing neurons of the locus coeruleus do change their discharge pattern with sleep-waking behavior, becoming more active in attentive wakefullness and exhibiting bursting discharges in REM sleep. However, we point out that this pattern of elevated unit firings during REM sleep reported by Chu and Bloom (1973) can also be found in many other non-catecholaminergic regions of the brain. Also, from the standpoint of responding during arousal, Bubenick and Monnier (1972) showed that individual cells of the locus coeruleus undergo changes in size with variations in sleep and wakefulness in rabbits. The nuclear diameter was smaller during sleep (with high delta activity) induced by stimulation of the "hypnogenic thalamic region". The size increased in sleep-resistant animals under influence of stress. This suggests that the activity of these specific locus coeruleus cells is altered during cortical arousal.

Arbuthnott et al. (1971) have observed that increased activity in the norepinephrine nerve terminals of the hypothalamus, preoptic area, and of the ventral part of the interstitial nucleus of the stria terminalis is involved in the maintenance of self-stimulation behavior. They found that electrical stimulation supporting self-stimulation behavior is accompanied by release of norepinephrine in specific areas of the brain along this particular pathway. They observed that lack of self-stimulation along the midline electrodes in the rat suggested that serotonin is not of importance in this behavior.

Stein and Wise (1969) demonstrated *in vivo* that norepinephrine can be released at central synapses by stimulation of the medial forebrain bundle system. Their data supported the idea that the release of norepinephrine at terminal sites of the medial forebrain bundle in the hypothalamus and limbic system was responsible, at least in part, for the positive reinforcement (self-stimulation) of behavior. Crow et al. (1972) implanted electrodes in the region of the locus coeruleus in rats and determined that a fiber pathway associated with the locus coeruleus and the mesencephalic route of the trigeminal nerve plays a critical role in self-stimulation. They hypothesized that the norepinephrine;containing system from the locus coeruleus is one of the two neural systems which can be activated to obtain electrical self-stimulation. Thus, activation of either of two catecholamine-containing pathways—a dorsal system arising from the locus coeruleus and releasing norepinephrine as a neurohumor, and a ventral system releasing dopamine and originating from the region around the interpeduncular nucleus—are important in self-stimulation. Recently Wise et al. (1973) showed that intraventricular administration of norepinephrine facilitated hypothalamic self-stimulation. Suppression of self-stimulation was obtained with intraventricular injections of serotonin. These and other findings supported the idea that behavior is facilitated by an alpha-noradrenergic "reward" system and suppressed by a serotonergic negative system and that these systems act reciprocally in the control of goal-directed behavior.

2. *Synchronizing Systems in the Brain*

Kostowski (1971a) electrically stimulated the mesencephalic reticular formation and pontine raphé and showed that these stimulations produced EEG synchronization. Kostowski et al. (1969) had previously shown that stimulation of the midbrain raphé in both rats and cats also produces EEG synchronization. They feel that synchronization obtained from the pontine reticular formation and mesencephalic reticular formation supports the idea that the raphé system is closely related to slow-wave sleep mechanisms. Kostowski et al. (1968) had stressed that the insomnia obtained by destruction of the raphé system in the rat resembles closely the insomnia induced by the acute inhibition of serotonin synthesis, thus providing a further argument for the role of serotonin in sleep. Morgane and Stern (1973b) have reported the same in cats. It is of interest to note that Dement et al. (1972) showed that with chronic PCPA treatment in cats the insomnia lasts only a few days even though serotonin levels remain markedly low. On the other hand, Polc and Monnier (1970) had previously shown that stimulation of the ponto-bulbar raphé in rabbits produces arousal. However, in those experiments the lowest frequency of stimulation used was 6 cycles per second. Kostowski showed that LSD strongly blocked the synchronization produced by brainstem stimulation and that the raphé stimulation effect was also abolished by reserpine. On the other hand, 5-HTP increased synchronization due to stimulation (low-frequency) of the brainstem.. He thus concluded that electrocortical synchronization seems to involve at least one serotonergic link.

Verzeano and Mahnke (1972) introduced serotonin by means of cannulae into the nonspecific thalamic nuclei of cats and monitored the electrical activity at the point of injection by means of microelectrodes. This agent changed the electrical activity to synchronization in a manner similar to that occurring in slow-wave sleep. On the other hand, the cholinomimetic carbamylcholine, injected through the same cannula at the same location when the synchronization by serotonin had been achieved, caused a complete desynchronization of the EEG waves and single unit activity, with a return to the pattern of a waking record. These investigators feel that these results support the hypothesis that some of the neuronal and synaptic systems concerned with arousal and wakefulness are cholinergic, while the neuronal and synaptic systems concerned with the induction of slow-wave sleep may be serotonergic. Cholinergic stimulation of the midline (non-specific) nuclei of the thalamus by Babb et al. (1971) desynchronized the surrounding areas and spread "epileptiform" discharges to the whole neocortex. These results are the first to indicate that injection of serotonin directly into a small thalamic neuronal network causes, within that network, synchronization at the gross EEG as well as at individual neuron levels. They also suggest that the thalamic mechanisms implicated in the control of synchronization and desynchronization may be based on the reciprocal activities of serotonergic and cholinergic neuronal systems. Along similar lines, Morgane and Stern (1973b) have reported that direct serotonin stimulation of the nucleus raphé dorsalis and medianus does not induce EEG or behavioral signs of sleep in cats but that following PCPA administration such raphé stimulation does induce cortical synchronization and behavorial sleep.

Sterman and Clemente (1962a, b; 1968) identified an EEG synchronizing zone in the base of the brain just rostral to the optic chiasm and have termed this region the basal forebrain synchronizing area. This zone consists of a rather complex network of neuron cell bodies and fibers, including the diagonal band of Broca. They found that stimulation of the ventral portion of the diagonal band was the most effective site for producing electroencephalographic synchronization. In order to produce synchronization the stimulation had to be bilateral and only high-frequency stimulation in these forebrain sites was effective in inducing sleep. They postulated (1962b) that the basal forebrain synchronizing influences and the reticular activating system might, in some manner, compete at the thalamic level, and that the relationship between the basal forebrain synchronizing zone and the midline thalamic systems requires further analysis. They also noted that the basal forebrain synchronizing area participates as a more general forebrain inhibitory system in behavior and that this zone has important functional connections with the cerebral cortex. The mechanism of these synchronogenic effects were not elucidated although relations between the basal forebrain and the anterior hypothalamus, medial thalamus, amygdala, hippocampus, and the brainstem were emphasized.

McGinty and Sterman (1968) later showed that large bilateral preoptic lesions produce complete sleeplessness in cats and that smaller lesions in this region result in a significant reduction of slow-wave sleep by 55-73% and REM sleep by 80-100%. Complete sleeplessness was followed by lethal exhaustion within a few days whereas incomplete sleeplessness persisted at maximum levels for 2-3 weeks. It is interesting that the suppression of sleep was characterized by a gradual onset during the first 1-2 weeks with a complete or partial recovery after 6 to 8 weeks. They noted that large symmetric lesions were required to produce sleeplessness, suggesting that sleep is facilitated by a relatively diffuse neural system. As to mechanism, they postulated that the brainstem reticular arousal system was released from antagonism by removal of basal forebrain structures. It is noteworthy that both slow-wave sleep and REM sleep appear in these studies to be dependent upon structures within the preoptic-basal forebrain region.

In a series of studies to elucidate fiber projections related to the mechanism of basal forebrain effects on sleep-waking behavior, Mizuno et al. (1968, 1969a, b) carried out a series of degeneration studies. In one study (1968), lesions involving the orbital gyrus inhibitory area was associated with preterminal degeneration bilaterally in the mesencephalic reticular formation. The degeneration was heaviest in the rostral midbrain with less in the caudal midbrain, pons, and medullary reticular nuclei. Following lesions in the orbital gyrus, degeneration was seen to join the medial forebrain bundle and could be traced to the lateral preoptic area. Orbito-thalamic fibers were followed through the anterior limb of the internal capsule and the internal medullary lamina. These fibers were found to terminate in the rostro-ventral part of the nucleus reticularis and ventralis anterior, and in the rostral parts of the intralaminar nuclei. They reach their terminations via the anterior thalamic radiation and the internal medullary lamina. In continuing studies Mizuno et al. (1969a, b) traced the medial forebrain bundle from the olfactory tubercle to the mammillary body, and from the preoptic area to the subthalamus, the central grey of the rostral midbrain and the midbrain tegmentum. Three projection pathways to the thalamus were observed: 1) the first courses in the stria medullaris via the inferior thalamic peduncle to terminate in the reticular nucleus, ventralis anterior, anterior ventralis, anterior dorsalis, parataenialis, medialis dorsalis, and habenularis lateralis; 2) the second pathway enters the internal medullary lamina via the inferior thalamic peduncle to distribute in the nucleus medialis dorsalis and in the intralaminar nuclei; 3) the third pathway to the thalamus ascends through medial hypothalamic areas to distribute fibers to the nucleus ventralis medialis and the midline nuclei. The orbital cortex projects to the thalamus via two pathways: 1) directly through the anterior thalamic radiation, and 2) indirectly through the medial forebrain bundle and the inferior thalamic peduncle via the olfactory tubercle, prepyriform region and lateral preoptic area. In summary, Mizuno et al. showed that the orbital cortex connects with the medial forebrain bundle mainly through the olfactory tubercle and preoptic zones, and is capable of achieving modulation of the activity of the limbic-midbrain circuit as well as the thalamo-cortical system.

One of the significant areas for study in the field of interactions of brainstem areas in sleep-waking behavior is the analysis of connections of the raphé system to the other synchronizing structures of the lower brainstem; for example, the area postrema and nucleus of the tractus solitarius. Studies of the interactions between the raphé system and locus coeruleus and the nucleus of the solitary tract or its afferents might lead to important advances in understanding the processes responsible for the onset of sleep. Bronzino et al. (1972) have shown a powerful serotonergic synchronizing influence to derive from this area but the pathways and mechanisms involved still remain largely unknown. Fuxe and Owman (1965), using the highly sensitive fluorescence technique, demonstrated catecholamines localized in nerve cell (not glial cell) bodies in the area postrema in rat, guinea pig, rabbit, cat, dog, and monkey and observed a dominance of catecholamine axons running in abundance just outside the area postrema. In the rat, nerve cells of the serotonin type were demonstrated. Interestingly, in the cat and rabbit nonfluorescing, as well as fluorescing, nerve cells were seen. They pointed out that most axon terminals from the area postrema entered the lateral reticular formation. As reviewed above, there is much evidence that the basal forebrain area (including the orbito-frontal cortex) plays an important role in the induction of cortical synchronization and, secondarily, in that of sleep. Since the pretreatment of cats with PCPA suppresses the EEG synchronizing effects of electrical stimulation of the basal forebrain area (Wada and Terao, 1970), this constitutes strong, but indirect evidence, that some serotonin terminals are involved in the presynaptic mechanism which mediates cortical synchronization. This might also explain why local stimulation with serotonin in this area also induces sleep (Yamaguchi et al., 1963, 1964). Jouvet feels the basal forebrain area to be mostly a strategic postsynaptic ensemble of neurons where the serotonin terminals act to trigger or "modulate" the neural mechanisms synchronizing the cortical activity. He has emphasized that this area should not be termed a hypothalamic "sleep" center" since lesions in the area produce a delayed onset (secondary) hypersomnia whereas raphé lesions produce an immediate long-lasting insomnia. However, Nauta (1946) has shown that lesions (knife cuts) in the caudal hypothalamus induce sleep while lesions in the preoptic areas induce chronic waking (in one animal for 13 days). Although he used the respective terms, "waking center" and "sleep center", Nauta carefully explained his concept of "centers" in terms of neural systems. Thus, he indicated that the medial forebrain bundle appears to be implicated in the transmission of impulses determining the sleep-waking rhythm. While no polygraphic records were taken in the 1946 Nauta study, it is hard to accept Jouvet's reasoning that the insomnia was a (1972c, p. 265) "nonspecific" effect and the animals "should have lived much longer" (like raphé lesioned animals). Nauta did have one animal that lived 13 days in "total" wakefulness so this question is still very much an open one.

3. Experiments Relating to the Monoamine Theory of Jouvet

As pointed out by Jouvet (1972c), the nervous system comprises many subsystems. Of course, the observation that highly limited and restricted brainstem lesions are able to suppress either sleep or waking is good reason to believe that certain of these systems are specialized to control the sleep-waking cycle. In considering the reticular formation in terms of histofluorescence mapping it is of considerable importance that the "unspecific" systems of the reticular formation are finally beginning to acquire some biochemical specificity.

Jouvet (1972a, b, c) has most prominently put forward the views that serotonergic neuronal systems are involved in slow-wave sleep mechanisms and that noradrenergic (and possibly cholinergic) systems are involved in REM sleep and waking. With regard to the serotonergic systems in the brain, Jouvet has pointed out that insomnias due to the lesion of serotonergic neurons, or due to inhibition of serotonin synthesis by drugs, have one common characteristic: the decrease of sleep is not followed by a subsequent rebound of sleep. This has suggested that the common mechanism in producing the decrease in sleep is a decrease of the turnover in central serotonergic neurons. Jouvet has also noted that insomnia may be induced by the activation of the ascending noradrenergic ponto-mesencephalic system either by direct stimulation of the mesencephalon, by nociceptive stimuli, by sleep deprivation, or by drugs such as amphetamine. What occurs is either a total insomina or a selective suppression REM sleep (by the sleep deprivation method) but never a selective suppression of slow-wave sleep. This insomnia is always followed by a rebound of slow-wave sleep and/or REM sleep, the intensity and duration of which are proportional to the duration of the insomnia. This factor suggests a possible regulation of the biosynthesis and turnover of serotonergic neurons by the increased activity of the "waking" system. He has noted that both forms of insomnia share one common characteristic, i.e., they can be suppressed by the inhibition of the synthesis of catecholamines by a-methyl-paratyrosine which decreases the turnover of central catecholaminergic neurons. Thus, catecholamine systems may relate to waking behavior.

Jouvet has shown that after lesions of the dorsal noradrenergic bundle at the level of the isthmus in cats there is a true hypersomnia, with significant increases in both slow-wave sleep and REM sleep for 4 to 5 days. In all these animals there is also an increase in forebrain 5-HIAA and tryptophan which parallels the decrease in norepinephrine. Interestingly, there was no significant change in forebrain serotonin or dopamine. These biochemical findings appear to suggest that the destruction of a bundle of ascending noradrenergic axons may have increased the turnover of some serotonin cells. Since terminals from noradrenergic neurons of the anterior part of the locus coeruleus are found in the anterior raphé (Loizou, 1969a), it is likely in Jouvet's experiments that the lesion of the isthmus may have suppressed an inhibitory control from noradrenergic ascending axons upon the anterior raphé system. True hypersomnia (increases of both slow-wave sleep and REM sleep) may then be the result of an increase in serotonin turnover.

In attempting to study the neurophysiological localization of the "executive" mechanisms of REM sleep the pontile origin of both ascending (fast cortical activity, PGO waves) and descending (inhibition of muscle tone, rapid eye movements) components of REM sleep has been demonstrated by several types of experiments. By carrying out various pontine transections Jouvet (1972c) has concluded that the anterior 2/3 of the lateral pons is the region most implicated in the "executive" mechanisms of REM sleep. He found that lesions in the dorso-lateral part of the pontine reticular formation totally suppressed REM sleep without interfering significantly with slow-wave sleep. Since norepinephrine-containing neurons of the dorso-lateral pontine tegmentum (groups A5, A6 and A7) are concentrated in the nucleus of the locus coeruleus, subcoeruleus, and adjacent nuclei, noradrenergic mechanisms have been implicated in REM sleep. Jouvet also found that bilateral lesions of the caudal part of the locus coeruleus (stereotaxic planes P3 and P4 in the cat) suppressed only the motor inhibition (atonia) which takes place during REM. During the first days after such lesions some permanent PGO waves were shown to occur but no REM sleep. Subsequently, around the 8-10th day types of so-called "hallucinatory behavior" occurred. Following such lesions the ascending components of REM sleep such as activated EEG, PGO activity, rapid eye movements, miosis, and total relaxation of nictitating membranes were present. Jouvet observed that after lesions of the caudal part of the locus coeruleus there are no significant alterations of endogenous monoamine content in either the mesencephalon or forebrain. He did, however, observe a 30 to 40% decrease or norepinephrine in the ventral pons and in the cervical spinal cord after such manipulations. These results make it appear that descending catecholamine neurons might be implicated in the control of the loss of muscle tone which occurs during REM sleep.

Jouvet also showed that a partial lesion located just rostral to the caudal part of the locus coeruleus decreases, but does not totally suppress, REM sleep. After a transitory increase of PGO activity during waking and slow-wave sleep the frequency of PGO activity during REM sleep was shown to decrease and this decrease was roughly proportional to the extent of destruction of these neurons and proportional to the decrease of REM sleep. More extensive bilateral lesions involving the caudal 2/3 of the locus coeruleus and nucleus subcoeruleus (ventral part of A6 and A5) definitively suppressed the occurrence of REM sleep. However, PGO activity was not suppressed completely and occasionally occurred during slow-wave sleep. This type of lesion induces roughly a 35% decrease of norepinephrine in the diencephalon and telencephalon without any change in serotonin or dopamine levels. Bilateral *total* lesions of the entire group of nuclei containing catecholamine neurons was shown to be followed by a decrease in waking and an immediate and permanent suppression of PGO activity and of REM sleep. This lesion causes a more significant decrease of noradrenaline in the mesencephalon, diencephalon, and telencephalon. In Jouvet's studies lesions in the anterior 1/3 of the locus coeruleus or of the ascending dorsal noradrenergic bundle at the level of the isthmus was associated with a temporary increase in slow-wave sleep and REM sleep lasting from 4 to 5 days without alteration of PGO activity. The decrease of norepinephrine in the telencephalon, diencephalon, and mesencephalon was accompanied by an approximately 30% increase of telencephalic 5-HIAA and tryptophan. In attempts to sharply localize the responsible brain areas, Jouvet's group has placed control lesions ventrally, medially, laterally, and caudally to the locus coeruleus neurons, i.e., in the entire group of vestibular nuclei, and noted that these do not result in significant alterations of slow-wave sleep, REM sleep or the amine content of the forebrain.

These data have led to the conclusion that neurons located in the dorso-
lateral area of the pontine tegmentum play a role in the execution of REM
sleep. From Jouvet's (1972a, c) analysis of his own lesion work it would appear that the most caudal part of the pontine catecholamine neurons are
related to descending mechanisms, whereas phasic PGO activity and fast
EEG activity appear to depend upon the neurons located in the caudal 2/3 of
the locus coeruleus area. Also, Jouvet's work purports to show that the
catecholamine neurons located in the anterior 1/3 of the locus coeruleus
complex does not seem to participate in the REM sleep mechanism, being,
apparently, concerned with the control of waking behavior. Of course, it is
emphasized that the coagulation technique is not selective enough to verify
that catecholamine neurons are the only ones responsible for the mechanisms
of REM sleep, since it is likely that "cholinergic" neurons which are also
concentrated in the locus coeruleus may play a significant role. Also, these
fine distinctions of the role of "thirds" of a nuclear complex such as the locus
coeruleus are simply beyond the resolution powers of lesioning procedures.
This is especially so in the cat where the locus is more of a "complex",
broken up by fiber systems (whereas in the rat is a tighter, better defined
"nucleus"). In none of Jouvet's published work does the histology bear out
this "microfractionation" of the coeruleus complex such as is implied
in his discussion of the roles of the anterior, middle, and posterior thirds
of this cellular assembly.

4. PGO Waves and LGN Activity

One of the most interesting "fractionations" of the REM state, relating to
chemical systems in the brain regulating specific components of this
phenomenon is that relating to PGO spike activity. This activity has come
under the closest scrutiny concerning pathways, chemistry, genesis, etc. To
date we can give the following summary of evidence indicating that PGO
activity depends upon some "pacemaker" system in the pontine tegmentum:

1) Pontine PGO activity persists during REM sleep in the chronic pontile
cat, but is absent in the LGN and visual cortex following pontine transection.

2) Dorsal prepontine transection of the brainstem suppresses PGO activity
in the lateral geniculate but not in the pons. Thus, the fiber systems from the
pacemaker to the LGN are interrupted but pontine PGO activity is intact.

3) Stimulation of the pontine reticular formation during REM sleep
triggers PGO's in the lateral geniculate nucleus, whereas the same
stimulation is not effective during either waking or slow-wave sleep.

4) Bilateral coagulation of the dorso-lateral pontine tegmentum at the level
of the locus coeruleus immediately suppresses cortical and lateral geniculate
PGO activity.

5) The Jouvet group has reported that microinjection of 6-
hydroxydopamine in the dorso-lateral pontine tegmentum subsequently
suppresses all PGO activity. Unfortunately, no histological findings are given
in this study.

In regard to this last point, Laguzzi et al. (1972) found that intraventricularly administered 6-hydroxydopamine is followed, after an initial period of agitation with cortical activation, by sedation which coincided with permanent discharges of PGO activity lasting 30 to 120 hr. The cortical activation and agitation were thought to be due to possible release of catecholamines since they were totally suppressed by pre-treatment with alpha-methyl-paratyrosine. Interestingly, this latter agent did not suppress the PGO discharges. Surprisingly, 6-hydroxydopamine produced marked depletions of both brain norepinephrine and serotonin levels. In chlorimipramine pretreated cats (serotonin system now protected), excitation was also induced by intraventricular administration of 6-hydroxydopamine, but it was of lesser intensity. These workers noted that in the period that secondarily follows injection of 6-hydroxydopamine (when both indoleamines and catecholamines were decreased), there was no significant alteration of the quantitative level of cortical synchronization, though this synchronization appeared during behavioral waking. REM sleep was diminished according to the dose of 6-hydroxydopamine administered (without chlorimipramine), with the frequency of PGO activity during REM permanently decreased by 50%, this decrease predominantly affecting the bursts of PGO activity. In the chlorimipramine pretreated animals given 6-hydroxydopamine there was no alteration of cerebral indoleamine levels while catecholamine levels were significantly decreased. In this group there was a significant (50%) and permanent increase of cortical synchronization. REM sleep returned to normal levels after 6 days, and decreased thereafter, but, most importantly, there was no alteration of the rate of PGO activity during REM sleep in this group, thus suggesting that the PGO disrupting effects of 6-hydroxydopamine (discussed above) were due to interference with serotonergic systems.

Descarries and Saucier (1972) reported that after administration of 6-hydroxydopamine intraventricularly there was a progressive disappearance of norepinephrine neurons in the locus coeruleus of the rat resulting from selective retrograde degeneration. Three months after injection the locus coeruleus was found to be absent and fluorescence microscopy confirmed the absence of norepinephrine perikarya in the brainstem of 6-hydroxydopamine-treated animals. In these studies it was pointed out that in regions more distant from the cerebral ventricles, such as the cerebral cortex, noradrenergic endings escaping the early effects of the drug are probably destroyed by rapid anterograde degeneration following damage to their axons along their course. Other projections arising from the locus coeruleus sustain the effect of the agent primarily in the dorsal noradrenergic bundle which runs close to the ventricle. Since intraventricular administration of 6-hydroxydopamine produces chemical lesions far removed from the ventricles this type of experiment has limited localizing capabilites such as, for example, revealing much of the function of the locus coeruleus specifically.

In the study by Descarries and Saucier no reports of the effects of these treatments on PGO activity were reported.

Jouvet and others have concluded that the PGO waves are under the control of a group of neurons located in the dorso-lateral part of the pontine tegmentum. The organization and trajectory of the ascending pathways mediating PGO activity is still obscure but components appear to run in the dorsal pontine and mesencephalic tegmentum. At least two main pathways can be assumed to ascend from the pontine "pacemaker" since the almost total destruction of both lateral geniculate nuclei does not suppress cortical PGO activity (Hobson et al., 1969). In these studies bilateral coagulation of the lateral geniculate nucleus and adjacent areas of the optic radiations was carried out in order to investigate whether the phasic electrical activity recorded from the cerebral cortex during desynchronized sleep was generated exclusively via a discrete ponto-geniculo-cortical fiber tract. Despite extensive damage of the subcortical areas of the visual system in cats, the cortical phasic activity was not abolished following these coagulations. Rather, the frequency of cortical waves remained the same as it had been prior to coagulation. These results indicate that the pathway transmitting the phasic activity is not discretely localized in the area of the LGN and optic radiations but is probably more diffuse at the thalamic level. Thus, the topography of the ponto-geniculate and ponto-occipital pathways have not been precisely mapped out. It is possible they are also part of a diffuse cholinergic system (see below under cholinergic system).

In further attempts to localize generator mechanisms for REM sleep phenomena, Jouvet (see 1972a, c) has shown that the cortical or lateral geniculate PGO's of REM sleep are not suppressed by retro-pontine transection or the total destruction of the vestibular or raphé nuclei. However, as noted, they were reported to be suppressed by prepontine transection or by coagulations of the dorso-lateral pontine tegmentum. Jouvet also showed that the lesion which suppresses PGO's following reserpine administration is similar to the lesion which suppresses the PGO's in sleep. Thus, he has proposed that it is likely that the pacemaker of PGO's after reserpine is the same as for PGO's in sleep.

According to Jouvet (1972c), the medial third of the locus coeruleus complex would correspond to the "pontine pacemaker" of PGO activity and may be responsible for both the *phasic* and *tonic* ascending components of REM sleep. From this area, catecholamine-containing axons might trigger isolated eye movements (terminals located in the oculomotor region of the pons and mesencephalon) or bursts of eye movements (terminals impinging upon the medial and descending vestibular nuclei) which occur during REM. The pathways and mechanisms responsible for activation of the cerebral cortex during REM sleep are not yet known, but it is unlikely that noradrenergic axons ascending in the dorsal noradrenergic bundle participate in the cortical activation of REM sleep, since after their destruction (which decreases cortical arousal) there is still cortical activation during REM sleep. PGO activity in the LGN during REM is also not affected by these lesions. As observed more fully below, some preponderance of evidence also favors cholinergic mechanisms in many aspects of cortical activation.

Bizzi and Brooks (1963a, b) have shown that groups of monophasic waves (7/sec) in the EEG appear synchronously in the pontine formation, the lateral geniculate nucleus (LGN) and occipital cortex during and shortly preceding the REM phase of sleep (PGO spikes). The geniculate potentials were shown to be triggered by low-frequency stimulation of the pontine reticular formation. They observed that a close temporal relationship exists, during the REM phase of sleep, between the PGO spikes of the LGN and visual cortex, and that only during this phase may the PGO waves be triggered by a pontine shock. They also pointed out that connections between the reticular neurons and lateral geniculate nucleus (the Scheibels, 1958) would not explain the long latencies of PGO waves triggered by electrical stimulation of the pontine reticular formation during REM sleep. Bizzi and Brooks (1963a, b) found that waves present in the pontine reticular formation and the lateral geniculate nucleus during REM sleep were synchronous. During REM sleep, low-frequency stimulation of the pons at the level of the nucleus reticularis pontis caudalis led to a response in the lateral geniculate nucleus which consisted of either a single wave or a group of two to three waves. These wave responses in the lateral geniculate nucleus appeared identical to spontaneous PGO spikes of REM sleep recorded from the same electrode. These studies, in addition to the finding that enucleation does not abolish PGO spikes, indicate that the PGO spikes recorded during REM sleep from the LGN are dependent upon an *extraretinal* input to this structure and that this activity may be a response to ascending impulses reaching the lateral geniculate nucleus from the pontine reticular formation. It was observed that pontine REM sleep waves could not, however, be produced by stimulation of the lateral geniculate nucleus. Also, Ogawa (1963) has shown that electrical stimulation of the midbrain reticular formation raises the rate of spontaneous discharge of lateral geniculate nucleus neurons and increases their ability to respond to intermittent light.

Various lesioning studies in the locus coeruleus complex by the Jouvet group have produced rather specific changes in REM sleep and PGO activity and these will be briefly reviewed here as they relate to possible mediating pathways and their chemistry. Roussel et al. (1967) showed that complete bilateral destruction of the locus coeruleus in the cat produces an important and selective diminution in norepinephrine levels in areas of the brain located in front of the pons, an effect accompanied by a suppression of REM sleep. They showed that almost total depletion (80-90%) of cerebral norepinephrine of the diencephalon and telencephalon brought about by such lesions do not provoke important changes in the generation of slow-wave sleep. In this study they carried out control lesions of the pontine tegmentum located immediately inside, outside, and caudad to the locus coeruleus, showing that these lesions do not produce changes in the state of sleep or in cerebral monoamines. Buguet et al. (1970) have postulated that the generator of the PGO spike is a noradrenergic neuron. Pointing to this hypothesis is the localization of the lesion suppressing the PGO which coincides with the topography of locus coeruleus neurons and to the suppressive action of 6-hydroxydopamine on the PGO. One problem in interpretating this study is that cholinergic neurons in the locus coeruleus were also probably lesioned by the neurotoxic effects of 6-hydroxydopamine. Buguet et al. (1970) observed suppression of PGO's by alpha-methyl-dopa, (which would form the false transmitter, alpha-methyl-norepinephrine) and a diminution of the PGO's and of REM sleep after the catecholamine antagonist, disulfiram. These findings agree with the hypothesis of the triggering of the PGO's by noradrenergic mechanisms. As noted above, ·according to a related hypothesis, it may be the deaminated metabolites of norepinephrine that trigger the PGO spikes (Jones, 1972), since reserpine (which triggers the PGO's) diminishes norepinephrine levels and (presumably) augments the deaminated derivatives. Also, the inhibitors of monoamine-oxidase augment the norepinephrine, diminish the deaminated derivatives, and suppress the PGO's. However, we have found that alpha-methyl-tyrosine, an inhibitor of catecholamine synthesis, does not reduce the rate or total number of PGO spikes which occur in REM sleep in the cat (Stern and Morgane, 1973b).

According to the hypothesis of the Jouvet group the triggering of PGO spikes at the pontine, geniculate or cortical level is controlled by two monoaminergically opposed mechanisms—one a catecholamine excitatory and the other a serotonergic inhibitory mechanism. Accordingly, the depolarization of the neurons would necessitate the removal of an inhibition exercised by serotonergic neurons since: 1) there is continuous triggering of PGO's when there is diminution of serotonin levels after lesions of the raphé or injection of PCPA; 2) there is immediate suppression of the PGO by injection of 5-HTP or monoamine-oxidase inhibitors (which augment serotonin at the level of the receptor). This serotonergic inhibition being removed, depolarization of the ponto-geniculate neuron or cortical neuron could then be provoked by the possible liberation of deaminated metabolites of norepinephrine located in a particular compartment.

Laurent et al. (1972) have attempted to more precisely define the topography of the generator of PGO spikes seen in waking after reserpine (PGO_R), elucidate their ascending pathways, and to explain their bilateral synchrony. Normally, the PGO_R spikes occur synchronously in the right and left LGN. In one series of studies they were able to induce asynchrony of the PGO_R by a median sagittal section of 10 mm at the level of the pontine tegmentum and by a section at the level of the supraoptic decussation. In further studies they attempted to localize the structures responsible for PGO_R. By producing sagittal sections, pontine and supraoptic, they were able to study the two hemispheres (half brains) each one showing autonomous PGO_R activity issued from an ipsilateral "generator". Two frontal partial hemisections in steps were carried out with the following results: the most rostral plane of section which leaves PGO_R intact was located in front of the caudal half of the reticularis pontis caudalis nuclei. The most caudal plane of section suppressing the PGO_R was found to be located just caudal to the nucleus reticularis pontis oralis. In other parts of this study, ponto-geniculate pathways were located. Coagulations made bilaterally at the level of the dorso-lateral part of the ponto-mesencephalic tegmentum suppressed the PGO_R without altering the phasic electrical activity recorded at the level of the nuclei of the sixth cranial nerve. In studying the general organization of the ponto-geniculate pathways of PGO_R they found that section of the supraoptic decussation and a frontal hemisection (or coagulation) in front of the right generator were necessary to suppress the PGO_R at the level of the right LGN. They felt then that the component of PGO_R activity on the left side represents the projection of pontine information by a left ipsilateral pathway. On the other hand, in the case of a hemisection in front of the right generator, the synchronous pairs of PGO_R's occurred at the level of the LGN's. The PGO_R thus represents the projection of the pontine information by the ipsilateral pathway for the left LGN, and then by the crossed pathways for the right LGN. They concluded that in intact cats the PGO_R (in pairs) are caused by the interaction of the ipsilateral and crossed pathways since sections of the supraoptic decussation (in which bilateral LGN recordings were made) revealed that the PGO_R's were separated by 80-90 msec (asynchrony). They felt that the persistence of activity of PGO_R after total cerebellectomy does away with any hypothesis of the pathways being exclusively ponto-cerebello-geniculate. They concluded that the topography of lesions suppressing PGO_R correspond with the catecholaminergic (intermediary) pathways originating from the area of the subcoeruleus nucleus and crossing the midline at the level of the supraoptic decussation.

Jones (1972), by a variety of pharmacological manipulations, came to the conclusion that two roles of norepinephrine in the states of vigilance may be identified by anatomical and biochemical differentiation. She pointed out that norepinephrine-containing cells of the pontine and mesencephalic reticular formation may be involved in cortical activation of waking through the release of norepinephrine and the cells of the pontine tegmentum, which contain both norepinephrine and monoamine oxidase, may be involved in PGO spiking and REM sleep through the release of deaminated metabolites of norepinephrine. Increase in levels of norepinephrine, produced pharmacologically by administration of its precursor and inhibition of its metabolic inactivation, led to an increase in behavioral arousal and electrographic waking. This increase in waking was not in every case paralleled by an increase in PGO spiking or REM sleep. Spiking and REM sleep were increased by inhibition of COMT (catechol-o-methyltransferase), decreased by inhibition of amine reuptake mechanisms, and suppressed by inhibition of MAO. These results appear to implicate norepinephrine in the mediation of waking and of deaminated metabolites of norepinephrine in the generation of PGO spiking and REM sleep.

In these studies, inhibition of MAO by 3 different inhibitors led to the total suppression of PGO spiking and REM sleep for varying lengths of time depending upon the inhibitor. Jones interpreted these results as pointing to the indispensible role of MAO in PGO spiking and REM sleep. The progressive return of PGO spiking and REM sleep following the administration of these two inhibitors suggested a progressive accumulation of sufficient amounts of newly formed MAO and, concurrently, of deaminated metabolites. The deaminated metabolites of norepinephrine released from cells containing both norepinephrine and MAO in the dorso-lateral pontine tegmentum appear to be involved in PGO spiking and REM sleep. Jones emphasized that two different catecholaminergic systems have been delineated in the brainstem of the cat and implicated in two different roles of waking: 1) a noradrenergic system whose cell bodies are located in the pontine and mesencephalic reticular formation and which is responsible for cortical activation; and 2) a dopaminergic system whose cell bodies are located in the substantia nigra and which is responsible for activation of the extrapyramidal system. She concluded that the involvement of catecholaminergic neurons, dopaminergic and noradrenergic, in arousal mechanisms has been supported by this pharmacological study.

It is of interest that Brooks et al. (1972) carried out a study of the effects of serotonin depletion and correlated this with PGO activity in cats. In one study they depleted the brain of serotonin by systemic administration of reserpine and compared this with the temporal course of PGO-wave activity induced by similar reserpine treatment. They found a good correlation between the initial decrease in serotonin throughout the brain and the appearance of PGO activity. During recovery, however, serotonin levels remained low at the time when regulation of PGO-wave activity began to return to normal. In a second study reserpine was infused into the 4th ventricle and this caused changes in PGO activity similar to systemically administered reserpine. Serotonin levels, measured at the time when PGO waves appeared following infusion of reserpine into the 4th ventricle, were significantly depressed only in the pons. These investigators felt these results to be consistent with the hypothesis that monoaminergic neurons exert a tonic inhibitory influence at the brainstem level which serves to regulate or "gate" REM-type PGO waves. In these studies no measures of catecholamines were carried out so the results provided no direct indication regarding the relative importance of serotonin and catecholamines in the genesis of PGO activity following reserpine administration. Serotonin appears more implicated in this process, however, since administration of the serotonin precursor 5-hydroxytryptophan suppresses PGO activity after reserpine. Also, following PCPA treatment, waves resembling PGO's are induced. Most important, from the standpoint of morphological localization, the ventricle infusion experiments indicate that the influence of reserpine on PGO waves is probably exerted at the level of the brainstem, caudal to the diencephalon. These experiments indicate that reserpine acts at a lower brainstem level since PGO waves appeared in the lateral geniculate and marginal gyrus at a time when serotonin levels were close to normal in both structures and significantly depressed only in the pons. Brooks et al. feel this experiment reveals the site at which the normal regulation of REM-type PGO waves probably takes place. In the framework of the monoamine-gating hypothesis their results suggest that the gating neurons act upon some brainstem structure and, since a variety of evidence has placed the pacemaker which triggers REM-type PGO waves in the latero-dorsal part of the pontine tegmentum, then monoaminergic neurons may exert their tonic inhibitory influence directly upon this pacemaker. This, of course, is consistent with the finding that stimulation of the pacemaker area normally evokes REM-type PGO waves only during REM sleep.

In a study to determine the neurochemical bases of the PGO waves Jacobs et al. (1972) produced "functional homologues" of REM sleep PGO waves during waking and were able to block these with atropine. In a related study, Henriksen et al. (1972) showed that, following REM sleep deprivation, atropine blocked the occurrence of PGO waves during REM sleep. They concluded that an active cholinergic mechanism underlies the production of these waves. We (Stern and Morgane, 1973b) have shown that catecholamines do not apparently play an important role in the production of PGO waves since inhibition of catecholamine synthesis (by alpha-methyl-tyrosine) in the cat did not alter the rate of PGO-wave discharge during REM sleep despite a marked reduction in the level of brain catecholamines. It should also be noted that Matsuzaki et al. (1968) reported that an intravenous injection of the cholinomimetics eserine or pilocarpine induced loss of neck EMG activity, REM and PGO waves in the pons of cats with mesencephalic or pontine transections. These effects were also blocked by pretreating with atropine. These workers also showed that eserine had the same effect if the transection was made even more caudally, i.e., at the mid-pontine level. Also, Magherini et al. (1971) reported that intravenous injections of eserine produced eye movements and associated PGO waves in a variety of brainstem structures (including the vestibular nuclei, oculomotor nuclei, medial longitudinal fasciculus and surrounding reticular formation) in cats with transections at the precollicular level. Magherini et al. (1971) further reported that bilateral lesions of the medial and descending vestibular nuclei, in decerebrate cats, abolished eserine-induced bursts of eye movement and bursts of PGO waves. Administration of eserine did not, however, elicit the single eye movements or single PGO waves that occur in isolation during REM sleep and during the period of slow-wave sleep immediately preceding it. On the basis of these data these authors concluded that the bursts of both PGO waves and eye movements are mediated by a cholinergic mechanism that is dependent on the integrity of the medial and descending vestibular nuclei. These authors proposed that bursts of REM were dependent on cholinergic processes, whereas in the Henriksen et al. (1972) study, such bursts were seen following large doses of atropine which blocked the occurrence of bursts of PGO waves. These latter authors interpreted this as suggesting that these two types of phasic PGO events, previously thought to be mediated by the same neurochemical mechanism, can be pharmacologically dissociated.

Review of a few key studies relative to the chemistry of the LGN neurons is important at this time. It has been shown that acetylcholine, norepinephrine, and serotonin are all capable of producing both facilitation and depression of LGN neurons when directly applied by iontophoretic techniques (Satinsky, 1967). Mostly, however, there appears to be facilitation by acetylcholine and norepinephrine, and depression by serotonin. Shute and Lewis (1963) have demonstrated histochemically (see below) a cholinesterase-containing pathway ascending from the brainstem to the LGN and the Swedish group have described ascending noradrenergic and tryptaminergic pathways originating in the brainstem and running to LGN. Further, electrical stimulation of the midbrain reticular formation has been shown to result in alteration of LGN neuron activity. Thus, the brainstem appears to be the origin for many amine systems (cholinergic, adrenergic, and tryptaminergic fibers) running to the LGN. Phillis et al. (1967a) have presented evidence that both catecholamine and serotonin-containing nerve terminals in the lateral geniculate nucleus are inhibitory transmitters. They have pointed out that the ascending fibers are very thin, i.e., about 1-2 microns in diameter. They also observed that acetylcholine has a predominantly excitatory action on cells in the lateral geniculate nucleus and that the cholinergic/-monoaminergic balances might be expected to control the level of excitability of this nucleus.

Curtis (1972) has noted that there is histochemical evidence for a projection from the brainstem to the lateral geniculate nucleus from the locus coeruleus and raphé nuclei and that these projections are very small unmyelinated axons. Guillery and Scott (1971) have described a system of very fine axons, which appear to be beyond the resolution power of the light microscope, and make axosomatic contacts with cells throughout this nucleus. They have suggested that these may constitute an input from the brainstem which, by virtue of the synaptic location, could exercise considerable influence over the firing pattern of the cells. There is pharmacological evidence for amine-containing fibers to the LGN from the brainstem, including cholinergic fibers systems (see below). Many of these are so small that they have been missed in conventional degeneration type studies. It appears that the silver methods have apparently failed to stain the catecholamine and serotonin pathways originating in the brainstem. It is also possible that some of these chemical pathways may actually be resistant to silver staining. However, Bowsher (1970) has been able to trace reticular projections to the lateral geniculate nucleus in the cat using Nauta degeneration techniques. He found that small lesions placed in the region of the nucleus of the posterior commisure were most effective in producing degeneration in the lateral geniculate nucleus. Whether these are chemical systems concerned with PGO activity remains to be determined.

Although most of the cholinergic systems relating to sleep-waking activity are discussed in a separate section (below), it is essential that they also be introduced here in relation to chemistry of LGN mechanisms and relations with monoamine systems. In further studies, Phillis et al. (1967b) presented evidence suggesting that acetylcholine is the transmitter released by terminals of nerves of the reticular formation projecting to the LGN. They showed that many geniculate neurons are excited by acetylcholine and that the facilitatory effects of stimulation of the reticular formation on the responses of these cells could be abolished by the application of cholinergic antagonists. They further observed that, in addition to the cholinergic projection system, other non-cholinergic excitatory pathways may project from the mesencephalon to the LGN as well as at least one inhibitory system. It seems probable that inhibitory effects of reticular stimulation are mediated by monoaminergic projection systems.

The most detailed discussion of the pharmacology of thalamic and geniculate neurons has been given by Phillis (1971). In his review it was emphasized that cholinergic agents have predominantly excitatory effects on LGN neurons while serotonin is predominantly inhibitory and norepinephrine excites 70% of the lateral geniculate neurons. In another study Deffenu et al. (1967) determined acetylcholine and serotonin levels by bioassay in the lateral geniculate bodies, superior colliculus, and occipital cortex of cats transected at the midpontine pretrigeminal level. They noted that the geniculate acetylcholine content does not seem influenced by visual deafferentation but instead is affected by the degree of activation of the cats themselves. These results suggested that a large part of acetylcholine present in the lateral geniculate body might be related to fibers originating from the reticular formation.

Influences of the reticular activating system on the LGN have been repeatedly demonstrated (Bizzi and Brooks, 1963a).Evidence showing the importance of sleep and wakefulness on the responsiveness of LGN units to flashes of modulated sine-wave light have been presented (Maffei and Rizzolatti, 1965; Maffei et al. 1965). According to Angel et al. (1965), stimulation of the mesencephalic reticular formation produces an enhancement of excitability of the optic fibers entering the LGN. Stimulation of the mesencephalic reticular formation in the cat with pretrigeminal transection facilitates also the late part of the evoked responses of the superior colliculus to stimulation of the optic nerve (Marchiafava and Pepeu, 1966). However, the large number of pathways connecting the superior colliculus with other brain regions may offer an explanation for the limited changes of acetylcholine levels found in the different groups of animals investigated. Although there is evidence that stimulation of the cerebral cortex may affect the response of LGN neurons, it is more likely that the differences in acetylcholine content of the LGN depend upon variations of activity of cholinergic fibers originating from the reticular formation and impinging upon geniculate neurons. Evidence in favor of this hypothesis is: 1) there are fairly numerous afferents from the thalamus and from the mesencephalic reticular formation to the ventral part of the LGN in the cat (Szentagothai, 1963); and 2) there is a moderate content of cholinesterase activity in the same ventral part of the LGN (see below). Moreover, histochemical (Krnjević and Silver, 1965; Shute and Lewis, 1967) and pharmacological data, discussed below under cholinergic systems, demonstrates an important cholinergic component in the ascending activating pathway from the midbrain reticular formation.

Matsuoka and Domino (1972) studied the effects of various agents on activity of single lateral geniculate neurons in the acute cat. Most of these cells increased their response to ipsilateral optic tract and midbrain reticular formation stimulation. Nicotine and physostigmine significantly increased the spontaneous firing rate of single geniculate neurons, and physostigmine enhanced their poststimulus discharge rate to optic nerve stimulation. The effects of midbrain reticular formation stimulation were further enhanced by physostigmine. They concluded that a major cholinergic facilitatory system exists which influences lateral geniculate neurons and that this involves the reticular formation. Their data showed that physostigmine enhanced unit response to optic tract stimulation. Although it is obvious that acetylcholine cannot be the excitatory synaptic transmitter released at optic nerve terminals by orthodromic volleys, they thought it still may act as a facilitatory modulator, especially from the reticular formation. It is interesting that Phillis et al. (1967a) suggested that inhibitory effects of reticular stimulation were mediated by a monoaminergic projection system and the facilitatory effects of reticular stimulation were mediated by a cholinergic system. Matsuoka and Domino's data do support the hypothesis of a cholinergic modulatory system which appears to be mostly facilitatory.

Collier and Mitchell (1966) studied the central release of acetylcholine during stimulation of visual pathways and concluded that two ascending cholinergic systems may be associated with spontaneous release of acetylcholine in the visual cortex evoked by stimulation of the eyes by light and by direct stimulation of the lateral geniculate body. These were a nonspecific reticulo-cortical pathway which they felt responsible for the EEG arousal response and a more specific thalamo-cortical pathway associated with augmenting and repetitive after-discharge responses. The first system was thought to be concerned with the small but widespread increase in acetylcholine release from the cortex following stimulation of the visual pathway while the second system could give rise to the larger increases evoked from the primary receiving areas of the cortex.

In concluding this section, it is of some interest to note that the dorsal nucleus of the lateral geniculate body appears to exclusively receive monoamine terminals whereas the ventral nucleus of the lateral geniculate appears to receive cholinergic terminals. Many regions, including the striatum and limbic forebrain structures, appear to receive both types of chemical innervation. The extent of overlap of these two systems in the brain is not well known and there is no direct evidence that monoamine/acetylcholine synapses exist. Nevertheless, from these types of studies it can be seen that chemical anatomy can shed considerable light on the intricacies of chemical organization of neural systems.

5. *Experiments of the Italian Group*

Many heroic lesioning experiments have been carried out in hope of localizing and circumscribing the brain areas concerned with sleep-waking behavior. A few key ones, bearing especially on problems related to neural circuitry, will be discussed. Zanchetti (1967), attempted to localize the "pacemaker" mechanisms of REM sleep which Jouvet hypothesized as being located in the pons. By electrolytic destruction several areas were ruled out in these studies including the dorsal and ventral nuclei of Gudden, the nucleus centralis superior of Bechterew, the nucleus raphé dorsalis and nucleus raphé pontis, the nucleus reticularis tegmenti pontis of Bechterew, the locus coeruleus and the nucleus subcoeruleus. Zanchetti, in commenting upon the lesions of the Jouvet group, noted that in each instance the lesion involved the nucleus reticularis pontis caudalis and, in some animals, the nucleus reticularis pontis oralis. Jouvet had originally claimed that the neurons responsible for REM sleep should be included within the limits of the nucleus reticularis pontis caudalis, in particular. Rossi et al. (1963) also had obtained data that pointed to the middle pons as the presumed location of the neurons involved in the induction of REM sleep. Zanchetti showed that the nucleus reticularis pontis caudalis was completely intact in five of seven cats in which REM sleep was abolished by other pontine lesions and that this nucleus could, therefore, be excluded as the REM sleep pacemaker. Of the various brainstem structures examined in this study, only the nucleus reticularis pontis oralis could not be excluded as a possible site of REM sleep neurons. Zanchetti's data indicate that the neurons responsible for induction of REM sleep are located within the limits of the nucleus reticularis pontis oralis, more precisely in its middle one-third, in an area which extends both medially and laterally. He has noted that it is possible that the raphé nuclei at this level are also involved, although their destruction were without effect on REM sleep when the adjacent reticular nucleus was spared. Histological control in many of these experiments, however, leaves much to be desired. Camacho-Evangelista and Reinoso-Suárez (1964) have shown that lesions in the area of the nucleus reticularis pontis oralis produce EEG synchronization whereas lesions in the pontine and caudal midbrain tegmentum, dorsal, lateral, and caudal to the lesions producing synchronization, resulted in EEG activation. Their findings also indicate that in the rostral part of the pons there are structures responsible for EEG activation, since their destruction gives rise to synchronization. They have concluded that these structures are the nucleus reticularis pontis oralis and nucleus reticularis ventralis, since synchronization was found only when the lesions destroyed a sufficient area of these nuclei. Rossi (1963) had originally pointed out that the inhibitory influence leading to the "deeper phase" of sleep takes origin from the neurons of the rostral part of the nucleus reticularis pontis caudalis and the caudal part of the nucleus reticularis pontis oralis. It would appear that attempts to make such fine distinctions by lesioning procedures, which lack this degree of resolution power, are not clarifying these issues satisfactorily.

It is important to point out that Carli et al. (1963) have shown that interruption, at different levels, of the ascending or descending limb of the limbic-midbrain circuit does not prevent the occurrence of electrographic aspects of REM sleep. None of these lesions interfered with the appearance of desynchronized EEG patterns throughout episodes of REM sleep. EEG desynchronization could also be seen during wakefulness following complete interruption of the limbic-midbrain connections. These lesions, likewise, did not prevent the appearance of theta rhythm in the hippocampus. Zanchetti (1967) summarized the results of the Italian workers as also showing that the ascending pathways, through which the pontine pacemaker of REM sleep influences neo-cortical and hippocampal activity, remain unknown and theorized that these pathways are likely to be widely scattered throughout the tegmentum. Candia et al. (1967) observed that, contrary to the results seen after transecting one-half of the rostral pons, unilateral partial lesions of the rostral pons, involving either "specific" or "non-specific" structures, do not prevent the appearance of desynchronized EEG patterns of REM sleep in the ipsilateral hemisphere in cats. This effect, however, was obtained by lesions of the medial as well as lateral tegmental structures of the midbrain. Their findings might be interpreted as indicating that there is not a single pontine structure, or clustered group of structures, of crucial importance for the EEG desynchronization of REM sleep. Indeed, their work could be interpreted as indicating that the whole rostral pons appears to contribute to the EEG desynchronizing influence and that this influence runs rostrally through the midbrain tegmentum without following any known fiber pathways.

Moruzzi (1972), in a comprehensive and analytical review of the literature, especially from the point of view of the Italian school, has discussed the importance of midbrain hemisection experiments, emphasizing the ipsilateral arrangement of the ascending activating pathways. The striking

EEG asymmetries, with marked tendency toward synchronized activity ipsilateral to lesions, is summarized by him as due to the withdrawal of ascending activating influences. The EEG asymmetry produced by midbrain hemisection in the mid-pontine pretrigeminal animal preparation have led Moruzzi to the following conclusions: 1) that the activating influence, or at least the part of it which appears to be critically important for the maintenance of the waking state, arises above the pretrigeminal transection; 2) that the abolition of the sleep-waking cycle is due to an imbalance of antagonistically oriented structures in the brain; and 3) that the recovery of the cycle in the chronic preparation is due mainly to compensation of this imbalance.

The strictly unilateral synchronization phenomenon might appear as a surprising finding if one considers that the EEG manifestations of wakefulness and arousal are always bilateral. The EEG activation of the entire neocortex is, in fact, the usual result of any *unilateral* stimulation of the reticular formation (Moruzzi and Magoun, 1949). Only occasionally was a strictly ipsilateral disappearance of slow cortical rhythms obtained by stimulating the medullary reticular formation on one side in their large series of studies. Moruzzi has emphasized that a distinction should be made between the tonic and phasic activation underlying, respectively, the state of wakefulness and the phenomenon of enhanced arousal. He feels that experiments on EEG asymmetries show that a tonic flow of activating reticular impulses reaches each hemicerebrum through predominantly ipsilateral channels. At the level of the upper midbrain, in other words, the ascending reticular system is separated into two major channels, one to each half of the forebrain. However, cross connections are likely to be present, and functionally very important, both at the level of the brainstem and the hypothalamus. These connections, which clearly exist, may well explain why the entire brain is usually awake or is normally aroused as a whole.

In general, Moruzzi (1972), has summarized a vast and often conflicting literature dealing with lesions and transection experiments and drawn two major conclusions: 1) the ascending reticular system and a group of neurons lying in the posterior hypothalamus are endowed with a tonic activating influence and are probably concerned with the maintenance of wakefulness; and 2) the lower brainstem and the basal forebrain area contain structures with opposing functions, which exert a tonic deactivating influence and lead ultimately to sleep. Moruzzi emphasizes that lesion and stimulation experiments show that the structures which appear to be directly and critically responsible for both sleep and wakefulness, and for the alteration between these states, are localized in the diencephalon. These are primarily in the anterior and posterior hypothalamus and in the basal forebrain. He notes that the sleep-waking cycle does not arise within, but is strikingly controlled by, the ascending system of the brainstem. This control, which is both tonic and phasic in nature, is only one aspect of a much wider problem: that there are different levels of "activation" that are required for different levels of behavior.

6. *Interaction of Amine Systems in the Brain*

In narrowing the brainstem sites potentially involved in sleep-waking behavior it is essential to eliminate certain critical areas. Thus, Jouvet and Delorme (1965) showed that destruction of the nuclei of the raphé (dorsalis and pontis), of the dorsal and ventral nuclei of Gudden, of the medial two-thirds of the nucleus reticularis pontis oralis and nucleus reticularis pontis caudalis, of the nuclei tegmenti pontis of Bechterew, of the nucleus centralis superior of Bechterew, all allow cortical activation to persist along with a diminution of muscle tonus during sleep. They noted that lesions destroying the locus coeruleus, on the other hand, led to an immediate and marked suppression of REM sleep. In additional studies, Petitjean and Jouvet (1970) have shown that limited lesions of the isthmic region (junction of mesencephalon and pons) produces a significant augmentation of slow-wave sleep and REM sleep in the cat. This hypersomnia is accompanied by a lowering of cerebral norepinephrine and an augmentation of tryptophan and of 5-HIAA levels. These chemical changes suggest that an augmentation of the turnover of serotonin is responsible for increased slow-wave sleep. It is possible that this augmentation of serotonergic activity is due to the removal of some inhibitory control exercised by a group of noradrenergic neurons located at the anterior part of the pons.

The "executive" mechanisms of REM sleep would, according to Jouvet's synthesis (1972c), appear to be triggered from the caudal two-thirds of the locus coeruleus complex (the principal nucleus of the locus coeruleus), the ventro-medial component of the locus coeruleus, the subcoeruleus, and possibly the nucleus parabrachialis medialis. Jouvet's experiments indicate that the caudal one-third of the locus coeruleus may be responsible for the catecholamine mechanisms involved in the control of total inhibition of postural muscle tonus. Such a control may be quite direct since heavy projections from the area of the locus coeruleus to the accessory nerve responsible for the innervation of the neck muscles have been demonstrated by Olson and Fuxe (1971). This control may be exerted, in part, via the reticulo-spinal tract of the bulbar reticular formation (Fig. 16).

Jouvet (see 1972a, c) has claimed that "total" lesions of the raphé system completely suppress REM sleep and strongly decrease slow-wave sleep. He notes that destruction of the anterior part of the raphé (nucleus raphé dorsalis and nucleus raphé centralis) induces a state of permanent arousal during the first 2 to 3 days but REM sleep still appears (without preceding slow-wave sleep) periodically for 5 to 10 percent of the time. These data suggest that the anterior raphé neurons are probably related more to slow-wave sleep mechanisms than to REM. On the other hand, destruction of the "caudal" raphé (nucleus raphé pontis and nucleus raphé magnus) was

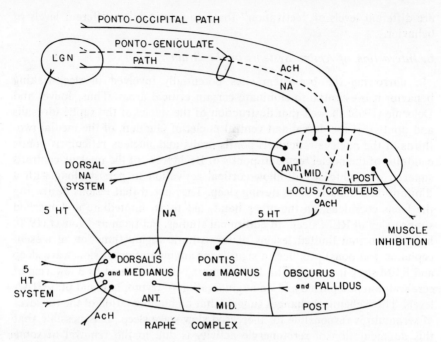

Fig. 16. Schematic representation of possible routes of interaction between divisions of the raphé complex and locus coeruleus described in text. Well developed noradrenergic (NA) terminals have been shown to synapse with serotonergic (5-HT) cells in the anterior raphé (dorsalis and medianus). These raphé nuclei project forward in the medial forebrain bundle as described. Cholinergic projections from these same areas are indicated (AcH). Reciprocal internuclear connections link the various divisions of the raphé (Ant., Mid., and Post.). The locus is divided into the three divisions described by Jouvet, with projections from the middle raphé (and possibly posterior raphé) synapsing on a cholinergic neuron before finally entering the middle-third division of the locus coeruleus. It is likely that the dorsal noradrenergic pathway encompasses projections from both the anterior (ant.) and middle (mid.) divisions of the locus coeruleus although these are shown as two groupings on this figure.

followed by almost complete disappearance of REM sleep, whereas slow-wave sleep was decreased to only 40% of control levels. From this work Jouvet has concluded that the caudal raphé neurons may represent the "priming" serotonin neurons which project to the dorso-lateral part of the pontine tegmentum (locus coeruleus) where the "executive mechanisms" of REM sleep are located (Fig. 16).

Jouvet has championed the view that serotonin neurons located mostly in the rostral raphé (nucleus raphé dorsalis and nucleus raphé medianus) are involved in behavioral and EEG aspects of slow-wave sleep while the middle (nucleus raphé pontis, nucleus raphé magnus) and caudal raphé (nucleus raphé pallidus, nucleus raphé obscurus) are responsible for the "priming" of REM sleep, these latter two groups sending fibers to the caudal two-thirds of the locus coeruleus complex, i.e., to the region of the locus coeruleus responsible for the "executive" mechanism of REM sleep. The ascending and descending pathways of the serotonin systems are not yet mapped out with the same precision as the catecholamine pathways but, as noted in this review, most ascending fibers appear to follow the medial forebrain bundle in close proximity to ascending noradrenergic and dopamine neurons. The serotonin bundle exists in the midbrain tegmentum, since lesions in this area, especially in the limbic midbrain area (Morgane and Stern, 1972), selectively decrease telencephalic serotonin. It is also possible that some descending serotonergic pathways to the spinal cord may contribute to the modulation of postural muscle tone during slow-wave sleep. Thus, in Jouvet's scheme of things, caudal raphé neurons play a role in "priming" REM sleep mechanisms whereas rostral raphé neurons may be involved in behavioral and EEG aspects of slow-wave sleep.

Jouvet's group has shown that lesions of the catecholamine-containing cell bodies of the substantia nigra (group A9) produce a decrease in dopamine in the rostral brain and a behavioral state of akinesia and unresponsiveness. Some cats in which dopamine was markedly depressed, i.e., more than 90%, were almost comatose. Despite such depressed behavior a quantitatively normal EEG record of alternating sleep and waking activity persisted during the comatose state. These studies indicate that dopamine could play a role in behavioral alertness and motor coordination, presumably by way of the nigro-striatal system. On the other hand, dopamine-containing neurons do not significantly play a role in either synchronization or desynchronization since an almost total disappearance of dopamine from the telencephalon does not induce significant shifts in the EEG sleep-waking alternation. Jouvet has postulated that two mechanisms are implicated in the maintenance of waking: 1) a dopaminergic mechanism of the nigro-striatal system which is responsible for behavioral arousal and alertness and 2) a noradrenergic system originating in the anterior part of the dorso-lateral division of the pontine tegmentum and the mesencephalic reticular formation which appears to be responsible for the tonic cortical activation which usually accompanies waking. He postulates that this system does not play a role in the phasic cortical activation which accompanies external stimulation. It should again be emphasized that many cholinergic neurons are also intermixed with catecholaminergic neurons, particularly in the locus coeruleus and the substantia nigra (see below) but their role is still obscure.

With regard to the noradrenergic pontine "waking" system, these neurons, according to Jouvet (1972c), are situated in the anterior part of the locus coeruleus. They send axons to the noradrenergic bundle which ascends near the central gray matter, and collaterals to the anterior part of the raphé system (Loizou, 1969a, b; Maeda, 1970; Olson and Fuxe, 1971). These neurons ascend in the mesencephalon, at the hypothalamic level comprising the more dorsal (subthalamic) components of the medial forebrain bundle (Figs. 6 and 7) and contribute to the innervation of the telencephalon. The destruction of these cells of the dorsal noradrenergic pathway at the level of the isthmus is followed by a significant increase in both slow-wave sleep (presumably because anterior raphé inhibition is lifted) and REM sleep while biochemical analysis reveals a decrease of norepinephrine in the telencephalon and diencephalon and an increase of both tryptophan and 5-HIAA (indicating increased serotonin turnover). It is thus possible that some collaterals which project from the anterior part of the locus coeruleus may inhibit the rostral raphé system during waking (Fig. 16). These appear to tonically inhibit the anterior raphé system during waking, since their destruction is followed by transient hypersomnia. From the results of many studies, Jouvet has postulated that the catecholaminergic mesencephalic "waking" system corresponds to cell group A8 (dopamine-containing cells in the lateral mesencephalic reticular formation), which send numerous fibers to adjacent parts of the mesencephalic reticular formation. The destruction of this dopamine system decreases cortical arousal and is accompanied by a decrease of both dopamine and norepinephrine and a smaller decrease of serotonin (which indicates that serotonin fibers ascend close to this area). Following such lesions there was no increase in REM sleep and, thus, the result of the destruction of this group of mesencephalic catecholamine neurons is a decrease of EEG waking but not a true hypersomnia. From these data, it appears possible that these mesencephalic catecholamine (mostly dopamine) neurons are implicated in the maintenance of the tonic EEG activation mediated by the mesencephalic reticular formation rather than in a possible control of the raphé system. It is important to keep in mind that the A8 cell group projections are part of the nigro-striatal dopamine system. Also, as shown by numerous pharmacological experiments and determination of the release of acetylcholine, it is likely that cortical cholinergic mechanisms contribute the final common link mediating cortical arousal (see cholinergic section, below).

In summary, Jouvet has noted that two different forms of reductions of waking are possible: 1) true hypersomnia in which there are increases in both slow-wave sleep and REM sleep. A form of this was seen after localized lesions of the dorsal noradrenergic bundle at the ponto-mesencephalic junction. This hypersomnia was shown to be accompanied by an increase of telencephalic and diencephalic 5-HIAA suggesting an increased turnover in central serotonin and indicated that some noradrenergic neurons might control the synthesis of serotonin in the anterior part of the raphé system, and 2) another form of reduction of waking was due to an increase of cortical synchronization, which was observed after lesions of the mesencephalic catecholaminergic neurons (group A8 and the dorsal noradrenergic bundle). Jouvet has stressed that waking mechanisms are much more powerful than sleep-inducing mechanisms.

It is highly possible that serotonin/serotonin interactions occur in the raphé system via short inter-nuclear serotonergic axons linking the rostral, middle, and caudal raphé systems (Fig. 16). Moreover, there are well developed reciprocal relations between the raphé system and the locus coeruleus complex, since pathways and terminals originating from the raphé have been demonstrated streaming in the direction of and terminating in close vicinity to the locus coeruleus, and since medial fibers projecting from the locus coeruleus terminate in the raphé system (Loizou, 1969a, b; Olson and Fuxe, 1971). Since PGO activity, which presages (pre-REM PGO's) and accompanies REM sleep, appears to be associated with a decrease of serotonin in the terminals, it is possible that the terminals from the locus coeruleus may act upon serotonin cell bodies in a manner which suppresses the release of serotonin. Then the fast cortical activity observed during REM sleep might be due to the combined effects of ascending catecholaminergic and cholinergic mechanisms and the phasic decrease of serotonin release. Powerful inhibition of raphé units during REM has been shown by McGinty and Harper (1972) such that raphé units fired 2.6/sec in waking, 0.98/sec in slow-wave sleep and 0.13/sec during REM sleep. Alternations between slow-wave sleep and REM might well be related to the alternation between the release of serotonin in the synaptic cleft, its possible binding to the receptor, and its active reuptake, many of these effects regulated by locus coeruleus noradrenergic projections onto serotonergic units in the raphé. Since a subtotal insomnia of at least two weeks duration has been obtained after raphé lesions (Renault, 1967), it would appear that the onset of sleep has to be released by the active triggering of the serotonin sleep system (presumably via the locus coeruleus system) and not only by a possible circadian dampening of turnover of the catecholamine "waking" neurons. Along these same lines, it must be remembered that the reciprocity of connections between locus coeruleus and raphé means that raphé activity may modulate locus coeruleus firing. For example, the work of Brooks et al. (1972) indicated that monoaminergic systems from the brainstem may exert tonic inhibitory activity on the pontine pacemaker of REM phenomena. These may, in large part, arise from the raphé complex.

According to the monoamine theory of Jouvet, long-lasting cortical arousal requires the integrity of noradrenergic ascending neurons from the pontine or mesencephalic group, whereas local cholinergic cortical mechanisms probably enter into play at the cortical level. Phasic arousal would be mediated by the mesencephalic reticular formation. Waking behavior in this schema is under the control of the dopaminergic nigro-striatal system ascending in the medial forebrain bundle and the lateral hypothalamus. It is possible that behavioral and cortical arousal mechanisms may be completely separate (Nauta (1946) pointed this out in his early experiments on rats). It seems likely that the ventral noradrenergic pathways originating from the medulla and pons do not play important roles in waking behavior. Catecholamine and cholinergic (see review below) systems are likely involved in the so-called "executive" mechanisms of REM sleep and in the maintenance of tonic behavioral and EEG arousal. It is likely that at each level of organization in the brainstem, there is complex interaction between indoleamine, catecholamine, and cholinergic systems. Studies of interactions between these chemical systems can certainly be considered at the forefront in this field.

VI. THE CHOLINERGIC SYSTEMS

A. General Remarks

Pharmacological and biochemical evidence for cholinergic transmission in the central nervous system, while essentially indirect, now appears convincing. There is a large body of histochemical evidence of central cholinergic transmission based primarily on the distribution of acetylcholinesterase in the brain and spinal cord. Neurons of the peripheral nervous system that are known to be cholinergic contain high concentrations of acetylcholine (ACh), acetylcholinesterase (AChE), and choline acetylase (ChAc). The designation of a particular group of neurons in the central nervous system as "cholinergic" (or "monoaminergic") is considerably more difficult than in peripheral systems, chiefly because of the methodological problems of recovering and identifying the transmitter released only at their terminals following their stimulation.

From the methodological point of view, only AChE (and not ACh itself) can be localized histochemically at the present time, and it is obvious that this is not as direct a criterion of cholinergic function as would be the demonstration of the transmitter agent itself. Koelle (1969) has emphasized the close correspondence between quantitative values for ChAc and the intensity of histochemical staining for AChE at certain central tracts. The acetylthiocholine method (Koelle and Friedenwald, 1949), which was developed almost 25 years ago, remains the most specific histochemical procedure for the localization of AChE. In peripheral neurons AChE is distributed throughout the length of the axons and the same has been assumed centrally. The cholinergic system is revealed by a version of the thiocholine method originally devised by Koelle and Friedenwald for the detection of cholinesterase. As reviewed earlier, the monoaminergic systems can be visualized more directly since the monoamine transmitters themselves fluoresce under formaldehyde exposure. Shute and Lewis (1966) have noted in all the regions of the rat brain where monoamine-containing cells have been described, cells can be seen in thiocholine-incubated material that contains small amounts of AChE, and have postulated that this may indicate that monoaminergic neurons are "cholinoceptive". It is likely that the presence of AChE is not by itself sufficient evidence for the existence of a cholinergic pathway, but the absence of AChE activity is certainly a useful index of a non-cholinergic system. Also, it is generally seen that fibers rich in AChE do not form compact bundles in the central nervous system but rather comprise a relatively diffuse network of very fine fibers, in places complexly intermingled with other pathways. Thus, their specific isolation is extremely difficult and these systems have, therefore, been much more immune to manipulation by lesioning and stimulation procedures. Krnjević (1969) has noted that AChE-containing fibers are associated particularly with phylogenetically ancient regions of the brain. For example, he observes that the various "cholinergic" projections that ascend from the brainstem to the forebrain are predominantly related to the limbic system and striatum. He also points out that if cholinergic fibers are present in the central nervous system, they belong to a system of pathways that is distinct from the fast conducting tracts.

As a prerequisite to discussing possible cholinergic mechanisms in sleep-waking behavior it is essential to review the cholinergic circuits in the brain in some detail. Shute and Lewis (1966, 1967) and Lewis and Shute (1967) have made an extensive histochemical study of two major cholinergic systems in the brain, i.e., the ascending cholinergic reticular system and the cholinergic limbic system. Until these experiments there were no detailed maps indicating which nervous pathways in the brain are "cholinergic". In deciding which pathways in the brain should be regarded a cholinergic, these workers have assumed that central cholinergic neurons would, like those of the peripheral nervous system, contain the hydrolytic enzyme AChE in high concentration not only in the cell body, but also along the whole length of the axon, including the nerve terminals. The problem of determining the polarity of such fibers was greatly eased by the discovery that when AChE-containing tracts are lesioned, the interrupted ends of the axon differ on the two sides of the cut, i.e., the terminal portion becomes distended and varicose, and stains much more heavily for AChE than does normal fibers. In their studies of the ascending cholinergic reticular system, Shute and Lewis (1967) identified two major pathways, in this division; the dorsal tegmental pathway and the ventral tegmental pathway (see Fig. 17).

B. The Cholinergic Reticular System

1. The Dorsal Tegmental Pathway

Shute and Lewis (Fig. 17) defined this pathway as the system of cholinesterase-containing fibers which runs rostrally from the midbrain tegmentum and supplies the tectum, prectectal area, geniculate bodies, and thalamus, with some fibers also connecting with the globus pallidus. Essentially the dorsal tegmental pathway could be traced from the region of the nucleus cuneiformis of the midbrain (Fig. 17) which occupies a considerable area of the midbrain tegmentum, and, through its lower pole, connects with the pars compacta of the substantia nigra. This nuclear area essentially extends from the pons to the pretectal area. Since the cuneiform nuclear area is a main well-spring for the dorsal cholinergic tegmental pathway we will define it in more detail as follows: The term cuneiform nucleus covers a quadrangularly shaped area containing small to medium-sized cells with relatively few Nissl granules, and extends throughout essentially all of the midbrain from the lower border of the inferior colliculus to the rostral level of the superior colliculus (Olszewski and Baxter, 1954; Ziehen, 1920). Medially it is adjacent to the periaqueductal gray; laterally, to the medial lemniscus; and ventrally, it is bounded by the subcuneiform nucleus. The subcuneiform nucleus is a somewhat less dense cellular area than the cuneiform area and is distinguished further from it by clusters of larger cells and by less numerous glial satellites. It lies ventral to the latter area and medial

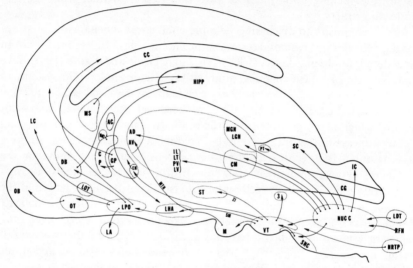

Fig. 17. Diagramatic representation of the ascending cholinergic reticular system of Shute and Lewis showing the two components of this system, i.e., the dorsal tegmental pathway and the ventral tegmental pathway. Note that the dorsal pathway emanates predominantly from the nucleus cuneiformis (Nuc C) of the mesencephalon and projects diffusely to the anterior (SC) and posterior (IC) colliculi, pretectal area (PT), medial (MGN), and lateral geniculate (LGN) nuclei (especially the ventral nucleus of the LGN), centre median (CM) and in- tralaminar thalamic nuclei (IL), several specific thalamic nuclei including the lateral ventral (LV) and posterior ventral (PV) nuclei, and the anterior thalamic nuclei, especially the antero- dorsal (AD) and antero-ventral (AV) groups. Note that the nucleus cuneiformis receives fibers from the latero-dorsal tegmental (LDT) area (including the locus coeruleus) and the reticular formation of the lower brainstem (RFH). The ventral tegmental pathway emanates mainly from the ventral tegmental area of Tsai (VT) and the substantia nigra (SNC) and projects primarily to the subthalamus (ST), zona incerta (ZI), hypothalamus and basal forebrain areas. These projections, in part, pass via the supramammillary bodies (SM), mammillary body (M), lateral hypothalamic area (LHA), lateral preoptic area (LPO) to the olfactory. tubercle (OT), nucleus of the lateral olfactory tract (LOT) and to limbic (LC) and other cortices. Direct fibers from this system supply the oculomotor nucleus (3). The entopeduncular nucleus (EN) and globus pallidus (GP) also receive direct fibers from this system, the latter, in turn, projecting to the caudate (C) and putaminal (P) formations, and nucleus accumbens (NA). Some con- nections, via the lateral preoptic area, are made with the diagonal band of Broca (DB) and medial septum (MS), the latter being the origin of cholinergic hippocampal (Hipp) afferents.

to the medial lemniscus and extends ventrally and ventro-caudally.

The cuneiform nucleus receives an input of cholinesterase-containing fibers from the reticular formation of the hindbrain and, most importantly, a powerful contribution from the latero-dorsal tegmental nucleus (locus coeruleus). After lesions of the nucleus cuneiformis there is a loss of staining in the inferior colliculus and in the deep layers of the superior colliculus as well as in the superficial and deep pretectal nuclei which normally receive a heavy innervation from the dorsal tegmental pathway. The centre median-parafascicular nuclear complex shows slight staining loss only, as does the medial geniculate body. In the thalamus the nuclei most affected are those which normally carry the heaviest innervation from the dorsal tegmental fibers, e.g., the intralaminar nuclei (marked loss of staining of the nucleus centralis lateralis), the inferior nuclei, the lateral thalamic nucleus, the postero-ventral thalamic nucleus, and the latero-ventral thalamic nucleus. Most fibers of the dorsal tegmental pathway were shown to traverse the reticular thalamic nucleus. This latter finding is particularly important when considering the projections of the midline thalamic system in the Golgi studies of the Scheibels (1966, 1967). As noted above, in those studies the thalamic synchronizing system projects rostrally through the reticular thalamic nucleus (Figs. 1, 2, and 4). At this point, while considering the thalamus, it is particularly pertinent to point out that there is highly selective staining of the intralaminar portions of the thalamus which stand out distinctly from specific thalamic nuclei. The studies of Olivier et al. (1970a) are most significant in this latter regard. They have made identifications of thalamic nuclei on the basis of their cholinesterase content in the monkey. The uneven distribution of cholinesterase was used as a criterion to delineate more precisely anatomical units within the thalamus. In general, lamellar nuclei showed a strongly positive reaction which permitted their division into three major groups: 1) the midline; 2) the intralaminar; and 3) the reticular and associated nuclei. On this basis, the midline group was shown to include the nucleus paraventricularis, the nucleus verticalis (centralis superior, intermedialis and inferior) and centralis densocellularis. On the other hand, the nucleus parataenialis, antero-reuniens, and reuniens were not thought to belong to the latter system. The intralaminar group was shown to be represented by a horizontal plate made up of the nucleus centralis medialis (rostrally) and the complex centrum medianum-parafascicularis (caudally) which extends latero-dorsally into the nuclei paracentralis, centralis lateralis, and centralis superior lateralis, and latero-caudally in the nuclei limitans and supra-geniculatus. The peripheral lameller nuclei also include the nucleus reticularis, which is prolonged caudally by the nucleus peripeduncularis, and nucleus geniculatis lateralis ventralis. Other nuclei of the anterior, medial, lateral and caudal territories of the thalamus were not readily identified in material prepared with the thiocholine technique. The uneven distribution of cholinesterase in the thalamus may, of course, have important functional implications for sorting out a possible "cholinergic" thalamic reticular system. This method thus can be used as a criterion to delimit anatomical and possibly functional units within the various thalamic fields. Until more systematic studies are done it is impossible at the present time to present a unified account of thalamic chemical neuronal assemblies and pathways.

2. The Ventral Tegmental Pathway

Shute and Lewis have applied the name "ventral tegmental pathway" to AChE-containing fiber systems (Fig. 17) which arise largely from the pars compacta of the substantia nigra and from cells of the ventral tegmental area of Tsai in the anterior mesencephalon. The ventral tegmental neurons are joined in their course by ascending fibers from the nucleus reticularis tegmenti pontis of Bechterew. The ventral tegmental fiber system enters the zona incerta, supramammillary region, and the lateral hypothalamic area, where there are many AChE-containing cells, and runs rostrally to the basal areas of the forebrain where they link with AChE-containing cells of the entopeduncular nucleus, globus pallidus, and lateral preoptic area (Fig. 17). Both the nigro-entopeduncular and nigro-striatal fibers form a part of the ventral tegmental system and these nigro-striatal "cholinergic systems" are important to note due to heavy emphasis in the literature on the nigro-striatal system being entirely a catecholaminergic (dopamine) complex involved in certain aspects of sleep-waking behavior (Jouvet 1972c). Shute and Lewis found that the mammillo-thalamic tract consists mainly of non-cholinergic fibers derived from the medial mammillary nucleus but also contains a number of ventral tegmental cholinergic fibers to the thalamic nuclei. Shute and Lewis have also shown that all cortical areas of the forebrain are innervated by systems of AChE-containing fibers which radiate laterally from the areas situated at the anterior end of the ventral tegmental pathway, especially the lateral preoptic area and globus pallidus. The olfactory cortex and olfactory bulb were shown to be supplied by cells primarily of the olfactory tubercle. The individual neurons of this entire system have large cell bodies and exceptionally long dendrites and are, therefore, thought to be capable of being activated by impulses from many different sources (see description of reticular characteristics, above). In general, this ventral tegmental pathway innervates, via cholinergic neurons, the caudate-putamen, nucleus accumbens, ventral part of the lateral amygdaloid nucleus, and the nucleus of the lateral olfactory tract.

The AChE-containing pathways of the forebrain are, therefore, thought to be derived, in large part, from the reticular formation of the brainstem and, also, especially in the case of the ventral tegmental fibers, from cell assemblies in the diencephalon and basal telencephalon which resemble reticular neurons in their form and staining characteristics. This latter is an important consideration since Leontovich and Zhukova (1963) and Nauta and Haymaker (1969), among others, consider the areas along the medial forebrain bundle system extending to the cortex as extensions of the reticular formation. Accordingly, Shute and Lewis have termed this cholinergic system the "ascending cholinergic reticular system" and have extended the concept of the "reticular formation" to include all the cell groups in the forebrain illustrated in Figure 17.

Shute and Lewis have assumed, based on the course and distribution of the AChE-containing fibers in the forebrain, that they form the anatomical basis of the ascending reticular activating system which is responsible for electrocortical arousal. It is of some interest to point out that the dorsal and ventral tegmental pathways described by them resemble very closely the thalamic and extrathalamic portions of the ascending reticular activating system described by Starzl et al. (1951) in the cat. In general, then, these mapping studies show that the cholinergic system of neurons has cortical terminals present diffusely over the neocortex and includes portions of the brainstem which have usually been considered a part of the reticular activating system. Some experimental confirmation for the hypothesis that the ascending cholinergic reticular formation is concerned with electrocortical arousal has been provided by the finding that high-frequency stimulation of the midbrain reticular formation in cats not only desynchronizes the EEG but also causes an increase in the output of ACh from the cerebral cortex (see below).

Shute and Lewis have pointed out that it is difficult to distinguish terminating axons from fibers of passage and that there are many regions where AChE-containing axons project onto nuclei consisting of cells rich in AChE, suggesting that the ascending cholinergic reticular system consists of a series of interconnected neurons which are cholinoceptive as well as cholinergic. Of course, the existence of a cholinergic component of the ascending reticular activating system does not necessarily mean that there is no other mechanism available for activating the cerebral cortex. There is evidence that mere blockage of cholinergic terminals at a cortical level is not sufficient to maintain a synchronized EEG since, when atropine is applied locally to the cortex or by intra-arterial injection, reticular stimulation is still capable of producing desynchronization. These physiological experiments are discussed in more detail below. Suffice it to note that while it is possible that the atropine dose was insufficient, an alternative interpretation is that noncholinergic corticopetal fibers, acting via the reticular thalamic nucleus, activate the cortex. This is discussed further below. It is of interest that the Scheibels (1966, 1967, 1970) have shown that the thalamic reticular nucleus is a type of filtering system through which fibers gathering to form the inferior thalamic peduncle (an important synchronizing system) pass on their way to the basal forebrain area.

As is well known, the reticular thalamic nucleus receives a powerful innervation from the nonspecific (midline and intralaminar) thalamic nuclei which bring about desynchronization of the EEG when stimulated at high-frequency but produce recruiting responses when the frequency of stimulation is low. It is likely that the pathway for recruiting responses probably does not involve a cholinergic link, since they are not abolished by atropine. It is most likely distinct from the pathway for electrocortical a-rousal, since recruiting responses are selectively depressed by the drug mephenesin which has no effect on arousal. Shute and Lewis reported earlier that the neurons of the non-specific thalamic nuclei do not themselves contain AChE (and so are presumably non-cholinergic) but newer work by Oliver et al. (1970a, b) indicates much of this complex is cholinergic. As will be discussed further below, in considering the anatomy of the ascending reticular formation, the desynchronization produced by high-frequency thalamic stimulation does not appear to be mediated by corticopetal projections of the reticular thalamic nuclei, but rather by an indirectly ascending cholinergic reticular system, either through fibers of passage which traverse the non-specific thalamic nuclei or, more likely, through projections of these nuclei back onto the tegmental reticular core and up the ventral leaf (see Figs. 1 and 4).

As reviewed above, among the nervous pathways which may exert an influence on the EEG are the widespread system of monoamine-containing fibers described by Dahlström and Fuxe (1964, 1965) and others. These fibers are heavily distributed to the hippocampal formation and medial cortex but have also been described as spreading to all areas of the cerebral neocortex. It is possible that the monoamine-containing system produces effects in the cortex which are opposite to those of the cholinergic system. Such an antagonism may well explain the EEG activation caused by large doses of reserpine, which depletes the brain monoamines. Hence, this agent may produce removal of an inhibitory influence on a cholinergic "arousal" mechanism. It is likely that cholinergic, monoaminergic, and possibly other neuronal chemical systems have regulatory functions in determining the level of excitation in different regions of the brain. The cholinergic system may mediate electrocortical arousal via the corticopetal radiations of the ascending cholinergic reticular system. As noted above, it is probable that behavioral arousal, on the other hand, may involve subcortical pathways, not all of which are cholinergic.

C. The Cholinergic Limbic System

The second major cholinergic system defined by Lewis and Shute (1967) is the cholinergic limbic system (Fig. 18). A variety of studies have shown a close functional relationship between the brainstem reticular formation and the hippocampal formation. It has been shown that stimulation of the midbrain reticular formation not only causes desynchronization of the cortical EEG, inhibiting slow rhythms and replacing them with high-frequency low-amplitude activity (4-7 cps in the cat), but also produces a synchronized hippocampal EEG, with slow-frequency, high-amplitude waves known as theta rhythm. It has been suggested that the hippocampus may itself modify

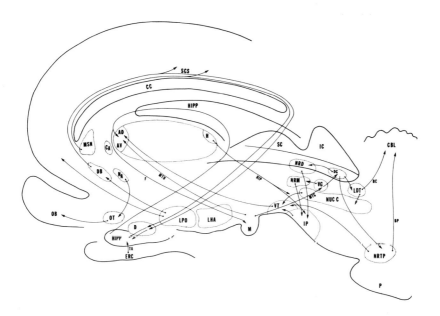

Fig. 18. Diagramatic representation of the cholinergic limbic system of Lewis and Shute. Fibers of one group in this system are afferent to the hippocampal formation passing from the medial septal nucleus (MSN) and nucleus of the diagonal band of Broca (DB) to the dentate gyrus (D), hippocampus (Hipp) proper (dorsal and ventral hippocampus), and subiculum. A second group of fibers pass from the antero-dorsal (AD) and antero-ventral (AV) thalamic nuclei to the retrosplenial and cingular areas, respectively (not shown). From the nucleus accumbens (NA) fibers of this system project to the olfactory tubercle (OT) and bulb (OB). Another group of neurons are afferent to the cerebellum, with fibers originating in the dorsal tegmental nucleus of a Gudden (DG) and thence projecting to the latero-dorsal tegmental nucleus (mainly locus coeruleus, LTD) and to cerebellum (CBL) via the brachium conjunctivum (BC). Another group of fibers from the dorsal nucleus of Gudden project directly to the nucleus reticularis tegmenti pontis of Bechterew (NRTP) and, via the brachium pontis (BP), to the cerebellum. One group of neurons of this cholinergic limbic system are afferent to the dorsal tegmental pathway component of the ascending cholinergic reticular system. These run from the dorsal tegmental nucleus of Gudden to the latero-dorsal tegmental nucleus and thence to the nucleus cuneiformis (Nuc C). A second group are afferent to the ventral tegmental pathway as follows: they run from the dorsal (DG) and ventral (VG) nuclei of Gudden, via the nucleus raphé dorsalis (NRD) and nucleus raphe medianus (NRM), to the interpeduncular nucleus (IP). Included in this group are projections from the habenular area connecting with the dorsal nucleus of Gudden and, through this, with the latero-dorsal tegmental nucleus, nucleus cuneiformis and substantia nigra. Also in this group are projections to the dorsal tegmental nucleus of Gudden, thence to the nucleus reticularis tegmenti pontis of Bechterew and, through this latter, to the ventral tegmental area of Tsai (VT). Other abbreviations: SCS = supracallosal stria; CC = corpus callosum; ERC = entorhinal cortex; TA = temporo-ammoniac fibers; P = pons; HIP = habenulo-interpeduncular tract; MTG = mammillo-tegmental tract; SC = superior colliculus; IC = inferior colliculus; H = habenula; MTH = mammilo-thalamic tract; M = mammillary body; LHA = lateral hypothalamic area; LPO = lateral preoptic area; CA = anterior commissure; F = fornix.

the activity of the reticular formation and, through it, modulate the activity of the cerebral cortex (Green, 1960). Apart from the fact that reticular influences largely reach the hippocampus via the septum, the mechanism by which the reticular formation and hippocampus are able to interact is unknown. Neurochemically, the fibers which arise from the medial septal nucleus and the nucleus of the diagonal band of Broca have been shown to be cholinergic and to supply the hippocampus proper, the dentate gyrus, and the subiculum.

Some evidence has accumulated indicating that the initial outflow from the hippocampus is non-cholinergic but that these non-cholinergic neurons impinge upon a number of nuclei whose cells are rich in AChE and which subsequently give rise to AChE-containing fibers. Thus, the mammillo-thalamic and mammillo-tegmental tracts, which arise from the medial mammillary nuclei and project, respectively, to the anterior thalamic nuclei and to the dorsal and ventral tegmental nuclei of Gudden, form second order neurons on the cholinergic pathways. These nuclei, which are presumabley cholinergic, project directly to medial cortical areas or to the olfactory bulb, or connect, via relays, onto the ascending reticular system. Thus, it appears that most of the anterior thalamic nuclei, which project onto the cingulate cortex, are cholinergic in type. The dorsal and ventral tegmental nuclei of Gudden are both innervated by mammillo-tegmental fibers and both come under powerful influences of the hippocampal-fornix projection system. The cells of both nuclei are rich in AChE and AChE-containing fibers emanating from the dorsal tegmental nucleus can be seen in normal material to project to the latero-dorsal tegmental nucleus (nucleus dorsolateralis tegmenti or locus coeruleus) and to the nucleus reticularis tegmenti pontis of Bechterew.

The latero-dorsal tegmental nucleus (locus coeruleus) sends cholinesterase-containing fibers not only to the cerebellum but also to the nucleus cuneiformis (Fig. 18). Thus, the hippocampal-tegmental projection is linked with the dorsal tegmental pathway of the ascending cholinergic reticular system. Also, a continuous chain of cholinesterase-containing neurons can be traced from the dorsal and ventral tegmental nuclei of Gudden, via the nucleus raphé dorsalis and medianus (which also contain AChE) to the interpeduncular nucleus. This latter nucleus contains large amounts of AChE and these AChE-containing neurons connect largely with those of the ventral tegmental area of Tsai. It is interesting that, unlike the axons of the dorsal and ventral tegmental neurons, the fibers which make up the mammillary peduncle do not contain AChE, and so are thought to be non-cholinergic. Most of the evidence, then, is that the projections of the dorsal and ventral tegmental nuclei of Gudden onto the interpeduncular nucleus, and through this nucleus onto the AChE-containing neurons of the ventral tegmental area of Tsai, provide a powerful cholinergic link between the hippocampal-fornix projection system and the ventral tegmental pathway. Since the interpeduncular nucleus projects onto cholinergic neurons of the ventral tegmental area of Tsai, the habenulo-interpeduncular tract can be regarded as providing an additional route by which the hippocampus can act on the ventral tegmental pathway.

In summary, the term "cholinergic limbic system" can be applied to groups of AChE-containing neurons which are intimately related to the hippocampal formation and its projection pathways in the forebrain and midbrain (Fig. 18). As shown by Lewis and Shute (1967) the cholinergic limbic system consists of two groups of nuclei: the nuclei of group 1 are afferent with respect ot the hippocampal formation. Those of group 2 are innervated by the hippocampal system and project primarily to the medial cortex, cerebellum, and nuclei of the ascending cholinergic reticular system. The neurons of the interpeduncular nucleus, which contain AChE, appear to form a major link between the cholinergic limbic system and the ventral tegmental pathway of the ascending cholinergic reticular system.

Since hippocampal afferents whose cell bodies are located in the nucleus of the diagonal band of Broca lie along the course of the ventral tegmental pathway of the ascending cholinergic reticular system it has been speculated that these neurons may play some role in determining the electrical activity of the hippocampus during arousal. It must be kept in mind, however, that cholinergic fibers are not the only afferent projections to the hippocampus traveling via the septum and fornix. For example, there is an extensive innervation by the monoamine-containing fibers which arise from cells of the midbrain lying dorsal and lateral to the interpeduncular nucleus (see below and Figs. 3, 18, and 19). These monoaminergic fibers do not have the same distribution in the hippocampal complex as those of the cholinergic system. For example, Lewis and Shute (1967) have pointed out that monoaminergic terminals appear to relate more closely to apical dendrites of pyramidal cells of the hippocampus whereas cholinergic terminals relate to the basal dendrites of pyramidal cells. These differences in connectivities of chemical circuits may have important, but as yet undertermined, functional significance.

Shute and Lewis have emphasized that, in general, cells rich in AChE are not found at the sites of monoamine-containing cells, although there are some exceptions. of special interest being that of the nucleus locus coeruleus and the substantia nigra. It is interesting that monoamine-containing fibers in the diencephalon have a similar course to that of AChE-containing fibers in the ventral tegmental pathway. However, Shute and Lewis have also pointed out that the distribution of monoaminergic and cholinergic terminals at subcortical levels is not identical. More work is obviously needed to study the innervation densities of hypothalamic and other neuronal assemblies with respect to these two major chemical systems. It is obvious that there are many areas in which cholinergic and monoaminergic systems overlap and probably interrelate. For example, cell groups A4, A5, A6, and A9 stain extremely heavily for AChE and may thus be regarded as cholinergic as well as noradrenergic. In Shute's latest review on cholinergic systems (1970) he notes that the ascending AChE-containing fibers in the lateral hypothalamus form part of the extrathalamic portion of the ascending reticular activating system.

In another study of the functional role of the nigro-neostriatal dopamine neurons Andén et al. (1966a) observed that the neostriatum contains a high concentration of ACh and AChE and noted that it is highly likely that the

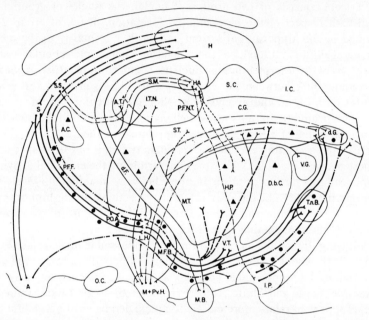

Fig. 19. Schematized representation of the limbric forebrain-limbic midbrain reciprocating circuitry illustrating (black dots) points from which sleep was induced by direct cholinergic stimulation in the cat. Arousal was produced by cholinergic stimulation of the sites indicated by black triangles. Loci immediately above and below the medial forebrain bundle were stimulated with cholinergic agents using the exploring cannula technique. Note the close correspondence of the sleep loci with the trajectory of the MFB system. Lesions behind a cannual system from which sleep was induced blocked the sleep-evoking action of cholinergic agents as did atropine placed in a cannula posterior to sleep-positive cannula placement. Other abbreviations: H=hippocampus; HA=habenular nucleus; SC=superior collicus; IC=inferior colliculus; CG=central gray; dG=dorsal tegmental nucleus of Gudden; ST=subthalamic region; VG=deep tegmental nucleus of Gudden; TnB=central tegmental nucleus of Bechterew; Db-C=decussation of brachium conjunctivum; IP=interpeduncular nucleus; VT=ventral area of Tsai; HP=habenulointerpeduncular tract; MB=mammillary body; M+PvH=medial and periventricular hypothalamic regions; OC=optic chiasm; A=amygdaloid nucleus; MFB= medial forebrain bundle; MT=mammillothalamic tract; dF=descending fornix column; LH=lateral hypothalamus; POA=preoptic area; PFF=precommissural fornix fibers; AC= anterior commissure; S=septum; SS=supracommissural septum; AT=anterior thalamic nucleus; ITN=intralaminar thalamic nuclear areas; PFNT=parafascicular nucleus of thalamus; SM=stria medullaris.

fibers containing AChE in the neostriatum (Koelle, 1954) represent true ACh nerve terminals. These workers found that the ACh fibers probably ascend uncrossed in the cerebral peduncle and in the internal capsule, since there is a severe loss of the ipsilateral AChE activity in the neostriatum after unilateral lesions at the junction between the mesencephalon and the diencephalon. They observed that it was likely that the cholinergic neurons to the neostriatum are functional antagonists of the dopamine system, pointing out that atropine and other cholinergic blocking agents are useful in the treatment of Parkinsonism. Naturally, the lesion may well have included an efferent pathway from the corpus striatum or another afferent neuron system to the neostriatum antagonistic to the dopamine system.

D. Acetylcholine Release Studies

Evidence has been accumulating for many years that the reticular formation influences acetylcholine levels in the cerebral cortex. Funderberk and Case (1951) suggested that cortical arousal is mediated via a cholinergic mechanism since they found that cortical arousal could be elicited with cholinomimetics and blocked by atropine. At that time, however, there was no evidence concerning the identity of possible cholinergic pathways, or the cells they might possibly innervate. There is a good deal of recent evidence on transmitter mechanisms in the cerebral cortex indicating that ACh is not the principal transmitter concerned in postsynaptic excitation or inhibition. In fact, the main excitatory transmitter is more likely to be an amino acid such as L-glutamate, while the main inhibitory transmitter is probably gamma-amino-butyric acid. The bulk of the evidence indicates that ACh seems to be associated with relatively slow ·and prolonged excitatory effects involving only a certain portion of cortical neurons. ACh has long been considered a good neurotransmitter candidate responsible for the desynchronization or activation of the cortical EEG during arousal responses. That desynchronized activation can be reproduced readily in experimental animals by intracarotid injection of ACh was shown by Bonnet and Bremer (1937) and later confirmed by Rinaldi and Himwich (1955a, b). This form of cortical activation occurs even in the collicular transected preparation and is thus not dependent upon the brainstem, but rather has a direct cortical action.

Krnjević (1967) also has pointed out that some cortical cells are innervated by cholinergic nerve fibers that are probably related to the arousal mechanism. In his earlier work he showed that the distribution of AChE in the forebrain shows a rather characteristic pattern which corresponds well with the distribution of ACh-sensitive cells. He found that a diffuse cholinergic network appears to be present in the deeper cortical layers where it closely invests many of the pyramidal cells. Further, most of the network was thought to probably be made up of ascending fibers with a subcortical origin. Along the lateral and frontal aspects of the hemisphere, these fibers were traced down to the external capsule and the deeper region of the striatum, while those in the upper and medial regions appeared to arise from the septum and fornix. Lesions in the forebrain showed that the various fibers do indeed ascend to the cortex, but it was not possible to exactly establish the situation of their cells of origin. The cells could be in the septum or the lenticular nucleus, or they might be further back in the midbrain reticular formation which, as shown by Shute and Lewis, send AChE-containing projections to the forebrain. Krnjević and Silver (1965) demonstrated the subcortical origin of the cholinergic radiation to the cortex in an ontogenetic study of the development of AChE-containing fibers. They showed very clearly that the neocortex is free of AChE throughout its earlier development, whereas the striatal and septal primordia contain AChE from the earliest stages onward. AChE-containing fibers from these areas grow progressively into the pallium and invade the cortex at a relatively late stage. From these various kinds of evidence, it appears that the deeper and older layers of the cortex receive a cholinergic innervation originating from the basal and relatively ancient portions of the forebrain. This innervation may be the forebrain extension of a cholinergic reticular system present throughout much of the brainstem. Via this system of fibers, the older parts of the brain may exert some control over the cerebral cortex.

Most of the recent evidence is consistent with the original hypothesis of Funderburk and Case (1951). A continuous, possibly multisynaptic, system of cholinergic fibers extends from the level of the midbrain to the cortex, passing through the striatum and the septum and provides a diffuse innervation for the neurons in the deeper cortical layers. The excitability of these cells would thus depend upon the rate of release of ACh by the ascending fibers. Desynchronization of the EEG in arousal could result from a marked increase in random spontaneous activity, which would prevent the synchronized activation of cortical cells by thalamic volleys. It is possible that the rhythmic thalamic activity may itself be influenced by similar ascending cholinergic pathways. Many details of cortical innervation by the cholinergic system need to be worked out. For the present the following may be noted: AChE-staining fibers are found ramifying throughout the various layers of the intact cortex although the majority occur quite deep in relation to the pyramidal cells of layer 5 and the polymorph cells of layer 6. These branches originate from a system of fibers which form a predominantly tangential system running beneath the cortex (Krnjević and Silver, 1965). Other fibers appear to reach the cortex from the corpus striatum and septal areas, which systems may be directly comparable with those described by Shute and Lewis (1967). Various observations on isolated cortical slabs strongly suggest that there are *both* intrinsic and extrinsic components of the cortical cholinergic system: an intracortical system which may originate in the polymorph cells of layer 6, and an extracortical system from the corpus striatum and septal area.

Krnjević (1967) has emphasized that there is a continuous, possibly multisynaptic system of cholinergic fibers extending from the level of the midbrain to the cortex, passing through the striatum and the septum. These fibers appear to provide a diffuse innervation for the neurons in the deeper cortical layers. The excitability of these cortical cells appears to depend upon the rate of release of ACh by the ascending fibers. Desynchronization of the EEG in arousal could result from a marked increase in random spontaneous activity, which would prevent the synchronized activation of cortical cells by thalamic volleys. He speculated that it is possible that the rhythmic thalamic activity may itself be influenced by similar ascending cholinergic pathways.

It is well known that behavioral arousal and cortical electrographic arousal can be dissociated pharmacologically. For example, eserine can elicit cortical arousal without greatly alerting the behavior of an animal. A comparable dissociation can be induced by appropriate lesions in the brainstem (Feldman and Waller, 1963). These observations suggest that other areas of the brain also play a vital role in the mechanism of sleep and arousal and that if cholinergic pathways are also involved, they may have different pharmacological properties resembling many ACh-sensitive cells in various subcortical regions. If studies of the release of ACh in the cerebral cortex is an indication of its functional role then these should be examined in some detail with respect to anatomical correlations. Pepeu and Mantegazzini (1964) showed that the amount of cortical ACh may be related to the degree of activity of the reticular activating system. They found that a midbrain hemisection in a midpontine pretrigeminal cat preparation causes an asymmetry in the EEG, with a marked increase in the ACh content of the cortex from the synchronized hemisphere, and suggested that the increase in ACh is related to the decrease of nervous activity caused by the hemisection. They concluded that the EEG activated pattern of the pretrigeminal preparation is maintained by a tonic barrage of impulses arising in the rostral portion of the pons. The midbrain hemisection would then produce ipsilateral sleep with the decrease of the number of activating impulses impinging upon the cerebral cortex. They felt that it was conceivable that the resting state of ascending fibers during the EEG synchronization leads to accumulation of ACh in these fiber endings or in the cortical neurons or both. Pepeu (1972) has shown that in the cat, if the reticular formation is disconnected from the cortex by means of a transection at the collicular level, the ensuing EEG synchronization is associated with a higher cortical ACh content than that found in cats with an intact activating system showing EEG desynchronization. He has provided data suggesting that the pathways responsible for the release of ACh evoked from the primary receiving area is the more specific thalamo-cortical pathway associated with augmenting and repetitive after-discharge responses. Smaller increases in ACh output observed in other parts of the cortex were thought to be due to stimulation of the nonspecific reticulo-cortical pathways. It was also shown that unilateral lesions which destroy most of the septum caused a 23% decrease in ACh content of the whole brain, whereas bilateral lesions of the fimbria and of the hippocampus resulted in a 31% decrease in brain ACh.

Further proof that ACh may be involved in desychronized cortical activation and in the arousal response comes from experiments in which the rate of liberation of acetylcholine from the cortical surface has been measured in states of sleep and wakefulness, either following brainstem lesions, anesthesia, or during natural states of sleep and waking. By the use of these methods it has been found that the rate of liberation of ACh from the surface of the cerebral cortex varies systematically with the state of alertness of the animal (Kanai and Szerb, 1965; Krnjević, 1967; Phillis and Chong, 1965), i.e., high rates of liberation of acetylcholine during arousal. Jasper and co-workers (1965, 1967, 1969, 1971) have shown that ACh is not the mediator of primary specific afferent activation of the cerebral cortex but rather that it is related to nonspecific activation pointing out that the mediator(s) for specific afferents are as yet unknown. Certainly the release of ACh in the cerebral cortex is probably an indication of some significant functional role. It has been shown by Jasper (1969), Collier and Mitchell (1966), Kanai and Szerb (1965) and Phillis and Chong (1965), among others, that ACh release into the cortex is very much increased following stimulation of afferent pathways or the midbrain reticular formation. These results have widely been interpreted as being consistent with the possibility that an ascending cholinergic system mediates cortical arousal.

Some experimental confirmation for the hypothesis that the ascending cholinergic reticular formation is concerned with electrocortical arousal has been provided by the finding that high-frequency stimulation of the midbrain reticular formation in cats not only desynchronizes the EEG but also causes a 5- to 6-fold increase in the output of ACh from the cerebral cortex (Kanai and Szerb, 1965). The increase in ACh output in those studies still occurred when electrocortical arousal was prevented by systemic atropine.The effect of the atropine, therefore, was to block the post-synaptic effects, at cortical levels, of the acetylcholine released as the result of reticular stimulation. The finding that atropine blocked the EEG signs of arousal without affecting the increase in ACh output indicates that the enhanced output of ACh was not the result of a general increase in neural activity in the underlying cortex during EEG arousal. The simplest interpretation of the action of atropine on the EEG is that it blocks the postsynaptic effect of ACh in the cortex where, as has been shown by Krjnević (1967, 1969) and Phillis's group (1965, 1967a, b), it also antagonises the stimulating effects of electrophoretically applied ACh. The work of Kanai and Szerb (1956) also demonstrates that cholinergic pathways are part of at least two distinct cortical systems. One is the specific corticopetal system producing increased ACh release in the sensory area and the second is a nonspecific system involved in the EEG arousal response, producing increased ACh release in a wide area of the cortex. As reviewed, this widespread cholinergic system has been demonstrated histochemically by Shute and Lewis, who found important cholinergic tracts ascending from the midbrain tegmentum to the cortex and to other parts of the forebrain. The pathways involved in cortical arousal and increased ACh output may be different since the two phenomena do not always vary in parallel fashion when the reticular formation or other subcortical areas are stimulated (Szerb, 1967). It is interesting that retinal, lateral or medial geniculate stimulation also increased the release of ACh in the primary receiving areas of the cortex which favors the view that, besides nonspecific cholinergic corticopetal pathways, there also exists specific cholinergic sensory pathways. Thus, ACh may then be involved in the phasic arousal which accompanies sensory stimulation. In these studies, Szerb concluded that the projections responsible for EEG activation and increased cortical ACh release originate in the mesencephalic tegmentum. Spontaneous, afferent or electrical stimulation of this area was found to activate two pathways. However, the two projections were shown to follow divergent paths on their way to the cortex, since they could be stimulated or blocked selectively. Atropine, for instance, blocked only EEG activation but not the increased ACh output due to reticular formation stimulation. He observed that it is likely that the cholinergic pathways associated with the specific afferent and the diffuse ascending system are distinct and should probably serve different functions. Khazan et al. (1967) have presented evidence that two typical cholinergic agents (eserine and neostigmine) were effective in suppressing the REM-blocking effect of chlorpromazine and imipramine, respectively. These findings thus support the proposed role of central cholinergic mechanisms in precipitating REM sleep.

In more recent experiments, with regard to ACh liberation from the cerebral cortex during sleep, Jasper and Tessier (1971) showed that the rate of liberation of free ACh from the surface of the cerebral cortex averaged 1.2 ng/min/cm of cortical surface during slow-wave sleep, 2.2 ng/min/cm during REM sleep, and 2.1 ng/min/cm during waking. They concluded that the rate of ACh release is related to the encephalographic pattern of desynchronized activation rather than to the behavioral responsiveness in their animals. Ilyutchenok and Gilinsky (1969) demonstrated the existence of an inhibitory cholinergic synapse in the cerebral cortex by showing that topical application of the ACh antagonists benactyzine and atropine abolishes the inhibition of spontaneously active cortical neurons induced by stimulation of the reticular formation. In these studies the electroencephalographic arousal reaction produced by stimulation of the reticular formation was also abolished.

Jordan and Phillis (1972) have provided evidence for a system of intracortical cholinergic neurons which make direct inhibitory contacts with neurons in the superficial layer of the cortex in cats. Phillis and York (1967) proposed that ACh is an inhibitory transmitter in the cerebral cortex and presented evidence to show that the inhibition of cortical neurons evoked by repetitive stimulation of various regions of the brain, including the adjacent cortical surface, was mediated by ACh. This inhibition was blocked by atropine. The studies of Jordan and Phillis (1972) lend support to the assertion that cholinergic inhibitory synapses are present in the more superficial layers (layers 2, 3, and 4 of the cerebral cortex). Such a distribution of cholinergic inhibitory terminals would be consistent with the finding that the highest concentrations of ACh in the cerebral cortex of the cat are found in layers 2, 3, and 4. It is apparent that the inhibition described by Jordan and Phillis is mediated by the intracortical cholinergic interneurons.

Probably some of the most direct evidence for existence of cholinergic (or cholinoceptive) systems in the brain are those dealing with direct chemical stimulation with cholinergic agents. Hernández-Peón et al. (1962, 1963) mapped out several hundred loci in the cat brain from which cholinergic stimulation induced sleep. In these studies, micro-amounts of cholinergic crystalline material inserted along the trajectory of the medial forebrain bundle and its extensions induced, with latencies of 1 to 5 min, behavioral and electrographic signs of sleep. This comprehensive series, when plotted on brain maps, followed so closely the limbic forebrain-limbic midbrain circuit that the two practically overlap (Fig. 19). The polarity of this cholinoceptive system was shown to be descending, in the sense that lesions in the medial forebrain bundle posterior to the chemical cannula system blocked the sleep-inducing effects, whereas lesions placed anterior to the cannula did not have such an effect. Also, atropine placed in the medial forebrain bundle system posterior to the cannula blocked cholinergic induction of sleep. Thus, Hernández-Peón et al. concluded that this constituted a descending cholinergic hypnogenic system which might function by inhibiting the mesodiencephalic activating system. The distinct possibility that this same system corresponds to the basal forebrain inhibitory system outlined by Sterman and Clemente (1962a, b, 1968) has seemed a definite possibility, but little work on the descending systems has been done in recent years. Their role in sleep-waking behavior remain obscure. Shute (1970) also has discussed the work of Hernández-Peón et al. (1962, 1963) regarding the descending cholinergic system. He notes that a descending cholinergic pathway is unlikely because the AChE containing fibers of the medial forebrain bundle are all ascending. Shute thinks that it is more probable that there is a non-cholinergic descending inhibitory pathway containing relays in which transmission can be modified by an ascending cholinergic input. Cordeau and Mancia (1959) and Cordeau et al. (1963) also induced sleep in cats by direct cholinergic stimulation of the brain. In further studies along these lines, Matsuzaki et al. (1967, 1968) demonstrated that it is probable that cholinergic mechanisms in the central nervous system are involved in inducing REM sleep in the mesencephalic (pre-collicular) cat. They showed that the induction of REM sleep by cholinergic-potentiating agents is due to their central effects and not to peripheral ones. The most effective agent in inducing REM sleep was found to be physostigmine.

E. Hippocampal Theta Rhythm

It is now relevant to discuss hippocampal rhythms and their mode of generation with regard to amine systems in the brain, particularly in relation to cholinergic mechanisms. Although the hippocampal record commonly shows theta rhythm when the neocortical EEG is of the alert or active type, fast activity only is thought to occur in unanesthetized animals confronted with a novel unconditioned stimulus, as part of the so-called "startle response" (Grastyán et al.,(1959). Fast, low-amplitude activity can, in fact, be produced experimentally in the hippocampus by stimulating the medial septum (Torii, 1961). The same result can be obtained from stimulation of the medio-ventral tegmentum and lateral hypothalamic area, areas traversed by cholinergic neurons of the ventral tegmental pathway, which appears to connect with the cholinergic neurons of the diagonal band and septum. It is extremely interesting that fast activity produced in this way is abolished by atropine (Longo, 1956). It is noteworthy that fast activity resulting from reticular stimulation or administration of eserine can survive septal lesions. This must mean either that fast hippocampal activity can be produced by cholinoceptive projections onto the hippocampus which do not traverse the septum, e.g., those from the entorhinal cortex, or that some of the septal neurons responsible escaped damage. Destruction in the septal region would need to be very extensive to involve all cells from that area to the hippocampus. Theta rhythm, unlike fast activity, is always abolished by septal lesions. It is possible that at the level of the septum the monoaminergic supply to the hippocampus, which arises more caudally in the brainstem, forms a more compact and, therefore, more vulnerable bundle than the cholinergic fibers. One major cholinergic output from the hippocampus passes either directly or through a relay in the mammillary nucleus to elements of the cholinergic limbic system which connect directly with the medial cortex or, through links with the ascending cholinergic reticular system, with the lateral cortex of the cerebral hemispheres. These connections provide a means by which the hippocampus can influence electrical activity in other regions of the forebrain, as in arousal.

The role of the septum in relation to hippocampal theta activity (hippocampal arousal pattern) was first demonstrated in the rabbit by Green and Arduini (1954). They found that theta rhythm in the hippocampus, elicited by nonspecific stimuli which simultaneously aroused the animal, could be abolished by septal lesions. They also observed that hippocampal theta rhythm could be triggered by impulses originating from stimulation of the medial septum. A somewhat similar hippocampal synchronized rhythm, which could be evoked by administration of eserine and amphetamine, was also abolished by septal lesions (Mayer and Stumpf, 1958). In contrast, Brücke et al. (1959) inhibited the hippocampal arousal pattern by electrical stimulation in the medial septal region. Other work showed that procaine injection into the septum also blocked synchronized patterns of the hip-

pocampus induced by physostigmine. Since all these changes were associated
with medially placed lesions and stimulations, it has been assumed that the
medial region of the septum is the pacemaker for the synchronized pattern
found in the hippocampus and other brain structures. Von Euler and Green
(1960), showed that repetitive stimulation of the septum may drive the theta
rhythm in the hippocampus. It was found by Petsche and Stumpf (1960) that
the area most intimately associated with the hippocampal theta rhythm was
in the septal part of the nucleus of the diagonal band. They further postulated that the septum serves as a last relay to the hippocampus from the
brainstem reticular system which could initiate or influence hippocampal
theta rhythm.

Green and Arduini (1954) noted that, during the transition from
drowsiness to alertness, hippocampal arousal rhythms usually preceded those
of the neocortex, while with behavioral changes in the reverse direction the
hippocampal theta rhythm associated with arousal was suppreffsed before
the appearance of neocortical "sleep spindles". These time sequences suggest
that the hippocampus may be concerned in initiating reticular activity
associated with the alert state. Green and Arduini (1954) have demonstrated
in the rabbit, cat, and monkey that the afferent inputs from the activating
system in the brainstem to the hippocampus, which induced hippocampal
arousal activity (theta rhythm), were conveyed from the midbrain tegmentum
through the lateral hypothalamus, septum, precommissural and dorsal
fornices. It is interesting that Green (1957) found that, in hip-
pocampectomized cats, electrocortical arousal was difficult to produce by
reticular stimulation and, unlike the arousal obtained in normal animals,
lasted only for the duration of the stimulus. He also emphasized that hippocampal stimulation does not usually lead to generalized neocortical
desynchronization. In addition to effects on arousal it is possible that
neurons from the anterior thalamic nuclear group to the medial cortex, those
of nucleus accumbens to the olfactory tubercle, those of the ascending
cholinergic reticular system, and those neurons that are afferent to the
ascending cholinergic reticular system, are related to processes of learning
and memory. Thus, neurons to the dorsal tegmental pathway from the dorsal
tegmental nucleus and those from the dorsal tegmental and deep tegmental
nucleus, as well as the raphé dorsalis and nucleus raphé medianus to the
interpeduncular nucleus, and from the dorsal tegmental nucleus to the
substantia nigra and ventral tegmental area, may all be involved in the
reputed role of the hippocampus in learning and memory. Green (1964) has
pointed out that it is likely that hippocampal effects on memory processes are
achieved by influences acting on parts of the brain external to the hippocampus rather than as an intrinsic property of the hippocampus itself.

It has also been postulated by Shute and Lewis that the effects of
cholinergic and monoaminergic systems on the hippocampal activity may, in
some degree, be opposed to one another. Such a point of view has been

favored by reports that hippocampal neurons are facilitated by ACh whereas those which show sensitivity to either norepinephrine or serotonin are depressed. Also, the firing rate of hippocampal cells is accelerated by cholinomimetic drugs such as eserine. There is some evidence in favor of the monoaminergic system being primarily concerned with the production of theta rhythm. For example, Killam and Killam (1957) showed that theta rhythm is depressed by reserpine (which depletes the brain of monoamines) and slow hippocampal rhythms can be produced by electrical stimulation of the medial preoptic area, medial hypothalamic region, and the central grey matter of the dorso-lateral tegmentum of the midbrain (Torii, 1961). None of these areas, except the last, are sites of cholinergic cells, whereas some appear to coincide closely with monoaminergic pathways and cell groups, especially group A11. Although it has been shown that some cell groups in the hippocampus are active during theta rhythm (Green, 1964), the firing rate of other hippocampal cells may be depressed. Lewis and Shute (1967) have pointed out that it is possible that slow rhythms in the hippocampus are associated with a relatively low overall level of activity such as might result from an inhibitory innervation from the monoaminergic system. In favor of the cholinergic system playing some role in theta rhythm, is the fact that slow waves can be induced in the hippocampus by administering eserine so long as the septal area is intact (Green, 1964). It has also been claimed that neurons located in the medial part of the septum, which have been shown to be a source of cholinergic fibers supplying the hippocampus, act as a type of pacemaker and produce theta rhythm through their own slow rhythmical discharge. These neurons may themselves be influenced by the monoaminergic system, since monoaminergic endings have clearly been shown to end in the septum (Fuxe, 1965). Another possible role for cholinergic neurons of the medial septum and diagonal band of Broca may be to generate fast low-amplitude activity in the hippocampus. Such activity is superimposed on theta rhythm during moderate degrees of reticular stimulation and after administration of eserine, and replaces the theta rhythm when reticular stimulation is very strong. Hippocampal responses might in this manner be brought into line with those of the neocortex, where cholinergic projections are probably involved in the desynchronized, fast activity associated with unit firing which occurs during arousal.

In summary, it is noted that the medial septal and diagonal band portions of the limbic cholinergic system activate the hippocampal formation, and may be responsible for fast activity in the hippocampal EEG. Hippocampal theta rhythm, on the other hand, may well involve activity predominately of the monoaminergic systems. The connections of the limbic cholinergic system with the ascending cholinergic reticular system and with the medial cortex appear to enable the hippocampus to play a significant part in arousal and attention and possibly also in learning and memory.

In this section some conclusions about the cholinergic systems can be given. By judicious use of the histochemical method of Koelle (1954, 1969), it has been possible for various investigators to study the distribution of cholinesterase in the central nervous system. Two major cholinergic systems in the brain have been charted in some detail by use of this method. There is still some question whether AChE can be considered a reliable marker of cholinergic neurons, this latter point having been argued in some detail by Krnjević (1969) and Karczmar (1969) with no clearcut resolution of the matter. Karczmar (1969) has pointed out that the cholinergic system has been "overexploited". He mentions, for instance, that while some reticular neurons are cholinoceptive or perhaps even cholinergically innervated, and while cholinergic drugs markedly affect the reticular formation, the hypothesis that arousal results from the cholinergic mediation in the reticular formation should be taken with caution. He notes that the concentrations of substances, such as ACh and AChE, must be considered as secondary in importance compared with the patterns of synaptic organisation. This type of critique, however, could be applied to monoamine systems as well. Nevertheless, this consideration clearly points up the fact that histochemical tracing of neural circuits should be closely compared with studies of normal synaptological patterns (especially using Golgi methods), Fink-Heimer analysis of terminal degeneration and autoradiographic tracing of neuron pathways in working out the organization and function of these complex systems. Assuming that such due caution has been taken, it is stressed the methods elaborating the chemical identity of neurons and their projection systems have proven to be a most powerful tool.

VII. OTHER NEUROCHEMICAL SYSTEMS

Finally, only brief mention will be given to other potential chemical systems that may play important roles in organization of the vigilance states. Too little is known of these to integrate them systematically with the better mapped monoamine and cholinergic systems. In recent experiments Jasper et al. (1965) found that there was a significant increase in the rate of liberation of glutamic acid in animals maintained in the alert state (as judged by the EEG) compared to those in natural sleep or with continuous desynchronization of the EEG following high midbrain transection. Conversely, the rate of liberation of gamma-amino-butyric acid (GABA) was higher during sleep than during wakefulness, and, in fact, could not be measured if the animal was maintained alert by intermittent stimulation of the reticular formation. Also Jasper and Koyama (1967) found a significant change in the pattern of free amino acids liberated from the cortical surface during states of sleep and wakefulness. It is evident that one must consider changes in cortical amino acid liberation, especially glutamic acid, as well as release of ACh in the continuing search for chemical correlates of cortical activation related to sleep and wakefulness and possibly to states of arousal or attention.

Also, GABA, which has been proposed to act as an inhibitory transmitter substance in certain brain regions, shows, in regional uptake studies, that it is retained in different regions of the brain. Hökfelt and Ljungdahl (1971), using a similar autoradiographic technique as described for norepinephrine, have attempted to determine the cellular localization of exogeneous GABA in various brain regions. Diffuse accumulations of GABA grains over neuropil and well-defined accumulations of grains over certain cell bodies in the cerebellar and cerebral cortex and in the hippocampal formation have been found. They noted that it is premature to decide whether the cell bodies accumulating GABA could determine "GABA-neurons" or glial fields or maybe both. They also emphasize that if the first turns out to be correct, then it would be possible to map "GABA-neurons" in the brain and study their uptake mechanisms. At the present time it is impossible to identify GABA neuronal pathways in the brain in any systematic way. Their relations with other amine systems awaits further methodological development.

VIII. SUMMARY

Our task has been to describe in detail the chemical circuits in the brain as these may relate to the vigilance states and their various components—this has largely entailed description of the chemical maps drawn up by a wide variety of approaches, in particular defining these in relation to how their manipulation affects sleep-waking behavior and how these alterations correlate with changes in regional brain chemistry. With regard to the massive literature on the role of monoamines and acetylcholine in the regulation of sleep-waking activity, it is obvious that each of the observations, and particularly the conclusions drawn from them, could be challenged in one way or another. Depending on orientation, it might be noted that there have been several apparently contradictory and almost mutually exclusive hypotheses presented in this review. With all of this in mind, we will now summarize the organization of the principal chemical circuits in the brain as they relate to the role of the monoamines and acetylcholine in states of sleep and wakefulness.

A. Indoleamines

1. Serotonin

The serotonin neurons are mostly congregated in the raphé complex of nuclei in the medulla, pons, and mesencephalon. Neurons from the anterior group of raphé nuclei (linear nuclei, nucleus raphé dorsalis, nucleus raphé medianus, and nucleus centralis superior of Bechterew) largely overlie the limbic midbrain fields and project predominantly in a rostral direction, joining the medial components of the medial forebrain bundle at the hypothalamic level, and distributing to the entire basal forebrain area and diffusely onto the cerebral cortex. Neurons of the middle raphé group (nucleus raphé pontis and nucleus raphé magnus) project primarily to the surrounding reticular formation with some ascending and descending components, while nuclei of the posterior raphé group (nuclei raphé obscurus and pallidus) project primarily to the spinal cord.

A variety of lesion and pharmacological evidence indicates that serotonin is involved in the induction and maintenance of slow-wave sleep. Since slow-wave sleep normally appears to be a prerequisite for REM sleep, procedures which affect serotonin content of the brain will also eventually affect REM sleep. The main observations which have led to the relation of serotonin system to sleep are as follows:

1) Lesions of the raphé nuclei lead to a state of more or less permanent cortical desynchronization associated with behavioral arousal, i.e., to a definite shift toward waking in the sleep-wakefulness cycle. There is also a complete suppression of REM sleep if slow-wave sleep is decreased to less than 15% of recording time. Rough correlations exist between the extent of the raphé lesion, especially in the anterior raphé group, with the decrease in sleep time and the loss of serotonin in the forebrain. Involvement of just the rostrally projecting serotonergic systems in the medial forebrain bundle is not the whole story since various lesions in this system do not duplicate the picture seen after raphé lesions. Relations between the anterior raphé complex and the synchronizing system of the midline thalamus have not so far been satisfactorily demonstrated, although the effects of raphé lesions on slow-wave sleep (diminishing it) may relate to breaking facilitatory effects on thalamic midline synchronizing elements. In this regard, we have preliminary evidence of projections from the nucleus raphé dorsalis to the centre median-parafascicular complex in the rat (Morgane and Stern, unpublished).

Another morphological explanation that has been offered concerning the results of such midline raphé lesions suggests that the increase in waking time following these lesions is due to the interruption of ascending fibers originating in a "synchronizing" system of the caudal brainstem, which cross the midline through the raphé nuclei. Although this is one possibility, it certainly is not the sole explanation of these effects in view of the results obtained with other means of depleting the brain of its contents of serotonin.

2) Injection of PCPA (which depletes the brain of serotonin) in a variety of species is followed for the next few days by a gradual decrease in sleep time involving both slow-wave and REM sleep and produces an increased state of behavioral wakefulness and EEG activation. This effect lasts several days, following which the animal gradually returns to a normal sleep-waking pattern even when PCPA is administered chronically and serotonin levels are held low. During the height of the effect, when the animal shows the least sleep, injection of the serotonin precursor, 5-hydroxytryptophan, will trigger, in a few minutes, a state of slow-wave sleep followed by REM sleep which lasts a few hours before the animal returns to its sleepless condition. We have shown that anterior raphé lesions and PCPA administration

produce generally similar effects on sleep profiles, the PCPA effect being to produce significantly greater decreases in total sleep and percent of REM sleep to total recording time (Morgane and Stern, 1972b).

3) Reserpine is known to suppress slow-wave and REM sleep totally in the cat (in primates it elevates REM sleep), when given in a single dose of 0.5 mg/kg, the suppression lasting up to half a day. 5-Hydroxytryptophan, when given a few hours after reserpine, will restore slow-wave sleep but does not affect the suppression of REM sleep.

4) 5-Hydroxytryptophan, when injected intravenously, is followed within a few minutes by a state resembling slow-wave sleep which lasts several hours in cats. During this time REM sleep is totally suppressed and shows a rebound when the effect of the drug has passed. Also rats on tryptophan-free or tryptophan-rich diets show a significant change in their slow-wave sleep/REM sleep cycles, the former showing longer and the latter shorter cycles.

It seems that the presence of serotonin in the brain is a necessary condition for the patterns of sleep, both slow-wave and REM sleep, to become fully manifest. Its mode of action is not known but it seems unlikely that a metabolite of serotonin is the active agent since we have found that central administration of the tryptophols or 5-HIAA induces arousal, not sleep (Morgane and Stern, 1973b). From iontophoretic studies showing that serotonin is often inhibitory, the serotonin system could be thought of as some sort of "brake" on the neuronal elements promoting wakefulness. The chemical connectivities described above indicate that raphé neurons may directly inhibit cells in the locus coeruleus complex and influence waking via this system. This relationship also fits well with the view that serotonergic neurons inhibit the occurrence of PGO spikes. The effects of serotonin systems are, however, not limited to the lower brainstem reticular neurons since serotonin-containing terminals are widespread throughout most diencephalic and telencephalic formations.

2. Catecholamines

a. Norepinephrine. Norepinephrine-type neurons are present primarily in the medulla and pons and a few in the diencephalon, all being located in cell formations quite lateral to the midline. Projections from the locus coeruleus complex of the latero-dorsal pontine tegmentum appear to form the most well-developed rostrally projecting systems which innervate the diencephalon and telencephalon, overlapping to some extent the terminal areas of the serotonergic pathways. That these different chemical pathways may regulate different phasic and tonic components of REM sleep, as well as other aspects of the vigilance states, has been discussed. The main pathways projecting from the anterior locus coeruleus area may produce tonic EEG activation (also see dopamine section, below). Collaterals from the anterior locus coeruleus "waking" area, perhaps traveling in the dorsal noradrenergic bundle, may inhibit activity in the anterior raphé area thereby turning off the serotonin slow-wave sleep mechanisms generated there.

The bulk of the literature makes it appear that norepinephrine has a role primarily in processes concerned with waking, although dopamine systems have also been implicated in this regard (see below). The role of norepinephrine in waking processes is indicated by the following observations:

1) When norepinephrine is injected intravenously in acute "encéphale isolé" cats showing electrocortical synchronization, it induces desynchronization of the EEG and dilates the pupils in a state very much resembling wakefulness. The principal site of action appears to be neuronal assemblies situated in the rostral pons, since lesions placed here, and gradually advanced more and more rostrally, decrease and finally completely abolish the effectiveness of norepinephrine to desynchronize the EEG.

2) Lesions of the brainstem reticular formation in cats when selectively placed to destroy norepinephrine-containing neurons in the rostral pons, corresponding to groups A6 and A7 (coeruleus and subcoeruleus complex), are followed by a significant increase in the duration of electrocortical synchronization in the 24 hr. sleep-wakefulness cycle lasting for several days. The long-lasting cortical synchronization may or may not be accompanied by behavioral sleep and this dissociation between "cortical" and "behavioral" sleep is not seen if the lesion simultaneously reaches cell groups A8, A9 and A10, i.e., the dopamine-containing neurons of the lateral mesencephalic reticular formation, substantia nigra and ventral tegmental area of the mesencephalon. In such instance, the cats are comatose behaviorally when cortical synchronization is present. There appears to be a definite correlation between the number of norepinephrine-containing neurons destroyed, the increase in the daily duration of EEG synchronization, and the lowered content of norephinephrine in both telencephalic and diencephalic formations. REM sleep duration is not necessarily changed appreciably by such lesions but some secondary small decreases may sometimes be seen.

3) The effects on wakefulness of monoamine oxidase inhibitors, or reserpine, of alpha-methyldopa, and other drugs which affect monoamine stores in one way or another are not clear-cut because they effect all monoamines indiscriminantly, but to varying degrees. These drugs have been used extensively in animals for the study of their effects on REM which is often quite altered. Reserpine injected, i.p., in cats suppresses slow-wave sleep for 12 to 14 hrs and produces a stage which can be described as relaxed or quiet wakefulness, probably because it depletes all monoamine stores. However, intraventricular administration of reserpine does not depress sleep, but rather elevates REM time (Stern and Morgane, 1973a). Alpha-methyltyrosine, which blocks catecholamine synthesis, tends to reduce waking and

elevate slow-wave sleep and REM sleep, but the results are somewhat confusing in regard to REM. The excitation or raised level of arousal and decrease in total sleep time produced by amphetamine appears to be related to its effects on the liberation of norepinephrine, since this excitation is prevented by a blockade of norepinephrine synthesis such as that obtained by inhibition of tyrosine hydroxylase with alpha-methyl-tyrosine. In general, any procedure or drug which increases the amount of available norephinephrine will raise the arousal level while, conversely, decreasing the amount of available norepinephrine, appears to have a more tranquilizing effect.

4) Norepinephrine and amphetamines, when deposited directly into brain systems of acute and intact chronic cats, either in crystalline form or in solution, produce behavioral and electrocortical waking, sometimes accompanied by excitationa and increased motor activity. Several brain loci appear to be responsive, including the pontine and mesencephalic reticular formation, some regions of the hypothalamus, the preoptic region, and the nucleus ventralis medialis of the thalamus.

5) Dopa given intraperitonerally in cats is followed, after a latency of about 20 min, by a state of quiet wakefulness, with mydriasis and cortical desynchronization, which lasts several hours.

All of the above remarks relating to the role of norepinephrine in waking have had certain challenges posed to them. First, norepinephrine injected intraveneously does not produce wakefulness through a direct action on brainstem neurons—epinephrine aad norepinephrine do not cross the blood-brain barrier in any appreciable amounts except, perhaps, at the hypothalamic level. There are, however, some other regions which appear to escape the blood-brain barrier and these include the area postrema, and possibly the locus coeruleus. Additionally, it has been reported that following intravenous epinephrine infusion in cats, appreciable amounts of the drug can be found in cerebrospinal fluid. Another argument used against the direct action of intravenous norepinephrine on brainstem neurons notes that it is impossible to dissociate the arousal produced by intravenous norepinephrine for the concomitant rise in blood pressure. When such blood pressure changes are prevented, there is no arousal. Furthermore, when a rise in blood pressure is obtained through mechanical or by administration of vasopressin this is accompanied by electrocortical desynchronization. Finally, norepinephrine injected into the carotid artery does not always produce cortical desynchronization or is followed by electrocortical arousal only after relatively long latencies, i.e., a suffecient length of time for the drug to distribute itself through the entire circulation and be accompanied by a rise of blood pressure.

Secondly, another argument concerns the wakefulness or arousal obtained following injection of norepinephrine directly into the brain as being due to local pH changes, changes in osmotic pressure, mechanical stimulation, etc. It has been argued that the sites from which this effect can be obtained are too widespread in the brain and, therefore, this procedure has no localizing value for an arousal system. However, many experiments have controlled pH and local mechanical disturbances and so it should be also be mentioned that very often the local injection of ACh in the same regions and using identical techniques is followed by electrocortical synchronization and behavioral sleep.

Thirdly, Jouvet's results, where destruction of norepinephrine-containing neurons in the upper pons (locus coeruleus area) or lower mesencephalon, leads to decreased wakefulness (a change correlated to a decreased norepinephrine content in the brain) must also be cautiously evaluated, since the regions concerned have also been shown to contain high concentrations of cholinesterase-containing nuclei and pathways and have been described above as the origin of an ascending cholinergic system. The possible role of the concomitant destruction of this system has not been taken into account in most of the studies reviewed. This difficulty, of course, is present in all lesioning experiments, especially in the reticular core of the brainstem since it is, in practice, impossible to limit the lesion to a single functionally homogeneous neuronal population. It should be emphasized here that the so-called "chemical dissectors", such as 6-hydroxydopamine, 5, 6- or 5, 7-dihydroxytryptamine, etc., are likewise not as fully specific for particular chemical pathways as originally thought.

Finally, one additional argument, which generally runs counter to the role of norepinephrine in arousal, is the frequently quoted observation that when this substance is injected directly into the ventricular system of animals it produces, within a few minutes, a sleeplike state which has been variously described as similar to light anesthesia, lethargic or comatose behavior, lack of responsiveness, etc., a state which can last several hours. The apparent contradiction of these results with those obtained following other means of administering norepinephrine is difficult to resolve. What regions of the brain are reached by intraventricular injection are not known with any certainty. How deep the drug can penetrate from the surface of the ventricular walls within the time necessary for the sleep-like effect to become manifest is a moot point. The initial effect of intraventricular injection of norepinephrine is one of desynchronization followed, after some minutes, by synchronization of the EEG.

In summary, while it seems that much of the evidence is in favor of norepinephrine having a role in patterns of activity which accompany the waking state, many additional points regarding the role of this agent need to be clarified.

Role of Norepinephrine in REM Sleep. Apart from its role in wakefulness, norepinephrine appears also to be involved in aspects of REM sleep. The evidence for this, however, is often contradictory and is summarized as follows:

1) Bilateral lesions of locus coeruleus, a nucleus rich in norepinephrine-containing neurons, is followed by a total or subtotal disappearance of both the phasic and tonic events of REM sleep. There appears to be a rough correlation between the extent of the lesion, the decrease in REM sleep time, and the decrease of norepinephrine present in basal forebrain and telencephalic structures. However, it is important to keep in mind that the locus coeruleus is also rich in AChE, and little account has previously been taken of the cholinergic systems originating there in the various disturbances of sleep following its destruction.

2) In animals, drugs which interfere with norepinephrine synthesis selectively suppress REM sleep, for example, disulfiram which impairs the synthesis of norepinephrine from dopamine. Similarly, alpha-methyldopa selectively suppresses REM sleep, as well as the rebound phenomena which normally occurs after REM deprivation. It is probably metabolized to become a false transmitter and thereby reduces the norepinephrine content of the brain. Likewise, alpha-methyl-tyrosine which acts at the tyrosine hydroxylase level, suppresses REM in some species, but increases it in others.

3) Reserpine, given in large doses in cats, suppresses most manifestation of REM sleep for several hours. Conflicting reports exist as to whether during this time REM sleep reappears following injections of DOPA (which presumably replenishes norepinephrine stores). Also, eserine given after reserpine reverses the decrease in REM produced by reserpine. Thus, activation of a cholinergic mechanism may reverse reserpine's effects on REM sleep.

4) Rats which have been deprived of REM sleep for several days show an increased turnover of cerebral norepinephrine during the well-known rebound phenomena which follows REM deprivation. This may well be a nonspecific effect due to the stress involved in REM sleep deprivation.

Thus, the evidence in regard to catecholamines and REM sleep is involved and often contradictory. More detailed summaries may be found in King (1971), Hartmann (1970), and Jouvet (1972a,b,c). That specific chemical pathways (reviewed above) play a significant role in both phasic and tonic aspects of the REM state, however, is clear.

b. *Dopamine*   Very little literature exists on the role of dopamine in the regulation of sleep-waking cycles except in regard to its being a precursor of norepinephrine. Recently, experiments in which destruction of the ventral tegmental area of Tsai of the mesencephalon, lesions which include the pars compacta of the substantia nigra (cell group A9) and, possibly, A10 have produced akinetic and behaviorally comatose animals while leaving relatively intact the electrographic aspects of the sleep-waking cycle. In these animals, when the cortex is "electrographically awake" they appear incapable of manifesting the state of wakefulness behaviorally. The extent of the akinesia or depth of coma appears to be related to the decrease in dopamine content of the basal ganglia. The decrease in brain dopamine is associated with a more or less complete deficit in motor activity, apparently leaving intact the basic mechanisms involved in the sleep-waking cycle. It should also be noted, however, that reported lesions in the ventral tegmental area of Tsai also involved, to a large extent, cholinesterase systems which we have described above. The extent to which the destruction of this cholinergic system influences experimental observations is so far not elucidated.

B. Acetylcholine

Many lines of evidence suggest that acetylcholine is involved in states of wakefulness, slow-wave sleep, and REM sleep. It is emphasized that cholinesterase-containing neurons are present in several brainstem loci where they overlap, to a considerable extent, the monoamine-containing neurons. This overlap is such that it has been practically impossible to ablate one system while leaving the other intact. The rostral projections of the cholinesterase-containing neurons cover large territories of the forebrain and also overlap extensively with regions where monoamine terminals have been found.

Cholinergic mechanisms in the vigilance states may be briefly summarized as follows.

1) Acetylcholine when injected directly in various brainstem loci is followed by slow-wave sleep and sometimes by REM sleep episodes. These effects may last 4-5 hrs. or longer. Blocking the medial forebrain bundle behind a sleep locus prevents cholinergic induction of sleep.

2) The cortical desynchronization of wakefulness, whether occurring spontaneously or provoked by reticular formation activation or sensory stimulation, is accompanied by an increased release of acetylcholine in the cortex.

3) Anti-cholinergic drugs, such as atropine, produce a state of cortical synchronization resembling slow-wave sleep while leaving the animal behaviorally awake and sometimes over-excited. Atropine also usually abolishes REM sleep.

4) Anti-cholinesterases, for example eserine, seem to have mild effects on REM sleep, i.e., increasing REM sleep time, and possibly decreasing REM sleep latency.

Acetylcholine thus probably acts at different levels of the brainstem and seems to be involved in all three states of vigilance, probably interacting with the monoamine systems at various levels.

Cholinergic and cholinoceptive mechanisms in the brainstem and basal forebrain areas (along the limbic forebrain-limbic midbrain circuits) appear to promote slow-wave and possibly REM sleep. At the cortical level cholinergic systems seem to be involved in the electrocortical desynchronization of wakefulness. It remains to be seen whether they play a similar role in the desynchronization patters of REM sleep. Arguments relating to the two types of desynchronization (arousal states 1 and 2) have been given by Routtenberg (1968), but these are on tenuous grounds.

As noted, we have summarized the role of monoaminergic and cholinergic neuro-anatomical systems in sleep-waking behavior and very little has been said about the possible role of GABA and other amino acids in sleep and waking, yet various bits of experimental evidence exist indicating that they may also be involved in these processes. It is obvious that we are far from a complete understanding of the complex interactions of multiple chemical circuits in brain activity that occurs when an animal passes from wakefulness into sleep. Cordeau (1970) has stressed that we should stop thinking of wakefulness, slow-wave sleep and REM sleep as completely different states, each with its own system anatomically and biochemically well-defined, and with precise points of origin in the brainstem and traceable projections both rostrally and caudally. This search for a "localization of function" may not be applicable to sleep and waking processes, as indeed it is not for several other brain functions. Cordeau notes that we should think instead of sleep and wakefulness as "mixed" states in which all of the systems discussed in this review, and probably many others, are involved to a greater or lesser degree at various levels in the brainstem. In a similar vein Jouvet has summarized his views by noting that waking and slow-wave sleep appear to be under the control of two antagonistic serotonergic and catecholaminergic systems which probably interact with each other at different levels of the neuraxis. He observes that REM sleep, on the contrary, appears to depend on the synergistic or antagonistic influences of these two systems and, very likely, various cholinergic neurons. We might thus consider an animal as being either awake or asleep depending on the patterning of the activity in each and every one of these subsystems. There is a constant oscillation in a vigilance continuum between states of aroused waking and REM sleep. Even REM sleep, which in some respects seems to be at one end of the spectrum, appears to be a peculiar mixture of sleep and wakefulness. For example, is the dream some form of consciousness with the brain generating its own sensory input? On the other hand, during REM sleep, thalamo-cortical circuits seem to be cut off from the peripheral sensory input through active inhibitory processes and the somatic and vegetative spheres show their most marked sleep patterns. The suggestion that both cholinergic and noradrenergic mechanisms may be involved in wakefulness and REM sleep, and the observation that very often regions of the brainstem with norepinephrine-containing neurons also show large amounts of cholinesterase, may be somehow related, and the anatomical overlap not a mere coincidence.

Also, the so-called reticular systems and their projections have been called "diffuse" systems since they seem to affect the whole brain. They should possibly be thought of as "diffuse" in another sense, i.e., in the sense that, even if their highest concentration or density is in the core of the brainstem, where they may derive their tonic drive in normal conditions, they may also be omnipresent in the whole nervous system. What is being suggested here is that neural aggregates responsible for patterns of sleep or waking may be present at all levels of the brainstem in a sort of multi-tiered-type of organization with several substations projecting both rostrally and caudally, each substation reciprocally linked and providing positive or, most probably, negative feedback loops responsible for the so-called "reticular homeostasis" (Dell, 1963). This might explain, among other things, why electrical and chemical stimulation in so many brain loci can affect the states of sleep and waking in one way or another, or why telencephalic structures chronically separated from the reticular core of the brainstem may eventually show patterns approaching those of wakefulness.

The charting of four distinct chemical neuronal systems, i.e, the serotonergic, noradrenergic, dopaminergic, and cholingergic-containing neurons, is of great significance for correlating brain chemistry with anatomy and behavior such as sleep-waking states, among others. Attempts to individually manipulate these systems are taking place but it is extremely difficult to separate them by the lesioning technique, especially because of the extensive overlap of the systems. Hopefully, chemical lesions offer some opportunity to individually and selectively destroy particular elements and allow their individual roles to be determined, but so far these results are disappointing. Knowledge of their chemical anatomy at different levels in the brainstem has, however, facilitated their independent manipulation.

Waking, sleep, and dreaming are such infinitely complicated processes, involving so many interacting and overlapping neuronal fields, and subject to so many factors, that it would be entirely naive to incriminate only one or two transmitters in their mechanism, hence the need to begin to appreciate interactions among chemical systems at many levels in the brain. Future studies on interactions of chemical systems regionally will probably hold the key to the problem of unraveling the chemistry of the vigilance states.

This research was supported by Grants MH 0211 and MH 10625, National Institute of Mental Health.

REFERENCES

Aghajanian, G.K., Rosencrans, J.A., and Sheard, M.H. Serotonin: Release in the forebrain by stimulation of midbrain raphé. *Science 156*, 402-403 (1967).

Aghajanian, G.K. and Asher, I.M. Histochemical fluorescence of raphé neurons: selective enhancement by tryptophan. *Science 172*, 1159-1161 (1971).

Andén, N.E., Dahlström, A., Fuxe, K. and Larsson, K. Functional role of the nigro-neostriatal dopamine neurons. *Acta Pharmacol. Toxicol. 24*, 263-274 (1966a.)

Andén, N.E., Dahlström, A., Fuxe, K., Larsson, K. Olson, L. and Ungerstedt, U. Ascending monoamine neurons to the telencephalon and diencephalon. *Acta Physiol. Scand. 67*, 313-326 (1966b.)

Andén, N.E., Dahlström, A., Fuxe, K., Olson, L. and Ungerstedt, U. Ascending nonadrenaline-neurons from the pons and the medulla oblongata, *Experientia, 22*. 44-45, (1966c)

Anden, N.E., Carlsson, A., Dahlström, A., Fuxe, A., Hillarp, N.A. and Larsson, K. Demonstration and mapping out of nigro-neostriatal dopamine neurons *Life Sci. 3*, 523-530, (1964).

Andy, O.J. and Stephan H. *The Septum of the Cat*. C.C. Thomas, Springfield, Ill. 1964, pp. 84.

Angel, A., Magni, F. and Strata, P. Excitability of intrageniculate tract fibres after reticular stimulation in midpontine pretrigeminal cat. *Arch. Ital. Biol., 103*, 239-249 (1965).

Arbuthnott, G., Fuxe, K. and Ungerstedt, U. Central catecholamine turnover and self-stimulation behaviour. *Brain Res. 27*. 406-413 (1971).

Arbuthnott, G.W., Crow, T.J. Fuxe, K., Olson, L. and Ungerstedt, U. Depletion of catecholamines *in vivo* induced by electrical stimulation of central monoamine pathways. *Brain Res. 24*, 471-483. (1970)

Babb, T.L., Babb, M., Mahnke, J.H. and Verzeano, M. The action of cholinergic agents on the electrical activity of the non-specific nuclei of the thalamus. *Int. J. Neurol. 8*, 198-210 (1971).

Battista, A., Fuxe, K., Goldstein, M. and Ogawa, M. Mapping of central monoamine neurons in the monkey. *Experentia, 28*, 688-690 (1972).

Baumgarten, H.G. and Lachenmayer, L., 5, 7-Dihydroxytryptamine: Improvement in chemical lesioning of indoleamine neurons in the mammalian brain. *Zeit. Zellforsch. 135*, 399-414, (1972).

Bedard, P., Larochelle, L., Parent, A. and Poirier, L.J. The nigrostriatal pathway: A correlative neuroanatomical and neurochemical criteria in the cat and the monkey. *Exper. Neurol. 25*, 365-377 (1969).

Benetato, Gr., Uluitu, M., Bonciocat, C., Boros, I. and Dumitrescu-Papahagi, E. The effect of sectioning of the medial forebrain bundle on the serotonin content and functional capacity of the hypothalamic centers. *Rev. Roumainie Physiol. 4*, 3-12 (1967a).

Benetato, Gr., Uluitu, M., Bubuianu, E. and Bonciocat, C. The effect of sectioning of the medial forebrain bundle and of sodium diethylbarbiturate on the content in catecholamines and serotonin of the hypothalamus and rhinencephalic structures (amygdala and hippocampus). *Rev. Roumainie Physiol. 4*, 13-25 (1967b).

Bishop, G.H. The place of cortex in a reticular system. in; *Reticular Formation of the Brain*. H.H. Jasper, L.D. Proctor, R.S. Knighton, W.C. Noshay, and R. T. Costello, Eds., Little, Brown & Co., Boston, 1958, pp. 413-421.

Bizzi, E. and Brooks, D.C. Functional connections between pontine reticular formation and lateral geniculate nucleus during deep sleep. *Arch Ital. Biol. 101*, 666-680, (1963a).

Bizzi, E. and Brooks, D.C. Pontine reticular formation: Relation to lateral geniculate nucleus during deep sleep. *Science 141*. 270-271 (1963b).

Björklund, A., Falck, B. and Stenevi, U., Microspectrofluorimetric characterization of monoamines in the central nervous system: Evidence for a new neuronal monoamine-like compound. in, *Progress in Brain Research [Histochemistry of Nervous Transmission]*, Vol. 34, O. Eränkö, Ed., Elsevier, Amsterdam, 1971a, pp. 63-73.

Björklund, A., Falck, B. and Stenevi, U. Classification of monoamine neurones in the rat mesencephalon: Distribution of a new monoamine neuron System. *Brain Res. 32*, 269-285 (1971b).

Boakes, R.J., Bradley, P.B., and Candy, J.M. A neuronal basis for the alerting action of (+)-amphetamine. *Brit. J. Pharmacol. 45*, 391-403 (1972).

Bonnet, V. and Bremer, F. Action du potassium, du calcium et de l'acetylcholine sur les activités electriques spontanées et provoqueés de l'écorce cérébrale. *Compt. Rend. Seances Soc. Biol. 126*, 1271-1275 (1937).

Bowsher, D. Reticular projections to lateral geniculate in cat. *Brain Res. 23*, 247-249 (1970).

Bremer, F. Preoptic hypnogenic focus and mesencephalic reticular formation. *Brain Res., 21*, 132-134, (1970).

Briggs, T.L., and Kaelber, W.W. Efferent fiber connections of the dorsal and deep tegmental nuclei of Gudden. An experimental study in the cat. *Brain Res. 29*, 17-29 (1971).

Brodal, A. *The Reticular Formation of the Brain Stem. Anatomical Aspects and Functional Correlations.* Oliver & Boyd, Edinburg, Scotland, 1957, pp. 87

Brodal, A., Taber, E., Walberg, F., The raphé nuclei of the brain stem in the cat. II. Efferent connections. *J. Comp. Neurol. 114*; 239-259 (1960).

Brodal, A., Walberg, F. and Taber, E. The raphé nuclei of the brain stem in the cat. III. Afferent connections. *J. Comp. Neurol. 114*, 261-281 (1960).

Bronzino, J.D., Morgane, P.J. and Stern, W.C. EEG synchronization following application of serotonin to area postrema. *Amer. J. Physiol. 223*, 376-383 (1972).

Brooks, D.C., Gershon, M.D. and Simon, R.P. Brain stem serotonin depletion and ponto-geniculo-occipital wave activity in the cat treated with reserpine. *Neuropharmacology 11*, 511-520 (1972).

Brown, O.J. The nuclear pattern of the nontectal portions of the midbrain and isthmus in the dog and cat. *J. Comp. Neurol. 78*, 365-405 (1943).

Brücke, F., Petsche, H., Pillat, B. and Deisenhammer, E. Ein Schrittmacher in der medialen Septumregion des Kaninchengehirns. *Pfluegers Arch. Gesamte Physiol. 269*, 135-140 (1959).

Bubenick, G. and Monnier, M. Nucleus size variations in cells of the locus coeruleus during sleep, arousal and stress. *Exper. Neurol. 35*, 1-12 (1972).

Buguet, A., Petitjean, F. and Jouvet, M. Suppression des pointes ponto-géniculo-occipitales du sommeil par lésion ou injection *in situ* de 6 hydroxydopamine au niveau du tegmentum pontique. *Comp. Rend. Seances Soc. Biol. 164*; 2293-2298 (1970).

Camacho-Evangelista, A. and Reinoso-Suárez, F. Activating and sychronizing centers in cat brain: Electroencephalograms after lesions. *Science 146*, 268-270 (1964).

Candia, O., Rossi, G.F. and Sekino, T. Brain stem structures responsible for the electroencephalographic patterns of desynchronized sleep. *Science 155*, 720-722 (1967).

Carli, G., Armengol, V. and Zanchetti, A. Electroencephalographic desynchronization during deep sleep after destruction of midbrain-limbic pathways in the cat. *Science 140*, 677-679 (1963).

Chu, N. and Bloom, F. Norepinephrine-containing neurons: Changes in spontaneous discharge patterns during sleep and waking. *Science 179*, 908-910 (1973).

Clemente, C.D., Sterman, M.B. and Wyrwicka, W. Forebrain inhibitory mechanisms: Conditioning of basal forebrain induced EEG synchronization and sleep. *Exper. Neurol. 7*, 404-417 (1963).

Collier, B. and Mitchell, J.F. The central release of acetylcholine during stimulation of the visual pathway. *J. Physiol. (London) 184*, 239-254 (1966).

Cordeau, J.P. Monoamines and the physiology of sleep and waking. in, *L-Dopa and Parkinsonism*, A. Barbeau and F.H. McDowell, Eds., F.A. Davis Co., Philadelphia, 1970, pp. 369-383.

Cordeau, J.P. and Mancia, M. Evidence for the existence of an electroencephalographic synchronization mechanism originating in the lower brain stem. *Electroenceph. Clin. Neurophysiol. 11*, 551-564 (1959).

Cordeau, J.P., Moreau, A. Beaulnes, A. and Laurin, C. EEG and behavioral changes following microinjections of acetylcholine and adrenaline in the brain stem of cats. *Arch. Ital. Biol. 101*, 30-47 (1963).

Corrodi, H. and Jonsson, G. The formaldehyde fluorescence method for the histochemical demonstration of biogenic monoamines. A review on the methodology. *J. Histochem. Cytochem. 15*, 65-78 (1967).

Crosby, E. and Woodburne, R. The mammalian midbrain and isthmus regions. Part I. The nuclear pattern. General summary. *J. Comp. Neurol. 78*, 505-520 (1943).

Crow, T.J. and Arbuthnott, G.W. Function of catecholamine-containing neurones in mammalian central nervous system. *Nature 238*, 245-246, (1972).

Crow, T.J., Spear, P.J. and Arbuthnott, G.W. Intracranial self-stimulation with electrodes in the region of the locus coeruleus. *Brain Res. 36*, 275-287 (1972).

Curtis, D.R. Discussion of paper 'Nonretinal influences on the lateral geniculate nucleus' by J T. McIlwain, *Invest. Ophthalmol. 11*, 321-322 (1972).

Dahlström, A. and Fuxe, K. Evidence for the existence of monoamine-containing neurons in the central nervous system. I. Demonstration of monoamines in the cell bodies of brain stem neurons. *Acta Physiol. Scand. 62*,(Suppl. 232), 1-55 (1964).

Dahlström, A. and Fuxe, K. Evidence for the existence of monoamine neurons in the central nervous system. II. Experimentally induced changes in the intraneuronal amine levels of bulbospinal neuron systems. *Acta Physiol. Scand. 64*(Suppl. 247), 1-36 (1965).

Daly, J., Fuxe, K. and Jonsson, G. Effects of intracerebral injections of 5,6-dihydroxytryptamine on central monoamine neurons: Evidence for selective degeneration of central 5-hydroxytryptamine neurons. *Brain Res. 49*, 476-482 (1973).

Deffenu, G., Bertaccini, G. and Pepeu, G. Acetylcholine and 5-hydroxytryptamine levels of the lateral geniculate bodies and superior colliculus of cats after visual deafferentation. *Exper. Neurol. 17*, 203-209 (1967).

Dell, P. Reticular homeostasis and critical reactivity. in, *Progress in Brain Research (Brain Mechanisms)*, Vol. 1, G. Moruzzi, A. Fessard and H. Jasper, Eds., Elsevier Amsterdam, 1963, pp. 82-114.

Dell, P. and Vigier, D. Topographe des systèmes aminergiques centraux. in, *Colloques Nationaux du Centre National de la Recherche Scientifique*, Number 927, Editions du Centre National de la Recherche Scientifique, Paris 1970, pp. 17-32.

Dement, W.C., Milter, M.M. and Henriksen, S.J. Sleep changes during chronic administration of parachlorophenylalanine. *Rev. Can. Biol. 31*, 239-246 (1972).

Descarries, L. and Saucier, G. Disappearance of the locus coeruleus in the rat after intraventricular 6-hydroxydopamine. *Brain Res. 37*, 310-316 (1972).

Ernst, A.M. The role of biogenic amines in the extra-pyramidal system. *Acta Physiol. Pharmacol. Neerlandica 15*, 141-154 (1969).

Euler, C. von, and Green, J.D. Excitation, inhibition and rhythmical activity in hippocampal pyramidal cells in rabbit. *Acta Physiol. Scand. 48*, 110-125 (1960).

Falck, B., Hillarp, N.A., Thieme, G. and Torp, A. Fluorescence of catecholamines and related compounds condensed with formaldehyde. *J. Histochem. Cytochem. 10*, 348-354 (1962).

Feldman, S. and Waller, H. Dissociation of electrocortical activation and behavioral arousal. *Nature 196*, 1320-1322 (1962).

Fibiger, H.C., Lytle, L.D. and Campbell, B.A. Cholinergic modulation of adrenergic arousal in the developing rat. *J. Compar. Physiol Psychol. 72*, 384-389 (1970).

Funderburk, W.H. and Case, T.J. The effect of atropine on cortical potentials. *Electroenceph. Clin. Neurophysiol. 3,* 213-223 (1951).

Fuxe, K. Evidence for the existence of monoamine neurons in the central nervous system. IV. Distribution of monoamine nerve terminals in the central nervous system. *Acta Physiol Scand. 64* (Supp. 247), 37-85 (1965).

Fuxe, K. and Ljunggren, L. Cellular Localization of monoamines in the upper brain stem of the pigeon. *J. Comp. Neurol. 125,* 355-382 (1965).

Fuxe, K. and Owman, C. Cellular localization of monoamines in the area postrema of certain mammals. *J. Comp. Neurol. 125,* 337-354 (1965).

Fuxe, K., Hamberger, B. and Hökfelt, T. Distribution of noradrenaline nerve terminals in cortical areas of the rat. *Brain res. 8,* 125-131 (1968).

Fuxe, K., Hökeflt, T. and Ungerstedt, U. Localization of indolealkylamines in CNS. in, *Advances in Pharmacology,* Vol 6, Part A, S. Garattini and P.A. Shore, Eds., Academic Press, New York, 1968, pp. 235-251.

Fuxe, K., Hökfelt, T. and Ungerstedt, U. Morphological and functional aspects of central monoamine neurons. in, *International Review of Neurobiology,* Vol. 13, C.C. Pfeiffer and J.R. Smythies, Eds., Academic Press, New York, 1970, pp. 93-126.

Gerardy, J., Quinaux, N., Maeda, T. and Dresse, A. Analyse des monoamines du locus coeruleus et d'autres structures cérébrales par chromatographie sur couche mince. *Arch. Int. Pharmacody. Therap. 177,* 492-496 (1969).

Goldstein, M., Anagnoste, B., Owen, W.S. and Battista, A.F. The effects of ventromedial tegmental lesions on the biosynthesis of catecholamines in the striatum. *Life Sci. 5,* 2171-2176 (1966).

Grastyán, E. Lissak, K., Madarasz, I. and Donhoffer, H. Hippocampal electrical activity during the development of conditioned reflexes. *Electroenceph. Clin. Neurophysiol., 11,* 409-430 (1959).

Green, J.D. The rhinencephalon: Aspects of its relation to behavior and the reticular activating system.in, *Reticular Formation of the Brain.,* H.H. Jasper, L.D. Procter, R.S. Knighton, W.C. Nosháy and R.I. Costello, Eds., Little, Brown and Co., Boston 1957, pp. 607-619.

Green, J.D. The hippocampus. in, *Handbook of Physiology, Sec. 1, Neurophysiology,* Vol. 2, J. Field, H.W. Magoun and V. Hall, Eds., American Physiological Society, Washington, D.C. 1960, pp. 1373-1389.

Green, J.D. The hippocampus. *Physiol. Rev. 44,* 561-608 (1964).

Green, J.D. and Arduini, A. Hippocampal electrical activity in arousal. *J. Neurophysiol. 17,* 533-557 (1954).

Guillery, R.W. and Scott, G.L. Observations on synaptic patterns in the dorsal lateral geniculate nucleus of the cat; the C laminae and the perikaryal synapses. *Exper. Brain Res. 12,* 184-203 (1971).

Gumulka, W., Samanin, R. Garattini, S. and Valzelli, L. Effect of stimulation of midbrain raphé on serotonin (5-HT) level and turnover in different areas of rat brain. *Europ. J. Pharmacol. 8,* 380-384 (1969).

Hartmann, E. The D-state and norepinephrine-dependent systems. in, *Sleep and Dreaming,* E. Hartmann, Ed., Little, Brown & Co., Boston, 1970, pp. 308-328.

Harvey, J.A., Heller, A. and Moore, R.Y. The effect of unilateral and bilateral medial forebrain bundle lesions on brain serotonin. *J. Pharmacol. Exper. Therapeut. 140,* 103-110 (1963).

Havlicek, V. and Sklenovsky, A. The deactivating effect of catecholamines upon the electrocorticogram of the rat. *Brain Res. 4,* 345-357 (1967).

Heller, A. Neuronal control of brain serotonin. *Fed. Proc. 31,* 81-90 (1972).

Heller, A. and Moore, R. Effect of central nervous system lesions on brain monoamines in the rat. *J. Pharmacol. Exper. Therapeut. 150,* 1-9 (1965).

Heller, A. and Moore, R.Y. Control of brain serotonin and norepinephrine by specific neural systems, in *Advances in Pharmacology,* Vol. 6, Part A., S. Garatinni and P.A. Shore, Eds., Academic Press, New York, 1968, pp. 191-209.

Heller, A., Harvey, J.A. and Moore, R.Y. A demonstration of a fall in brain serotonin following central nervous system lesions in the rat. *Biochem. Pharmacol. 11*, 859-866 (1962).

Heller, A., Seiden, L.S. and Moore, R.Y. Regional effects of lateral hypothalamic lesions on norepinephrine in the cat. *Int. J. Neuropharmacol. 5*, 91-101 (1966).

Henriksen, S.J., Jacobs, B.L. and Dement, W.C. Dependence of REM sleep PGO waves on cholinergic mechanisms. *Brain Res. 48*, 412-416 (1972).

Hernández-Peón, R., G., Chavez-Ibárra, G. Morgane, P.J. and Timo-Iaria, C. Cholinergic pathways for sleep, alertness and rage in the limbic midbrain circuit. *Acta Neurol. Latinoamer., 8*, 93-96 (1962).

Hernández-Peón, R., Chavez-Ibárra, G., Morgane, P.J. and Timo-Iaria, C. Limbic cholinergic pathways involved in sleep and emotional behavior. *Exper. Neurol. 8*, 93-111 (1963).

Hobson, J.A., Alexander, J. and Fredrickson, C.J. The effect of lateral geniculate lesions on phasic electrical activity of the cortex during desynchronized sleep in the cat. *Brain Res. 14*, 607-621 (1969).

Hökfelt, T. and Ljungdahl, A.Uptake of [^{3}H] noradrenaline and gamma-[^{3}H] aminobutyric acid in isolated tissues of rat: An autoradiographic and fluorescence microscopic study. in, *Progress in Brain Research (Histochemistry of Nervous Transmission)*, Vol. 34, O. Eränkö, Ed., Elsevier, Amsterdam, 1971, pp. 87-102.

Hökfelt, T. and Fuxe, K. On the morphology and the neuroendocrine role of the hypothalamic catecholamine neurons. in, *Brain-Endocrine Interaction. Median Eminence: Structure and Function.* (International Symposium of Munich 1971), K.M. Knigge, Ed., Karger, Basel, 1972, pp. 181-223.

Horvath, F.E. and Buser, P. Thalamo-caudate-cortical relationships in synchronized activity. I. Differentiation between ventral and dorsal spindle systems. *Brain Res. 39*, 21-24 (1972).

Hubbard, J.E. and DiCarlo, V. Fluorescence histochemistry of monoamine-containing cell bodies in the brain stem of the squirrel monkey (*Saimiri sciureus*). I. The locus coeruleus. *J. Comp. Neurol., 147*, 553-566 (1973).

Hunter, J. and Jasper, H. Effect of thalamic stimulation in unanesthetized animals. *Electroenceph. Clin. Neurophysiol. 1*, 305-324 (1949).

Ilyutchenok, R. Yu. and Gilinsky, M.A., Anticholinergic drugs and neuronal mechanisms of reticulo-cortical interaction. *Pharmacol. Res. Commun. 1*, 242-248 (1969).

Jacobs, B.L., Henriksen, S.J. and Dement, W.C. Neurochemical bases of the PGO wave. *Brain Res. 48*, 406-411 (1972).

Jasper, H.H. Neurochemical mediators of specific and non-specific cortical activation. in, *Attention in Neurophysiology*, C.R. Evans and T.B. Mulholland, Eds., New York, Appleton-Century-Crofts, 1969, pp. 337-395.

Jasper, H.H. and Koyama, I. Rate of release of acetylcholine and glutamic acid from the cerebral cortex during reticular activation. *Fed. Proc. 26*, 373, 1967.

Jasper, H.H. and Tessier, J. Acetylcholine liberation from cerebral cortex during paradoxical (REM) sleep. *Science, 172*, 601-602, (1971).

Jasper, H.H., Khan, R.T. and Elliott, K.A.C. Amino acids released from the cerebral cortex in relation to its state of activation. *Science, 147*, 1448-1449 (1965).

Jones, B.E. Catecholamine-containing neurons in the brain stem of the cat and their role in waking. Thesis submitted to University of Delaware, 1969.

Jones, B.E. The respective involvement of noradrenaline and its deaminated metabolites in waking and paradoxical sleep: A neuropharmacological model. *Brain Res. 39*, 121-136 (1972).

Jones, B., Bobillier, P. and Jouvet, M. Effets de la destruction des neurones contenant des catécholamines du mesencéphale sur le cycle veille-sommeil du chat. *Comp. Rend. Seances Soc. Biol. 163*, 176-180 (1969).

Jonsson, G. Quantitation of fluorescence of biogenic monoamines demonstrated with the formaldehyde fluorescence method. in, *Progress in Histochemistry and Cytochemistry*, Vol 2, Gustav Fischer Verlag, Stuttgart, 1971, pp. 299-334.

Jonsson, G., Fuxe, K. and Hökfelt, T. On the catecholamine innervation of the hypothalamus, with special reference to the median eminence. *Brain Res. 40,* 271-281 (1972).

Jordan, L.M. and Phillis, J.W. Acetylcholine inhibition in the intact and chronically isolated cerebral cortex. *Brit. J. Pharmacol. 45,* 584-595 (1972).

Jouvet, M. Some monoaminergic mechanisms controlling sleep and waking. in, *Brain and Human Behavior,* A.G. Karczmar and J.C. Eccles, Eds., Springer-Verlag, New York, 1972a, pp. 131-161.

Jouvet, M. Veille, sommeil et rêve. Le discours biologique. *Rev. Med. 16-17,* 1003-1063 (1972b).

Jouvet, M. The role of monoamines and acetylcholine-containing neurons in the regulation of the sleep-waking cycle. in, *Ergebnisse der Physiologie, Vol. 64. Neurophysiology and Neurochemistry of Sleep and Wakefulness,* Springer-Verlag, Berlin, 1972c, pp. 166-308.

Jouvet, M. and Delorme, F. Locus coeruleus et sommeil paradoxal. *Comp. Rend. Seances Soc. Biol. 154,* 895-899 (1965).

Jouvet, M. and Jouvet, D. A study of the neurophysiological mechanisms of dreaming. *Electroenceph. Clin. Neurophysiol.* Supp. 24, 133-157 (1963).

Kanai, T. and Szerb, J.C. Mesencephalic reticular activiating system and cortical acetylcholine output. *Nature 205,* 80-82 (1965).

Karczmar, A.G. Is the central cholinergic nervous system overexploited? *Fed. Proc. 28,* 147-157 (1969).

Khazan, N., Bar, R. and Sulman, F.G. The effect of cholinergic drugs on paradoxical sleep in the rat. *Int. J. Neuropharmacol. 6,* 279-282 (1967).

Killam, E.K. and Killam, K.F. The influence of drugs on central afferent pathways. in, *Brain Mechanisms and Drug Action.* W.S. Fields, Ed., C.C. Thomas, Springfield, Ill. 1957, pp. 71-94.

King, C.D. The pharmacology of rapid eye movement sleep. in, *Advances in Pharmacology and Chemotherapy,* Vol. 9, S. Garattini, A. Goldin, F. Hawking and I.J. Kopin, Eds., Academic Press, New York, 1971, pp. 1-91.

Koelle, G.B. The histochemical localization of cholinesterases in the central nervous system of the rat. *J. Comp. Neurol.   100,* 211-235 (1954).

Koelle, G.B. Significance of acetylcholinesterase in central synaptic transmission. *Fed. Proc. 28,* 95-100 (1969).

Koelle, G.B. and Friedenwald, J.S. Histochemical method for localizing cholinesterase activity. *Proc. Soc. Exper. Biol. Med. 70,* 617-622 (1949).

Kostowski, W. The effects of some drugs affecting brain 5-HT on electrocortical synchronization following low-frequency stimulation of brain. *Brain Res. 31,* 151-157 (1971a).

Kostowski, W. Effects of some cholinergic and anticholinergic drugs injected intracerebrally to the midline pontine area. *Neuropharmacology 10,* 595-605 (1971b).

Kostowski, W., Giacalone, E., Garattini, S. and Valzelli, L. Studies on behavioral and biochemical changes in rats after lesion of midbrain raphé. *Europ. J. Pharmacol. 4,* 371-376, (1968).

Kostowski, W., Giacalone, E., Garatinni, S. and Valzelli, L. Electrical stimulation of midbrain raphé: Biochemical, behavioral and bioelectrical effects. *Europ. J. Pharmacol. 7,* 170-175 (1969).

Krnjević, K. Chemical transmission and cortical arousal. *Anesthesiology 28,* 101-105 (1967).

Krnjević,   K.   Central   Cholinergic   Pathways,   *Fed.   Proc.   28,*   113-120,   1969.

Krnjević, K. and Silver, A. A histochemical study of cholinergic fibres in the cerebral cortex. *J. Anat. 99,* 711-759 (1965).

Laguzzi, R., Petitjean, F., Pujol, J.F. and Jouvet, M. Effets de l'injection intraventriculaire de 6-hydroxydopamine. II. Sur le cycle veille-sommeils du chat. *Brain Res. 48,* 295-310 (1972).

Laurent, J.P., Cespuglio, R. and Jouvet, M. Délimitation des voies ascendantes responsables de l'activité ponto-géniculo-occipitale chez le chat. *Experentia 28,* 1174-1175 (1972).

Leontovich, T.A. and Zhukova, G.P. The specificity of the neuronal structure and topography of the reticular formation in the brain and spinal cord of carnivora. *J. Comp. Neurol.* *121*, 347-379 (1963).

Lewis, P.R. and Shute, C.C.D. The cholinergic limbic system: Projections to hippocampal formation, medial cortex, nuclei of the ascending cholinergic reticular system, and the subfornical organ and supro-optic crest. *Brain 90*, 521-540 (1967).

Lindsley, D.F., Barton, R.J. and Atkins, R.J. Effects of subthalamic lesions on peripheral and central arousal thresholds in cats. *Exper. Neurol. 26*, 109-119 (1972).

Loizou, L.A. Projections of the nucleus locus coeruleus in the albino rat. *Brain Res. 15*, 563-566 (1969a).

Loizou, L.A. Rostral projections of noradrenaline-containing neurones in the lower brain stem. *J. Anat. 104*, 593 (1969b).

Longo, V.G. Effects of scopolamine and atropine on EEG and behavioral reactions due to hypothalamic stimulation. *J. Pharmacol. 116*, 198-208 (1956).

Mabry, P.D. and Campbell, B.A. Serotonergic inhibition of catecholamine-induced behavioral arousal. *Brain Res. 49*, 381-391 (1973).

Maeda, T. Histochemical consideration on the relationship between monoamine oxidase and biogenic amines in the brain. *Advan. Neurol. 13*, 812-820 (1970) (in Japanese).

Maeda, T. and Pin, C. Organisation et projections des systèmes catécholaminergiques du pont chez le chaton. *Comp. Rend. Seances Soc. Biol. 165*, 2137-2141 (1971).

Maeda, T. and Shimizu, N. Projections ascendantes du locus coeruleus et d'autres neurones aminergiques pontiques au niveau du prosencéphale du rat. *Brain Res. 36*, 19-35 (1972).

Maffei, L., and Rizzolatti, G. Effect of synchronized sleep on the response of lateral geniculate units to flashes of light. *Arch. Ital. Biol. 103*, 609-622 (1965).

Maffei, L., Moruzzi, G. and Rizzolatti, G. Influence of sleep and wakefulness on the response of lateral geniculate units to sinewave photic stimulation. *Arch. Ital. Biol. 103*, 596-608 (1965).

Magherini, P.C., Pompeiano, O. and Thoden, U. The neurochemical basis of REM sleep: A mechanism responsible for rhythmic activation of the vestibulo-oculomotor system. *Brain Res. 35*, 565-569 (1971).

Magoun, H. "Discussion of chapter by H.W. Magoun: Ascending reticular system and wakefulness." in, *Brain Mechanisms and Consciousness,* J.F. Delafresnaye, Ed., Blackwell Publications, Oxford, 1954, p. 17.

Magoun, H.W. *The Waking Brain,* 2nd ed., C.C. Thomas, Springfield, Ill., 1969, pp. 188.

Mannen, H. "Noyau fermé" et "noyau ouvert". Contribution à l'étude cytoarchitectonique du tronc cérébral envisagrée du point de vue du mode d'arborisation dendritique. *Arch. Ital. Biol. 98*, 330-350 (1960).

Marchiafava, P.L. and Pepeu, G. Electrophysiological Studies of the tectal responses to optic nerve volleys. *Arch. Ital. Biol. 104*, 406-420 (1966).

Masaji, M., Okada, Y. and Shuto, S. Cholinergic agents related to para-sleep state in acute brain stem preparations. *Brain Res. 9*, 253-267 (1968).

Matsuda, Y. Effects of intraventricularly administered adrenaline on rabbit's EEG and their modifications by adrenergic blocking agents. *Jap. J. Pharmacol. 18*, 139-152 (1968).

Matsuda, Y. Effects of some sympathomimetic amines administered intraventricularly on rabbit's EEG. *Jap. J. Pharmacol. 19*, 102-109 (1969).

Matsuoka, I. and Domino, E.F. Cholinergic modulation of single lateral geniculate neurons in the cat. *Neuropharmacology, 11*, 241-251 (1972).

Matsuzaki, M., Okada, Y. and Shuto, S. Cholinergic actions related to paradoxical sleep induction in the mesencephalic cat. *Experientia 23*, 1029-1030 (1967).

Matsuzaki, M., Okada, Y. and Shuto, S. Cholinergic agents related to para-sleep state in acute brain stem preparations. *Brain Res. 9*, 253-267 (1968).

Mayer, Ch. and Stumpf, Ch. Die Physostigminwirkung auf die Hippocampus-Tätigkeit nach Septumläsionen. *Arch. Pharmakol. Exper. Pathol. 234*, 490-500 (1958).

McGeer, E.G., Wada, J.A., Terao, A. and Jung, E. Amine synthesis in various brain regions with caudate or septal lesions. *Exper. Neurol. 24*, 277-284 (1969).

McGinty, D.J. and Harper, R.M. 5-HT containing neurons: Unit activity during sleep. in, *Sleep Research, Vol 1,* M.H. Chase, W.C. Stern, and P.L. Walter, Eds. *Brain Information Service/Brain Research Institute, UCLA Los Angeles, 1972.*

McGinty, D.J. and Sterman, M.B. Sleep suppression after basal forebrain lesions in the cat. *Science 160,* 1253-1255 (1968).

McIlwain, J.T. Nonretinal influences on the lateral geniculate nucleus. *Invest. Opthalmol. 11,* 311-322 (1972).

Mitoma, CH. and Neubauer, S.E. Gamma-hydroxybutyric acid and sleep. *Experientia 24,* 12-13 (1968).

Mizuno, N., Sauerland, E.K. and Clemente, C.D. Projections from the orbital gyrus in the cat. I. To brain stem structures. *J. Comp. Neurol. 133,* 463-476 (1968).

Mizuno, N., Clemente, C.D. and Sauerland, E.K. Fiber projections from rostral basal forebrain structures in the cat. *Exper. Neurol. 25,* 220-237 (1969a).

Mizuno, N., Clemente, C.D. and Sauerland, E.K. Projections from the orbital gyrus in the cat. II. To telencephalic and diencephalic structures. *J. Comp. Neurol. 136,* 127-142 (1969b).

Mizuno, N. and Nakamura, Y. Direct hypothalamic projections to the locus coeruleus. *Brain Res. 19,* 160-163 (1970).

Monnier, M., Fallert, M. and Bhattacharya, I.C. The waking action of histamine. *Experientia 23,* 21-22 (1967).

Monti, J.M. Effect of recurrent stimulation of the brain stem reticular formation on REM sleep in cats. *Exper. Neurol. 28,* 484-493 (1970).

Moore, R.Y. and Heller, A. Monoamine levels and neuronal degneration in rat brain following lateral hypothalamic lesions. *J. Pharmacol. Exper. Therapeu. 156,* 12-22 (1967).

Moore, R.Y., Bhatnagar, R.K. and Heller, A. Anatomical and chemical studies of a nigro-neostriatal projection in the cat. *Brain Res. 30,* 119-135 (1971).

Moore, R.Y., Wong, S.R. and Heller, A. Regional effects of hypothalamic lesions on brain serotonin. *Arch. Neurol. 13,* 346-354 (1965).

Morest, K. A study of the area postrema with Golgi methods. *Amer. J. Anat. 107,* 291-303 (1960).

Morgane, P.J. Maturation of neurobiochemical systems related to the ontogenty of sleep behavior. in, *Sleep and the Maturing Nervous System,* C. Clemente, D. Purpura and F. Mayer, Eds., Academic Press, New York, 1972, pp. 141-162.

Morgane, P.J. and Stern, W.C. Relationship of sleep to neuroanatomical circuits, biochemistry, and behavior. *Ann. N.Y. Acad. Sci. 193,* 95-111 (1972).

Morgane, P.J. and Stern, W.C. Monoaminergic systems in the brain and their role in the sleep states. in, *Serotonin and Behavior,* E. Usdin and J. Barchas, Eds. Academic Press, New York, 1973a pp. 427-442.

Morgane, P.J. and Stern, W.C. Effects of serotonin metabolites on sleep-waking activity in cats. *Brain Res. 50,* 205-213 (1973b).

Morison, R. and Dempsey, E. A Study of thalamo-coritcal relations. *Amer. J. Physiol. 135,* 281-292 (1942).

Moruzzi, G. The sleep-waking cycle. in, *Ergebnisse der Physiologie,* Vol 64. *Neurophysiology and Neurochemistry of Sleep and Wakefulness,* Springer-Verlag, Berlin, 1972, pp. 1-165.

Moruzzi, G. and Magoun, H.W., Brain stem reticular formation and activation of the EEG. *Electroenceph. Clin. Neurophysiol. 1,* 455-473 (1949).

Nauta, W.J.H. Hypothalamic regulation of sleep in rats. An experimental study. *J. Neurophysiol. 9,* 285-316 (1946).

Nauta, W.J H. Discussion of chapter by H.W. Magoun: Ascending reticular system and wakefulness. in, *Brain Mechanisms and Consciousness,* J.F. Delafresnaye, Ed., Blackwell Scientific Publications, Oxford, 1954, p. 17.

Nauta, W.J.H. Hippocampal projections and related neural pathways to the mid-brain in the cat. *Brain 81*, 319-340 (1958).

Nauta, W.J.H., Henricus, G. and Kuypers, G.J.M. Some ascending pathways in the brain stem reticular formation. in, *Reticular Formation of the Brain*, Little, Brown and Co., Boston, 1958, pp. 3-30.

Nauta, W.J.H. and Haymaker, W. Hypothalamic nuclei and fiber connections. in, *The Hypothalamus*. W. Haymaker, E. Anderson and W.J.H. Nauta, Eds.., C.C. Thomas, Springfield, Ill., 1969, pp. 136-209.

Needham, C.W. and Dila, C.J. Synchronizing and desynchronizing systems of the old brain. *Brain Res. 11*, 285-293 (1968).

Nystrom, B., Olson, L. and Ungerstedt, U. Noradrenaline nerve terminals in human cerebral cortices: First histochemical evidence. *Science 176*, 924-926 (1972).

Ogawa, T. Midbrain reticular influences upon single neurons in lateral geniculate nucleus. *Science 139*, 343-344 (1963).

Olivier, A., Parent, A. and Poirier, L.J. Identification of the thalamic nuclei on the basis of their cholinesterase content in the monkey. *J. Anat. 106*, 37-50 (1970a).

Olivier, A. Parent, A., Simard, H. and Poirier, L.J. Cholinesterasic striatopallidal and striatonigral efferents in the cat and the monkey. *Brain Res. 18*, 273-282 (1970b).

Olson, L. and Fuxe, K. One the projections from the locus coeruleus noradrenaline neurons: The cerebellar innervation. *Brain Res. 28*, 165-171 (1971).

Olson, L. and Fuxe, K. Further mapping out of central noradrenaline neuron system: Projections of the subcoeruleus area. *Brain Res. 43*, 289-295 (1972).

Olszewski, J. and Baxter, D. *Cytoarchitecture of the Human Brain Stem*, Karger, Basel, 1954, pp. 199.

Parent, A. and Poirier, L.J. The medial forebrain bundle (MFB) and ascending monoaminergic pathways in the cat. *Can. J. Physiol. Pharmacol. 47*, 781-785 (1969).

Parent, A. Saint-Jaques, C. and Poirier, L.J. Effect of interrupting the hypothalamic nervous connections on the norepinephrine and serotonin content of the hypothalamus. *Exper. Neurol. 23*, 67-75 (1969).

Pepeu, G. Cholinergic neurotransmission in the central nervous system. *Arch. Int. Pharmacodyn. Therap. 196* (Supp.), 229-243 (1972).

Pepeu, G. and Mantegazzini, P. Midbrain hemisection: Effect on cortical acetylcholine in the cat. *Science 145*, 1069-1070 (1964).

Perenin, M.T., Maeda, T. and Jeannerod, M. Are vestibular nuclei responsible for rapid eye movements of paradoxical sleep? *Brain Res. 43*, 617-621 (1972).

Petitjean, F. and Jouvet, M. Hypersomnie et augmentation de l'acide 5-hydroxy-indolacetique cérébral par lésion isthmique chez le chat. *Comp. Rend. Seances Soc. Biol. 164*, 2288-2293 (1970).

Petitjean, F., Laguzzi, R., Sordet, F., Jouvet, M. and Pujol, J.F. Effets de l'injection intraventriculaire de 6-hydroxydopamine. I. Sur les monoamines cérébrales du chat. *Brain Res. 48*, 281-293 (1972)

Petsche, H. and Stumpf, Ch. Topographic and toposcopic study of origin and spread of the regular synchronized arousal patterns in the rabbit. *Electroenceph. Neurophysiol. 12*, 589-600 (1960).

Phillis, J. W. The pharmacology of thalamic and geniculate neurons. *International Review of Neurobiology*, Vol. 14, C.C. Pfeiffer and J.R. Smythies, Eds., Academic Press, New York, 1971, pp. 1-48.

Phillis, J.W. and Chong, G.C. Acetylcholine release from the cerebral and cerebellar cortices: Its role in cortical arousal. *Nature 207*, 1253-1255 (1965).

Phillis, J.W. and York, D.H. Cholinergic inhibition in the cerebral cortex. *Brain Res. 5*, 517-520 (1967).

Phillis, J.W., Tebecis, A.K. and York, D.H. The inhibitory action of monoamines on lateral geniculate neurones. *J. Physiol.* (London) *190*, 563-581 (1967a).

Phillis, J.W., Tebecis, A.K. and York, D.H. A study of cholinoceptive cells in the lateral geniculate nucleus.'J. Physiol. (London) 192, 695-713 (1967b).

Pin, C., Jones, B., and Jouvet, M. Topographie des neurones monoaminergiques du tronc cérébral du chat: Etude par histofluorescence. Comp. Rend. Seances Soc. Biol. 162, 2136-2141 (1968).

Pohorecky, L.A., Larin, F. and Wurtman, R.J. Mechanisms of changes in brain norepinephrine levels following olfactory bulb lesions. Life Sci. 8, 1309-1317 (1969).

Pohorecky, L.A., Zigmond, J.J., Heimer, L. and Wurtman, R.J. Olfactory bulb removal: Effects on brain norepinephrine. Proc. Nat. Acad. Sci. 62, 1052-1055 (1969).

Poirier, L.J. and Sourkes, T.L. Influence of the substantia nigra on the catecholamine content of the striatum. Brain 88, 181-192 (1965).

Polc, P. and Monnier, M. An activating mechanism in the ponto-bulbar raphé system of the rabbit. Brain Res. 22, 47-61 (1970).

Pujol, J.F., Mouret, J., Jouvet, M. and Glowinski, J. Increased turnover of cerebral norepinephrine during rebound of paradoxical sleep in the rat. Science 159, 112-114 (1968).

Pujol, J.F., Sordet, F., Petitjean, F., Germain, D., and Jouvet, M. Insomnie et métabolisme cérébral de la sérotonine chez le chat: Etude de la libération de la sérotonine mesurées in vitro 18 H apres destruction du système du raphé. Brain Res. 39, 137-149 (1972).

Ramón-Moliner, E. and Nauta, W.H.J. The isodendritic core of the brain stem. J. Comp. Neurol. 126, 311-336 (1966).

Renault, J. Monoamines et sommeils. Role du système du raphé et de la serotonine cérébrale dans l'endormissement. These de medecine, University of Lyon, 1967, pp. 140.

Rinaldi, F. and Himwich, H.E. Alerting responses and actions of atropine and cholinergic drugs. Arch. Neurol. 73, 387-395 (1955a).

Rinaldi, F. and Himwich, H.E. Cholinergic mechanism involved in function of mesodiencephalic activating system. Arch. Neurol. 73, 396-402 (1955b).

Rossi, G.F. Sleep inducing mechanisms in the brain stem. Electroenceph. Clin. Neurophysiol. Suppl. 24, 113-132 (1963).

Rossi, G., Minobe, K. and Candia, O. An experimental study of the hypnogenic mechanisms of the brain stem. Arch. Ital. Biol. 101, 470-492 (1963).

Roth, R.H. and Suhr, Y. Mechanisms of the γ-hydroxybutyrate-induced increase in brain dopamine and its relationship to "sleep". Biochem. Pharmacol. 19, 3001-3012 (1970).

Rothballer, A.B. Studies on the adrenaline-sensitive component of the reticular activating system. Electroenceph. Clin. Neurophysiol. 8, 603-621 (1956).

Rothballer, A.B. The effects of catecholamines on the central nervous system. Pharmacol. Rev. 11, 494-547 (1959).

Roussel, B., Buguet, A., Bobillier, P., and Jouvet, M. Locus coeruleus, sommeil paradoxal, et noradrénaline cérébrale. Compt. Rend. Seances Soc. Biol. 161, 2537-2541 (1967).

Routtenberg, A. The two-arousal hypothesis: Reticular formation and limbic system. Psychol. Rev. 75, 51-80 (1968).

Russell, G.V. The nucleus locus coeruleus (dorsolateralis tegmenti). Tex. Rep. Biol. Med. 13, 939-988 (1955).

Satinsky, D. Pharmacological responsiveness of lateral geniculate nucleus neurons. Int. J. Neuropharmacol. 6, 387-395 (1967).

Satinsky, D. Reticular influences on lateral geniculate neuron activity. Electroencephal. Clin. Neurophysiol. 25, 543-549 (1968).

Scheibel, M.E. and Scheibel, A.B. Structural substrates for integrative patterns in the brain stem reticular core. in, Reticular Formation of the Brain, H.H. Jasper, L.D. Proctor, R.S. Knighton, W.C. Noshay and R.T. Costello, Eds., Little, Brown & Co., Boston, 1958, pp. 31-68.

Scheibel, M.E. and Scheibel, A.B. Patterns of organization in specific and nonspecific thalamic fields. in, The Thalamus. D.P. Purpura and M.D. Yahr, Eds., Columbia University Press, New York, 1966, pp. 13-46.

Scheibel, M.E. and Scheibel, A.B. Structural organization of nonspecific thalamic nuclei and their projection toward cortex. *Brain Res. 6*, 60-94 (1967)

Scheibel, M.E. and Scheibel, A.B. Elementary processes in selected thalamic and cortical subsystems—The structural substrates. in, *The Neurosciences*. F.O. Schmitt, Ed., The Rockefeller University Press, New York, 1970, pp. 443-457.

Schlag, J.D. and Chaillet, F. Thalamic mechanisms involved in cortical desynchronization and recruiting responses. *Electroencephal. Clin. Neurophysiol. 15*, 39-62 (1963).

Sheard, M.H. and Aghajanian, G.K. Stimulation of the midbrain raphé: Effect on serotonin metabolism. *J. Pharmacol. Exper. Therapeut. 163*, 425-430 (1968a).

Sheard, M.H. and Aghajanian, G.K. Stimulation of midbrain raphé neurons: Behavioral effects of serotonin release. *Life Sci. 7*, 19-25 (1968b).

Shimizu, N. and Imamoto, K. Fine structure of the locus coeruleus in the rat. *Arch. Histol. Jap. 31*, 229-246 (1970).

Shute, C.C.D. Distribution of cholinesterase and cholinergic pathways. I. Evidence of cholinergic mechanisms. in, *The Hypothalamus*, L. Martini, M. Motta and F. Fraschini, Eds., Academic Press, New York, 1970, pp, 167-179.

Shute, C.C.D. and Lewis, P.R. Cholinesterase-containing systems of the brain of the rat. *Nature 199*, 1160-1164 (1963).

Shute, C.C.D. and Lewis, P.R. Cholinergic and monoaminergic pathways in the hypothalamus. *Brit. Med. Bull. 22*, 221-226 (1966).

Shute, C.C.D. and Lewis, P.R. The ascending cholinergic reticular system: Neocortical, olfactory and subcortical projections. *Brain 90*, 497-520 (1967).

Skinner, J.E. Electrocortical desynchronization during functional blockade of the mesencephalic reticular formation. *Brain Res. 22*, 254-258 (1970).

Skinner, J.E. Abolition of several forms of cortical synchronization during blockade in the inferior thalamic peduncle. *Electroencephal. Clin. Neurophysiol. 31*, 211-221 (1971).

Skinner, J.E. and Lindsley, D.B. Electrophysiological and behavioral effects of blockade of the nonspecific thalamo-cortical system. *Brain Res. 6*, 95-118 (1967).

Sladek, J.R. The distribution of catecholamine terminals within the mesencephalon, pons and medulla oblongata of the immature cat brain: A fluorescence microscopic study. Ph.D. Dissertation, University Microfilms, Ann Arbor, Michigan, 1971a, pp. 1-152.

Sladek, J.R. Differences in the distribution of catecholamine varicosities in cat and rat reticular formation. *Science 174*, 410-412 (1971b).

Sladek, J.R. Interspecies and age-dependent differences in the distribution of catecholamine varicosities within the brainstem reticular formation of the rat, gerbil and cat. *Anat. Rec. 172*, 407 (1972).

Sladek, J.R. and Hoffman, D.L. Differences in catecholamine distribution in the inferior olivary complex of various mammals. *Anat. Rec. 175*, 444-445 (1973).

Smelik, P.G. and Ernst, A.M. Role of nigro-neostriatal dopaminergic fibers in compulsive gnawing behavior in rats. *Life Sci. 5*, 1485-1488 (1966).

Starzl, T.E., Taylor, C.W. and Magoun, H.W. Ascending conduction in reticular activating system with special reference to the diencephalon. *J. Neurophysiol. 14*, 461-477 (1951).

Stein, L. and Wise, C.D. Release of norepinephrine from hypothalamus and amygdala by rewarding medial forebrain bundle stimulation and amphetamine. *J. Compar. Physiol. Psychol. 67*, 189-198 (1969).

Sterman, M.B. and Clemente, C.D. Forebrain inhibitory mechanisms: Cortical synchronization induced by basal forebrain stimulation. *Exper. Neurol. 6*, 91-102 (1962a).

Sterman, M.B. and Clemente, C.D. Forebrain inhibitory mechanisms: Sleep patterns induced by basal forebrain stimulation in the behaving cat. *Exper. Neurol. 6*, 103-117 (1962a).

Sterman, M.B. and Clemente, C.D. Basal forebrain structures and sleep. *Acta Neurol. Latinoamer. 14*, 228-244 (1968).

Stern, W.C. and Morgane, P.J. Serotonin and EEG spiking activity in the lateral geniculate nucleus. *Proc. 80th Ann. Convention, APA,* 837-838 (1972).

Stern, W.C. and Morgane, P.J. Effects of reserpine on sleep and brain biogenic amine levels in the cat. *Psychopharmacologia 28,* 275-286 (1973a).

Stern, W.C. and Morgane, P.J. Effects of alpha-methyl-tyrosine on REM sleep and brain amine levels in the cat. *Biol. Psychiat. 6,* 301-306 (1973b).

Szentagothai, J. The structure of the synapse in the lateral geniculate body. *Acta Anat. 55,* 166-185 (1963).

Szerb, J.C. Cortical acetylcholine release and electroencephalographic arousal. *J. Physiol.* (London) *192,* 329-343 (1967).

Taber, E., The cytoarchitecture of the brain stem of the cat. I. Brain stem nuclei of cat. *J. Compar. Neurol. 116,* 27-69 (1961).

Taber, E., Brodal, A., and Walberg, F. The raphé nuclei of the brain stem in the cat. I. Normal topography and cytoarchitecture and general discussion. *J. Comp. Neurol. 114,* 161-187 (1960).

Tebecis, A.K. and Maria, A. Dr. A re-evaluation of the mode of action of 5-hydroxytryptamine on lateral geniculate neurones: Comparison with catecholamines and LSD. *Exper. Brain Res. 14,* 480-493 (1972).

Torii, S. Two types of patterns of hippocampal electrical activity induced by stimulation of hypothalamus and surrounding parts of rabbit brain. *Jap. J. Physiol. 11,* 147-157 (1961).

Ungerstedt, U. Is interruption of the nigro-striatal dopamine system producing the "lateral hypothalamus syndrome"? *Acta Physiol. Scand. 80,* 35A-36A (1970).

Ungerstedt, U. Stereotaxic mapping of the monoamine pathways in the rat brain. *Acta Physiol. Scand.,* Supp. 367, 1-48 (1971a).

Ungerstedt, U. Introduction. in, *On the Anatomy, Pharmacology and Function of the Nigro-Striatal Dopamine System.* Kungl, Boktryckeriet P.A. Norstodt & Söner, Stockholm, 1971b, pp. 1-15.

Ungerstedt, U. Histochemical studies on the effect of intracerebral and intraventricular injections of 6-hydroxydopamine on monoamine neurons in the rat brain. in, *6-Hydroxydopamine and Catecholamine Neurons.* T. Malmfors and H. Thoenen, Eds., North-Holland Pub. Co., Amsterdam, 1971c, pp. 166-308.

Valverde, F. Reticular formation of the pons and medulla oblongata. A Golgi study. *J. Comp. Neurol. 116,* 71-100 (1961).

Valverde, F. Reticular formation of the albino rat's brain stem. Cytoarchitecture and corticofugal connections. *J. Comp. Neurol. 119,* 25-53 (1962).

Valverde, F. *Studies on the Pyriform Lobe,* Harvard University Press, Cambridge, 1965, pp. 131.

Velasco, M. and Lindsley, D.B. Role of orbital cortex in regulation of thalamocortical electrical activity. *Science 149,* 1375-1377 (1965).

Verhaart, W.J.C. *A Stereotactic Atlas of the Brain Stem of the Cat. Part I. Text,* F.A. Davis Co., Philadelphia, 1964, pp. 84.

Verhaart, W.J.C. *A Stereotactic Atlas of the Brain Stem of the Cat. Part II. Plates,* F.A. Davis Co., Philadelphia, 1964.

Verzeano, M. and Mahnke, J.H. Serotonin and thalamic synchronization. *Physiol. Behav. 9,* 649-653 (1972).

Villablanca, J. Electroencephalogram in the permanently isolated forebrain of the cat. *Science 138,* 44-45 (1962).

Villablanca, J. Permanent reduction in sleep after removal of cerebral cortex and striatum in cats. *Brain Res. 36,* 463-468 (1972).

Villablanca, J. and Schlag, J. Cortical control of thalamic spindle waves. *Exper. Neurol. 20,* 432-442 (1968).

Wada, J.A. and Terao, A. Effect of parachlorophenylalanine on basal forebrain stimulation. *Exper. Neurol. 28,* 501-506 (1970).

Weinberger, N.M., Velasco, M. and Lindsley, D.B. Effects of lesions upon thalamically induced electrocortical desynchronization and recruiting. *Electroenceph. Clin. Neurophysiol. 18*, 369-377 (1965).

Winkler, C. and Potter, A. *An Anatomical Guide to Experimental Researches on the Cat's Brain*, W.Versluys, Amsterdam, 1914.

Wise, D.C., Berger, B.D. and Stein, L. Evidence of alpha-noradrenergic reward receptors and serotonergic punishment receptors in the rat brain. *Biol. Psychiat. 6*, 3-21 (1973).

Wolman, M. A fluorescent histochemical procedure for gamma-aminobutyric acid. *Histochemie 28*, 118-130 (1971).

Yamaguchi, N., Marczynski, T.J. and Ling, G.M. The effects of electrical and chemical stimulation of the preoptic region and some nonspecific thalamic nuclei in unrestrained, waking animals. *Electroenceph. Clin. Neurophysiol. 15*. 154 (1963).

Yamaguchi, N., Ling, G.M. and Marczynski, T.J. The effects of chemical stimulation of the preoptic region, nucleus centralis medialis, or brain stem reticular formation with regard to sleep and wakefulness. *Recent Advan. Biol. Psychiat. 6*, 9-20 (1964).

Zanchetti, A. Brain stem mechanism of sleep. *Anesthesiology 28*, 81-99 (1967).

Ziehen, T. Centralnervensystem. in, *Handbuch der Anatomy des Menschen, vol. 4*, K. v. Bardeleben, Fischer, Jena, 1920.

ADDENDUM: Since the body of this paper was written, two additional, highly pertinent, papers have appeared that should be noted. In the first of these (Thierry, Blanc, Sobel, Stinus, and Glowinski, *Science 182:* 499-501, 1973) strong biochemical support for the existence of dopaminergic terminals independent of noradrenergic terminals in the rat cerebral cortex has been shown. In the second paper Norbin and Björklund (*Acta Physiol. Scand, Supp 388:* 1-40, 1973) concluded from a topographic study on monoamine neurons in human fetuses that the principles of monoamine neuron organization are similar in the rat and in man.

Advances in Sleep Research, Vol. 1
© 1974, Spectrum Publications, Inc.

CHAPTER 2

Phylogeny of Sleep

EDWARD S. TAUBER

This chapter constitutes an appraisal and reflection on sleep studies of inframammalian vertebrates in the light of evolutionary biology. Notwithstanding the growth of interest in the nature of sleep in the last 15 to 20 years, inframammalian sleep studies have been limited and have concerned themselves with determining whether or not sleep, including the existence of REM sleep, is present throughout the vertebrate phylum. Information on the nature of sleep has been acquired through behavioral and electrographic studies almost exclusively in mammals. The contributions of neurophysiology, neuroanatomy, and neurochemistry have also enlarged our understanding of sleep and its complexity. Nevertheless, no convincingly satisfactory definition of sleep is yet possible. For this reason, I will suggest the design of certain kinds of inquiries to illuminate how genetics and evolutionary biology might aid us in deepening our understanding of sleep.

To put matters in perspective, roughly 2400 species comprise the 19 orders of the class of mammals (Romer, 1963; Walker, 1964; Dowling, personal communication). However, there are at least 8600 species of birds and in the reptilian class, comprising 5 orders, there are about 5360 species, of which lizards number 3000 and snakes 2127. There are somewhat over 3000 species of amphibians, of which the salientia (anurans) alone comprise 2631 species. A modest estimate of the number of species of fishes is perhaps 40,000. It is therefore apparent that the class of mammals is conspicuously small in comparison with the other four classes of vertebrates. Yet the literature shows a preponderance of studies dealing with mammals. Between January 1, 1970 and the end of November, 1972, the National Library at Bethesday, Maryland, (Medline) retrieved 958 articles dealing with Rapid Eye Movement (REM) sleep. Of this number, only nine (less than 1 percent) dealt with REM sleep in inframammalian vertebrates, with an additional 27 titles dealing with non-REM sleep.

The dearth of attention to the comparative and phylogenetic aspects of sleep has been unfortunate because of at least one serious consequence; namely, a preclusion of the broadest possible base for the acquisition of new findings and hypotheses. The enthusiasm of investigators for further exploration of inframammalian species may have been dampened by the exciting discovery of REM sleep in man and mammals and its alleged absence or rudimentary nature in inframammalian species.

Other factors have also played a role in discouraging studies of lower animals: lack of familiarity with the species and frequent unavailability of the species. In addition, their ability to adapt to life under laboratory conditions is often precarious. Temperature, light-darkness factors, and specialized nutritional requirements present the investigator of lower order animals with unexpected and often insurmountable obstacles. Susceptibility to organisms not pathogenic to mammals introduces additional hindrances to the proper completion of a sleep study. Although the mammalian model of study has served mammalian investigation satisfactorily, it still falls short of being an ideal model for studying animals at a different level of phylogeny in that the sleep characteristics of inframammalian vertebrates need not be identical to those observed in mammals.

As one ascends the ladder of phylogeny one finds behavioral and/or electrographic evidence of sleep. It is at the level of mammals that a definitive compartmentalization of sleep and wakefulness achieves incontrovertible configuration. But what criteria will permit us to assert that the sleep-wakefulness cycle is clearly present in other taxa? As we shall see, evidence for its presence is accumulating for the avian class. What we know about sleep in respect of the classes of reptiles, amphibia, and fishes leaves much to be desired in terms of fact and interpretation.

The sleep pattern is differentiated in mammals into two categories: Slow Wave (non-REM) sleep and Rapid Eye Movement (REM) sleep. There are additional neurophysiological and neurochemical indices correlated with these two different sleep states. Earlier investigators sought to determine whether REM sleep or slow wave sleep occurred earlier in evolution. Since the evidence based on neuroanatomical and neurophysiological studies suggested that the brainstem played a significant role in the production of REM sleep (Jouvet, 1967, 1969), while slow wave sleep was allegedly correlated with more rostral structures in the brain, it was inferred that REM sleep arose earlier in evolution. This reasonable assumption was based on the fact that the brainstem is present in all vertebrates, while the cortex appeared later in evolution. However, this reassuring correlation encountered difficulties when REM sleep was found to be absent in certain inframammalian vertebrates (Hermann et al., 1964). Later studies indicated that REM sleep was present in certain birds, reptiles, and fishes (Klein et al., 1964; Tauber et al., 1966; Tradardi, 1966; Tauber et al., 1968; Tauber and Weitzman, 1969; Rojas-Ramirez and Tauber, 1970; Berger and Walker, 1972; Van Twyver and Allison, 1972).

At the present time, there is no unanimity of opinion with regard to these findings. The controversial aspect is not easy to resolve; however, the continued search for both REM sleep and slow wave sleep characteristics in inframammalian species is slowly progressing.

NEUROANATOMICAL AND NEUROPHYSIOLOGICAL BASIS FOR PHYLOGENY OF SLEEP

Certain neuroanatomical structures have been identified as subserving the two sleep states in mammals. Are similar structures present in inframammalian vertebrates? Roger Broughton (1972) has been active in directing attention to this central issue, and I will borrow heavily from his writings in this area, introducing at various points citations from additional readings. These anatomical substrates which serve to underlie slow wave and REM sleep, respectively, in the mammal may or may not be present in certain lower classes of vertebrates. As a result, there are several possibilities which have to be anticipated. The absence of a particular neural system or part could correlate directly with the absence of behavioral and/or electrographic evidence of a particular sleep state. On the other hand, a particular sleep state might be present but neural circuits different from those employed in the mammalian system would be responsible for positive behavioral and electrographic evidence of that particular sleep state. Thus for example, vision, which is controlled by midbrain mechanisms in lower animals, is predominantly under cortical control in mammals. One could not insist that the lack of a highly developed optic cortex in large families of birds, diurnal lizards, and many species of reef fishes would eventuate in their having vision not comparable to that of primates since in many respects their visual acuity is very highly developed.

Before reviewing the evidence for neuroanatomical structures subserving the two sleep states in inframammalian vertebrates, it will be useful to summarize briefly the electrographic and physiological mechanisms underlying the two sleep states in young human adults (Broughton, 1971).

Non-Rapid Eye Movement sleep occurs following sleep onset. This consists of Stage I (loss of alpha, presence of vertex waves and slow eye movements); Stage II consists of spindles and K-complexes on a low voltage background activity; and Stages III and IV reveal high-amplitude delta activity. Approximately every 90 minutes throughout the night, Non-REM is replaced with periods of REM sleep. Non-REM sleep reveals less delta patterning and the REM periods become generally longer and more intense as sleep progresses. When non-REM sleep shows increased delta activity there is slowing of cardiorespiratory rates, some reduction of muscle tone, and an increased threshold of arousal. In REM sleep on the other hand, electrocortical recording reveals low voltage theta activity, absence of spindles and K-complexes, and cardiorespiratory rate and blood pressure may become elevated and more variable; REM bursts, muscle twitching, significantly diminished muscle tone, and loss of deep tendon jerks are noted. Stage I accounts for approximately 5 percent of total sleep time while Stage II equals 50 to 55 percent, Stage III and IV 10 percent each and REM sleep approximately 20 to 25 percent. The sleep cycle in the newborn is much shorter than that observed in the adult; it is, however, at least 40 to 45 minutes. The percentage of deep Non-REM sleep and REM sleep are greater, with the latter approximately 50 percent of total sleep time. The REM state in infants may initiate sleep onset. With maturation, the sleep cycle lengthens and non-REM sleep tends to occur first. In the aged, sleep Stages III and IV tend to diminish; there is also a reduction in REM sleep. Total sleep time frequently decreases and sleep is often interrupted by episodes of wakefulness. Night sleep patterns in the aged are often modified by daytime napping, which must be taken into account.

The two types of sleep have been summarized (Broughton 1971) as follows:

> The waking state is maintained by tonic discharge of the subcortical arousal system, or so-called reticular activating system, located mainly in the mesencephalic tegmentum and posterior hypothalamus. It is now known that sleep onset is not passive but is due to active inhibition of the arousal system by at least two subcortical areas, one in the preoptic region of the hypothalmus, and the other in the pons. The dampening of ascending reticulocortical impulses leads to slowing of the EEG and, by idling of the unspecific thalamocortical pathways, to the sleep spindles. A decrease of reticulospinal activity explains the progressive diminution in muscle tone.
>
> In REM sleep, a marked central nervous system (CNS) upheaval occurs. Two lower brainstem centers discharge together, one triggering an ascending system, the other a descending system. The presence of two systems is stressed as their activities may be dissociated in various neurological conditions. The ascending system appears to have its onset in a restricted part of the pons, the *nucleus reticularis pontis caudalis.* By ascending pathways it is responsible for the EEG arousal and, due to phasic discharge superimposed upon a tonic one, the REM bursts, autonomic irregularity, myoclonic twitches and so-called *ponto-geniculo-striate* (PGO) spikes. The descending system has its onset in the neighboring *locus coeruleus* of the pons which, via connections to descending inhibitory reticulospinal pathways, gives rise to the areflexia and loss of muscle tone.

In order to provide the reader with some background in the comparative aspects of pertinent neural structures subserving sleep in inframammalian vertebrates, a brief review of some of the essential findings referable to sleep mechanisms in the mammal will be presented (Broughton, 1972). Since several chapters in this volume deal with the neuroanatomy and physiology of the sleep-waking state in considerable detail, the following description will be brief. Most of the evidence pointing toward the essential neural structures subserving sleep mechanisms has been acquired through stimulation, ablation, and pharmacological experiments. Rapid eye movement sleep (paradoxical sleep, rhombencephalic sleep) involves pontine reticular nuclei, both oral and caudal, which are responsible for tonic ascending discharges; phasic ascending discharges may be mediated by the medial and the descending vestibular nuclei. Descending motor inhibitory discharges are under the control of the locus coeruleus. The nuclei of the oculomotor system (N. III, N. IV, and N. VI), are significantly aligned with the vestibular nuclei via the medial longitudinal fasciculus and most probably accessory polysynaptic pathways. The rhinencephalon comprising amygdaloid nuclei and hippocampus along with pathways to the hypothalamus are also structures actively involved. The localization of synchronizing structures in the brainstem are not sufficiently well defined at resent to permit an unqeuivocal statement as to their location. This schema is admittedly simplistic since undoubtedly the participation of the entire brain is implicated in sleep and wakefulness.

PHYLOGENY: ITS IMPLICATIONS FOR AN UNDERSTANDING OF THE NATURE OF SLEEP

Since sleep research is concerned with the discovery of its origin and with locating which vertebrate representatives manifest sleep behavior, a background in the comparative aspects of vertebrates becomes essential. To obtain a complete and yet detailed understanding of an organism, it must be recognized that all parts of an organism do not evolve at the same rate, i.e., an entire organism is essentially a mosaic of primitive or ancestral and derived characters (Schaeffer, 1969). The terms "primitive" and "derived" as understood by biologists could have a bearing on many questions inherent in sleep research (e.g., REM, non-REM, and neurohumoral factors in relation to taxonomic groupings). The implications of this issue are dealt with in the mammaliansection where it is noted that REM sleep is present in placentals and marsupials, but not in the monotremes. In respect to fishes, Schaeffer (1969) gives the following operational illustration:

> For instance, certain characters that are primitive for the ray-finned fishes (actinopterygians) are derived in terms of the ancestral osteichthyan stock. On the other hand, the characters shared by early members of the three major osteichthyan groups (actinopterygians, crossopterygians, and dipnoans) presumably were present in their common ancestor and are therefore primitive for the class osteichthyes.

In order to acquire a grasp of the organization of the phyla in the vertebrate kingdom, I would like — as an example — to mention schematically the division dealing exclusively with the four living classes of fishes.

Class Agnatha
    Subclass Cyclostomata (cyclostomes)
        Petromyzon (lamprey)
        Myxine (hagfish)

Class Elasmobranchii (sharks and rays)
Class Holocephali (ratfishes)
  Chimaera (ratfish)
Class Osteichthyes (higher bony fishes)
  Subclass Actinopterygii (ray-finned fishes)
    Infraclass Chondrostei
      Acipenser (sturgeon)
      Polyodon (paddlefish)
      Polypterus (bichir)
    Infraclass Holostei
      Lepisosteus (gar)
      Amia (bowfin)
    Infraclass Teleostei
      Elops (tenpounder)
      Albula (bonefish)
      Clupea (herring)
      Perca (perch)
  Subclass Crossopterygii (lobe-finned fishes)
    Latimeria (living coelacanth)
    Rhipidistian stock (leading to the fish-amphibian transition)
  Subclass Dipnoi (lungfishes)
    Neoceratodus (Australian lungfish)
    Protopterus (African lungfish)
    Lepidosiren (South American lungfish)

Within this classification the most probable choice of species for study would come from the class Elasmobranchii, and the infraclass Teleostei which has by far the largest representation in recent times. The crossopterygian subclass consists of two subdivisions: the *Latimeria*, the recently discovered very primitive coelacanths, and the *Rhipidistian* stock, from which persumably the amphibians emerged; since the amphibians are tetrapods which have acquired the capacity for terrestrial adaptation, they are of particular importance for sleep research. Their early modifications consisted in the appearance of limbs, a mobile tongue for catching and swallowing prey, and the stapes. Furthermore, these early tetrapods seem to show modifications of the cerebellum in line with the transition from fin movement to limb movement. These particular terrestrial adaptations bring to mind immediately the types of motor phenomena that one might anticipate emerging during sleep. Terminal twitchings of the limbs are well known; there is now evidence that (the stapes) middle ear muscle activity shows phasic activity during REM sleep, (Pessah and Roffwarg, 1973) and recently Flanigan et al. (in press) have provided strongly presumptive evidence of tongue movements in their reptilian studies. It is tempting to suspect that the phasic activity demonstrable in REM sleep has undergone evolutionary modifications over time but that some of the most primitive motor mechanisms are still retained during the state of brain activation.

Modern views concerning speciation and evolutionary lineages have brought to light newer and more reliable ways of understanding taxonomic trends. G.J. Nelson (1969) has pointed out that approximately 98 percent of the species of recent chordates occupy two evolutionary lineages, apparently related, but having separate histories back to at least the Devonian period. He indicates that one lineage comprises "the mammals, birds, crocodiles, lizards, snakes, rhynchocephalians, caecilians, frogs and probably also the salamanders, lungfishes and coelacanths, and possibly even the bichirs and reedfishes: in short, the land vertebrates and their relatives among fishes. The second lineage includes the sturgeons, paddlefishes, gars, bowfins, and among the Teleosts (numerous representatives) but in short, the vertebrates commonly called actinopterygians. Some 21,000 species occupy the former group; and the latter group may be estimated between at least 18,000 and 40,000 species." (Nelson, 1969).

These two groups as evolutionary lineages are stated to have a historical reality. The interrelationships of the included species are in some instances controversial, but Nelson points out that although the relationships of some mammal groups are obscure, nevertheless all mammals are related among themselves. Relationship in this sense is equated with evolutionary relationship due to common ancestry. Thus all recent species of mammals most probably have a common ancestor and form a monophyletic group. Furthermore, the latest ancestor common to all mammals probably did not give rise to any recent species of birds, snakes or anything else but mammals. "Somewhat less well established but generally accepted relationships are that between birds and crocodiles and that among lizards, snakes and rhynchocephalians. Finally, relationships hardly established at all are those of the turtles, caecilians, frogs, salamanders, lungfishes and coelacanths." Nelson informs us of many more extremely interesting and valuable data to which the reader could refer. Nelson also warns against certain biases with respect to evolutionary progress, since the temptation of man is to overvalue his own position in a discussion of vertebrate evolution (Nelson, 1969).

HOMOLOGY

In studying comparative and evolutionary aspects of sleep, the concept of homology acquires a great significance morphologically and functionally with respect to the structures and functions implicated in sleep. Although the term "homology" can be defined briefly: "Homology means common ancestry" (Bock, 1969a), what constitutes a homologous structure or function may present formidable difficulties. Bock proposes the following formal definition of homology: "Homologous features or conditions of features in two or more organisms are those that can be traced back phylogenetically to the same feature or condition in the immediate common ancestor of these organisms." He states further that homology is defined in terms of phylogeny but that the definition of phylogeny can still be independent: "Phylogeny is the lineages of animals and plants resulting from their descent through time. Organisms evolve and leave a trail of phylogeny behind them."

The term "homologous" can be used appropriately in a relativistic sense. Thus, the wings of birds and the wings of bats are regarded as homologous in terms of tetrapod forelimbs, or the cerebellar hemispheres of man and the chimpanzee are homologous as mammalian or primate conditions. However, the application of the term "homology" becomes progressively more valuable the more exclusively and narrowly these features can be defined. Thus, for example, if the sleep record of a chimpanzee and of man were more similar than that of man and the gorilla, the term "homologous" could not be applied with respect to the sleep records of the man and the chimpanzee unless it could be demonstrated that there is a closely shared ancestral linkage. The issue however is still not a simple one, for particular structural or functional features could be similar by way of independent origin in unrelated phyletic lines (parallelism), or the sharing process could be a result of convergent evolution. Unfortunately, what is not homologous is much more reliably determined than what could be homologous. Nevertheless, as Broughton (1972) has indicated the search for homologous neural structures subserving sleep mechanisms is essential.

SLEEP STUDIES IN SUBMAMMALIAN VERTEBRATES

This section will be devoted to discussing the sleep findings in submammalian vertebrates. The number of studies in this area is small, so that an excursion into the possible origin and evolution of sleep behavior and its neurophysiological and neuroanatomical correlates remains speculative.

The sleep researcher is obliged to live with an uncomfortably large amount of scientific uncertainty. The enigmas confronting the biologist's efforts to deal with the fossil record, ancestral lineages, homologies, speciation, and so forth, do not set the stage too reassuringly for sleep investigations. Although it is imprecise to organize the classes of vertebrates into a simple ascending ordinal sequence where the fishes initiate the history of vertebrate evolution and are then closely followed by the amphibia, reptiles, birds and mammals, nevertheless, for the purposes of exposition, such a plan may prove satisfactory.

Fishes

A search of the literature reveals that behavioral observations of fishes in "sleep," let alone in states of inactivity, are scanty. One reason is the absence of adequate electrophysiological and telemetering devices appropriate to scientific inquiry in a water medium. Apart from a number of separate descriptive reports concerning states of inactivity, the most valuable fish studies have been written by Weber (1961), and more recently by Starck and Davis (1966).

Weber's studies were conducted at the Berlin Aquarium and at other leading European aquaria. His article discusses the posture and resting niches of approximately 200 different species of fishes. He states that during quiescence or sleep fish generally place their fins smoothly against their bodies, but not infrequently the fins may also be extended away from the body. Generally speaking, genuine sleep is accomplished when the animal has no fear of enemies and can find protection in a secure hiding place. The exceptions to this generalization are occasionally seen in specimens retained in captivity. Broadly speaking, fishes are always prepared to respond to danger in order to fight or flee. He points out that although sensitivity to stimuli is exquisite, this sensitivity is diminished in unambiguous sleep. He supports this statement by relating how he was able to deal roughly with certain fishes before bringing them to a state of alertness. Unambiguous sleep is characterized by definite sleeping positions. Fishes may lie flat against a rock or in the sand, or they may wedge themselves head down into a crevice. Some species wedge themselves head up. Generally, the species of fishes which tend to hide often require several minutes of stimulation, for example, powerful illumination, before they leave their resting place. It is not uncommon for a fish to sleep under an overhanging ledge, appearing pressed up like a balloon against the ceiling.

Weber reminds us that except for a few sharks, the eyes of fishes have neither lids nor nictitating membranes. Fishes which stir up the ground or break the water in leaving it, such as Periophthalmus, loaches, the eel (*Anguilla canariensis Val.*), and the lungfish (*Protopterus annectens Owen*), have so-called spectacles (transparent tissue protecting the cornea).

The majority of fish are diurnal. Deep sea fish, as well as the eel, flat fish, and catfish belong to the nocturnal group. Most pelagic fishes avoid contact with solid bodies while most bottom fish are strongly inclined to hide between plants and rocks, in crevices and tunnels, or dig themselves into the sand or mud.

Evidence at hand suggests that conventionally defined sleep is seen predominantly in marine species. Weber indicates that many species of marine fishes which bury themselves in the sand leave the mouth and an eye exposed to the water. He observes that certain labrids are in a sleeping position when the eyeball is rotated to a point where the iris is not visible. This finding suggests how a fish is able to protect himself from optic stimulation.

His experience with sharks was limited. However, he mentions that one of the species, *Galeorhinus canus,* living in the North Sea, belongs to the perpetual swimmers, who are on the move all their life. He queries whether some of these perpetual swimmers might not be able to sleep even while swimming.

Some species of sharks have eyelids, as mentioned above, while certain genera exclusively possess the nictitating membranes. He mentions one shark, *Ginglymostoma cirratum*, which sleeps during the daytime within rock crevices and remains undisturbed by divers. The data suggest that the arousal threshold is high since this shark can be roughly grabbed by the tail before he awakens and very speedily swims away.

Nocturnal fish tend to remain in dark places during the daytime but with the onset of darkness begin their predatory activities. Certain nocturnal species, however, seem to be inactive even at night. Catfish are alleged to show fairly well defined rest-activity periods. Practically all species of cichlids fall into that group of fresh water fish in which rest can be clearly observed. In nature, most of the fresh water fish indigenous to the streams of Germany revealed no definitive sleep. Weber has made the interesting observation that *Idus idus* distribute themselves beneath the water surface in the Berlin Aquarium, while members of the same species lay on the sandy bottom in the Antwerp Aquarium. He indicates that this is an astonishing finding in that the resting habits of other species tend to be the same despite change of habitat.

Weber goes on to state that not all fish of the sea and inner waters reveal behavioral differences by day and night. Aside from the above-mentioned shark species there are other fish which never rest and which presumably swim while asleep. He mentions in particular the mackerel, *Scomber scombrus*, the tuna fish, *Thunnus thynnus*, and arowina, the sword fish *Osteoglossum bicirrhosum*, a fresh water giant from Brazil and the Guianas. Two species of sturgeons, *Acipenser sturio* and *A. ruthenus*, have not been seen to rest.

Numerous observations have been made of the number of gill beats per minute which indicate a definite diminution during the transition to rest. The rate in the dwarf catfish went from 40 to 30 per minute, in the cod from 60 to 25 per minute, in the goldfish (*Carassius auratus*) from 175 to 40 per minute, and in the *Epalzeorhynchus kalopterus* (Asian Cyprinid) from 19 to 10 per minute from the active to the quiet state. (Weber, 1961).

Of particular interest to the sleep researcher concerned with homeothermy and slow wave sleep are the studies by Carey (1973) of two groups of warm blooded fishes, the tunas and the mackerel sharks. Members of these families of fishes possess an unusual vascular network, the "rete mirabile," which is specialized in some way to serve the purpose of thermoregulation. The rete mirabile refers to the vascular distribution in warm-blooded fishes. Whereas in cold-blooded fishes the major blood vessels course along the vertebral column and radiate out to the small vessels, in the warm-blooded fishes the cutaneous vessels carry most of the blood, and from there the blood supply is shunted to the muscles. Carey found that at a water temperature of 5°C, the body temperature of the bluefin tuna registered 26°C. At a water temperature of 35°C, the temperature of the fish was almost 34°C. Thus the bluefin tuna has to a large extent mammalian-like thermoregulatory control. The other members of the tuna family as well as the mackerel sharks reveal unquestionably the capacity for adjusting their body temperatures significantly above water temperatures, although not precisely in line with that observed in the bluefin tuna. The tunas and mackerel sharks are among the fastest and most powerful predators in the sea. We recall that the former group are teleosts while the latter group belong to the elasmobranchs. These two unrelated groups of fishes reveal by their specialized capacity to raise their body temperatures an adaptive advantage of increased swimming speed by virtue of the extra power available to them from warm muscles. As will be noted subsequently in this chapter, it has been proposed that slow wave sleep and homeothermy could be significantly correlated (Van Twyver and Allison, 1972). A study of these species of fishes would aid us in determining whether homeothermy and neural structures, alleged to serve slow wave sleep, reveal a significant correlation.

In the continued search for biological correlates of the sleep patterns from a phylogenetic standpoint, Allison et. al. (1972) have proposed that the evolution of paradoxical sleep in the mammalian lineage might be linked to the development of viviparity in the early therian mammals. This speculation would oblige us to be familiar with which classes, orders, and species of vertebrates give birth to living young. Romer indicates that "in various sharks and rays the fertilized eggs are retained in the mother's reproductive tract, and develop there so that the young are born alive. (A limited number of reptiles and nearly all mammals have similarly developed this procedure.)" In addition to the cartilaginous fishes a small number of teleosts and amphibians are viviparous (Romer, 1970). It is hoped that some of these avenues of inquiry that have been put forth might stimulate investigators interested in sleep from a comparative and phylogenetic standpoint.

To my knowledge, the only polygraphic study of sleep of fishes was carried out by Peyrethon and Dusan-Peyrethon (1967). They implanted 25 tenches (*Tinca tinca*, a species of cyprinid) during their period of inactivity (from October to May). They recorded cerebral activity, EMG, respiration (gill movement) and ECG. They claimed that there was no evidence of variations in cerebral activity in any of the states of activity and rest and paradoxical (REM) sleep was not found.

A study was carried out by the author in collaboration with Elliot D. Weitzman (Tauber and Weitzman, 1969) of certain Bermuda reef fish involving detailed behavioral and physiologic observations during the activity-inactivity cycle of two families of foveate reef fish, (wrasses: *Irideo bivittata*, and parrot fish, *Scarus guacamaia, Scarus vetula, Scarus coeruleus, Sparisoma viride, Sparisoma abildgaardi, Sparisoma squalidum, Sparisoma croicensis, Sparisoma aurofrenatum*). Observations of eye movements, respiratory rate, fin and body movements, and color patterns were made on fish maintained in sea water tanks under a natural 24 day-night lighting as well as in a controlled light-dark laboratory regimen. During the dark phase prolonged diminution of activity, an irregular respiratory rate, and decreased responsiveness to alerting stimuli occurred manifested by a tolerance to handling. Independent (non-conjugate) eye movements were clearly present during periods of prolonged behavioral inactivity. For several hours all species of parrot fish had at least two to four eye movements for 30 second periods while inactive. The tanks in which the fish were placed were screened off so that the experimenter could make observations under very diminished illumination. While at the Bermuda Biological Station, Doctor Robert Johannes, on a diving expedition, made several underwater observations of the eye movements of a sleeping surgeon fish (*Acanthurus coeruleus*). In addition, complete inactivity of numerous species of fishes was noted in the Bermuda aquarium during nighttime observation. A puddingwife (*Halichoeres radiatus*) with head and one eye exposed above the sand in its tank was observed to have bursts of eye movement activity.

During the last year and a half, blueheads (*Thalassoma bifasciatum*), Spanish hogfish (*Bodianus rufus*), and puddingwife (*Halichoeres radiatus*), species of wrasses (family Labridae), were under observation in hundred-gallon tanks in which a 12 hour light-dark cycle was employed. Several of the fishes lived under this lighting regimen for three to four months whereas others died after several weeks and were then replaced. Once darkness super-vened and sleep oocurred, it was possible to touch these fishes for periods up to several minutes and to raise them almost to the surface of the water in the tank before they would awaken and rapidly swim off. Observations of eye movements were difficult to obtain, but when the eye was clearly discernable, frequent eye movements could be noted as the fish lay on the sand or under the sand, providing the head was appropriately exposed (Tauber and Briggs, unpublished data).

Broughton (1972) has indicated that in cyclostomes, plagiostomes, teleosts, and ganoids, the brain and the brainstem in particular evolve rapidly in respect to the possible neural structures subserving sleep mechanisms. There is claimed to be present a reticular formation and definitive reticular nuclei such as the nucleus reticularis inferior (vagal region), a nucleus reticularis medius (level of the vestibular nerve), nucleus reticularis superior in the midbrain region, and a nucleus reticularis mesencephali extending from the level of the oculomotor nucleus to the posterior commissure. These are small in number in lampreys but increase in number in cartilaginous and bony fishes. The medulla of teleosts contains two large Mauthner cells with descending pathways for the control of tail movemeets. In addition, there are primary and secondary connections with the lateral line and vestibular nuclei, the cerebellum, the sensory nucleus of the fifth nerve, and the superior colliculus. A raphé grouping of the reticular cells is not present at any level, although scattered cells lie in the raphé region in certain car-tilaginous and bony fishes. A locus coeruleus has not been clearly recognized.

The lateral line and vestibular systems with their nuclei show marked development in the higher fishes. The following vestibular nuclei are present in teleosts: the descending, the lateral, superior, and the so-called tangential vestibular nuclei. A medial vestibular nucleus is not present. Therefore the various anatomical centers allegely responsible for mammalian sleep are not fully present in fishes (Broughton, 1972).

Can one draw any reliable inferences concerning neural structures in fishes in relation to sleep in fishes? If we assume that sleep is present in certain families of teleosts (for example, parrot fish) but is not present in certain other families of teleosts (for example, cyprinids) can we assume that there are significant differences in their respective neural structures? One of the simplest assumptions that could be made is that there are certain requisite neural structures? One of the simplest assumptions that could be made is that there are certain requisite neural structures without which behavioral sleep is impossible. Broughton has indicated that one does not find the full complement of anatomical centers responsible for mammalian sleep in the fish. He suggests, however, that it is conceivable that certain fish might be able to enter a state comparable to quiet sleep through the medium of pre-optic inhibition of the brainstem reticular formation. He is able to extend the speculation to the possibility of there being phasic discharges transported by the vestibular and ocular neural circuits inducing a state similar to active or REM sleep despite the absence of the locus coeruleus. In the report on Bermuda reef fish (Tauber and Weitzman, 1969) it was concluded that not only was behavioral sleep present but also that the type of sleep observed was associated with continuous rapid eye movements. These findings in the reef fish may represent the earliest present evidence from a phylogenetic stand-point of REM sleep with its tonic and phasic components.

If one considers environmental conditions in the broadest sense as determinants of sleep patterns similarly to the fruitful manner in which such studies have been conducted by Bert (Bert and Collomb, 1966; Bert et. al., 1967, 1970, a, b) and Pegram (Pegram et. al., 1969) for primates, it is most likely that additional knowledge would accrue on the subject of sleep in fishes. It is my own impression, however, that lower vertebrates tolerate modifications of environmental conditions very poorly. This seems to be particularly the case for marine species. Many of the fresh water fishes would of course be much easier to deal with under experimental conditions, but convincingly discriminable rest-activity cycles similar to those observed in certain marine species have not been reported for fresh water fish. A further disadvantage is that the visual-oculomotor system of the majority of fresh water species is less highly developed than that in marine species.

In attempting to examine the role of different environmental challenges upon the sleep patterns of animals, (Allison and Van Twyver, 1970), active, powerful predators sleep more deeply than do animals who are preyed upon. These latter animals are alleged to sleep more fitfully for survival reasons, so as to be able to take flight easily. One can suspect that predator/prey relationships for terrestrial animals and animals of the sea, in particular the littoral species of fishes, share certain similarities of challenge. Pelagic species, on the other hand, occupying huge expanses of open waters, require different modes of adaptation for survival. Competition for food could be extremely challenging. However, one could imagine that with adequate camouflage or great speed, many fishes might survive surprisingly well. It would be interesting to know much more about how the numerous species of perpetual swimmers, such as certain species of sharks, rays, and mackerels, among others, deprived of the usual rest time provided by sleep, manage to avoid becoming preyed upon. It would be of considerable interest to determine whether some form of sleep, such as microsleep, exists for this group of fishes. It will also be of great value to study the possible sleep patterns of the warm-blooded fishes mentioned above, particularly in respect to the relationship of homeothermy and slow wave sleep.

Although there is clear evidence of behavioral sleep in numerous species of fishes (Weber, 1961), the switch to wakefulness may occur extremely quickly under some conditions of stimulation. There may be a specialized neural switching mechanism which requires only a relatively light stimulus to instantly awaken the fish. This possibility makes us continue to examine how we conceptualize the arousal threshold. Under some conditions the amplitude of the stimulus may be the sole determinant in producing arousal. Under other conditions a selective factor may be more important than the amplitude of the input signal.

Amphibians

The first description of in vivo brain potentials in amphibians was reported by Gerard and Young (1937) for *Rana catesbiana and Rana pipiens.* These early workers recorded various patterns of electrical activity depending upon the brain area selected. Segura and de Juan (1966) carried out a study over a period of two years of the EEG pattern of chronically implanted nonanaesthetized or freely moving toads (*Bufo arenarum Hensel*). Seasonal variations in the spontaneous electrical activity of the brain, as well as in the EEG responses to sudden changes in illumination were found. During spring and summer they detected "alpha-like" rhythm over the olfactory bulb and forebrain in over 90 percent of their recordings. At that time of year, during inactivity, spindles were very prominent. Simultaneously a striking increase in frequency and voltage of recorded brain potentials, as well as a high sensitivity to changes in illumination were observed. During the winter despite maintenance of the same environmental conditions "alpha-like" discharges were present in only 6.6 percent of recordings. In addition, spindles were completely abolished and there was a definite reduction in the evoked responses to changes of lighting.

The first studies of sleep-wakefulness behavior in amphibians were conducted in Hobson's laboratory (Hobson, 1967). He observed that the bullfrog, *Rana catesbiana*, revealed neither electrographic criteria nor threshold criteria for sleep in the laboratory and that this species appears to maintain vigilance at rest during daytime hours in the field. He subsequently studied several species of tree frogs (Hobson, et. al., 1968) of the genus Hyla in order to compare and contrast the findings obtained under laboratory conditions. *H. squirella* and *H. cinerea*, nocturnally active species, appeared to be in a resting state by day. Unless directly stimulated, these specimens were immobile and the eyes were closed. If stimulation was sufficiently intense the posture was modified, the eyes were open, and they would occasionally leap to a neighboring plant. The author inferred that the elevation of arousal threshold was sufficient to permit one to state that these frogs demonstrated behavioral sleep. A different species, *H. septentrionalis*, manifested similar behavior in nature however the behavior of these specimens in the laboratory differed from that seen in the field. They tended to be inert and nonreactive unless heavily stimulated and therefore appeared to be constantly asleep or "torpid." Following persistent stimulation however the full complement of motor responses was evoked. Activity or alertness and inactivity or torpor, and their accompanying electrographic manifestations in hylids were similar to those observed in ranids. EEG synchronization was associated with activity and alertness while torpor was associated with a relatively low-voltage fast EEG. Of importance was the observation of a close positive correlation between EEG synchronization and respiratory rate. Muscle tone did not change with respect to the state of torpor nor was there evidence of ocular motility. Hobson concluded that the tree frogs in contrast to the bullfrog revealed a type of behavioral sleep more clearly resembling mammalian behavioral sleep.

McGinty and Lucas (1972) selected the tiger salamander (*Ambystoma tigrinum*) for their study of sleep in amphibians. Behavioral activity in the tiger salamander is characterized by an elevated head, locomotion, biting at food, and withdrawal movements. The quiescent periods are manifested solely by inactivity and a lowered head. They reported no eye movements other than blinks during quiescence. The EEG characteristics of their adult specimens revealed low-voltage nonsynchronous waves similar to that seen during wakefulness in mammals. The EEG did not show any persistent alterations in frequency or synchrony associated with the one or the other behavioral condition. They did note, however, that there was a small increase in amplitude during periods of arousal or orienting behavior. A brief period of synchronization following respiration was noted, similar to that found in the frog. These authors carried out a power-spectral analysis of the EEG in order to locate the beginnings of synchronizing and desynchronizing processes. Contrasting larval forebrain with adult forebrain EEG recordings, they noted that amplitude was lower in the former than in the latter. They also reported that synchronization and amplitude elevations associated with respiration and orienting were absent. They were able to define regular cycles of activity and inactivity by quantifying the frequency of body movements. They obtained a 4 hour ultradian rest-activity cycle in either light or dark periods within the 24 hour day. Since equivalent cycles were noted from August through November, the authors point out that it is intrinsic and distinct from circadian and seasonal variations. They concluded that the salamander manifests the same behavioral appearance of sleep in a cyclic fashion as do higher verterbrates. Furthermore, they are of the opinion that the observed behavioral events in the salamander must be the precursors of quiet sleep, despite the fact that the EEG criteria associated with mammalian sleep do not appear. No evidence for active REM sleep was found in this amphibian.

Returning to the question of neural structures in the amphibian brain, Broughton (1972) states that the reticular nuclear groupings present in cyclostomes, plagiostomes, teleosts and ganoids are not generally present in the amphibian brain. The larval-tailed amphibians have a Mauthner cell. This cell is absent in tailless anurans. There are no main reticular nuclei although there are scattered reticular cell groupings near the oculomotor nerve nuclei. Raphe groups and the locus coeruleus are absent. Although there is no evidence of descending or medial vestibular nuclei, superior vestibular nuclei, tangential vestibular nuclei, and homologues of the lateral vestibular nuclei are found. As Broughton has indicated, active sleep would seem inconceivable in the absence of reticular pontine nuclei, medial and descending vestibular nuclei, and the locus coeruleus. It would also seem equally improbable to predict the presence of quiet sleep in the absence of raphé nuclei and other brainstem reticular nuclei.

It has been emphasized above that the number of sleep studies in amphibians is still so limited that it is difficult for this reviewer to draw any formal conclusions about their sleep. Behavioral and electrographic criteria referable to active (paradoxical) sleep present no challenge since both the frogs and the salamander do not reveal it. Whether one can define a sleep state despite the absence of slow waves (even though such electrical patterns are not to be expected in the amphibian brain), is an open question. Perhaps further studies in amphibians will allow us to avoid arbitrariness as well as prematurity of decision. An initial approach to the resolution of the question of sleep in amphibians might consist of acquiring a wider familiarity with the types of amphibian adaptation. Of the three orders of amphibians (Gymnophiona, Caudata, and Salientia), the Salientia offer the most promising representatives for study, both because of their worldwide distribution, and the large number of species. Except for the exclusively waterless desert areas and the coldest areas of the globe, frogs and toads are found in the warmest climates and in cold regions such as the high Andes, Himalayas, Alaska, and certain parts of the Arctic circle. Certain highly poisonous species found in the families Bufonidae and Dendrobatidae whose skin secretions are so lethal as to discourage predation might be valuable for sudy. Many members of both families and in particular the "arrow-poison" group must be rarely confronted with enemies. Undisturbed sleep, at least in mature specimens, might be expected.

It would appear from various ecological analyses (Allison and Van Twyver, 1970) that in the mammalian class at least, the "good" sleepers consist of animals that are powerful, can defend themselves successfully and can find a safe place of concealment, such as a den or burrow. The "poor" sleepers among the mammals are surface dwellers who rely primarily on vigilance and the capacity for flight. In the case of amphibians, it is of course impossible to present with accuracy a fair assessment of their success in concealing themselves since they are objects of prey desired by fishes when they are in the larval stage, and by reptiles, birds, and mammals when they reach maturity. Thus, in attempting to determine which species might have maximum chances of survival, it would seem reasonable to assume that the highly poisonous members in a class of vertebrates otherwise defenseless would possess a valuable protective adaptation.

It was pointed out previously that among the more important somatic modifications observed in the emergence and evolution of tetrapods was the development of the tongue. Certainly in anurans the tongue is very important despite the fact that there are some species that are tongueless. One might anticipate that the elegantly precise tongue movements called for in anurans would be reflected in those areas of the brainstem responsible for its control. As a consequence it would be valuable for electrographic implantations to place electrodes in the neural tissues extending behind the level of the vagal accessory complex into the cervical region of the spinal cord in order to monitor its activity during different behavioral states. The salamanders and frogs do not have a hypoglossal nerve despite evidence of its presence in the ancestors of tetrapods. It is stated that its absence in frogs and salamanders represents one of the degenerate characters of these animal orders. (Romer, 1970).

The technical problems associated with chronic implantations of the tongue may not be too formidable since its root attachment is at the base anteriorally of the lower jaw in frogs and toads. The search for evidence of phasic activity in these lower vertebrates is worth pursuing in that motor correlates of these neural discharges during sleep have so far not been found. It is conceivable that tongue movements might be present during periods of quiescence or quiet sleep.

If behavioral sleep is absent in the amphibian class, and if electrographic evidence of sleep is also lacking, the absence of a neural substrate subserving sleep would be perfectly reasonable. If, on the other hand, the existence of behavioral sleep is validated in the absence of correlated electrographic evidence, then one is confronted with a puzzling question. It would imply that other neural mechanisms must be responsible for mediating physiological sleep. It seems inconceivable to conclude that there are no definitive neuroanatomical and neurophysiological correlates of behavioral sleep, even if those substrates are not the same as those found in birds and mammals.

Reptiles

Among the various schemata for classifying vertebrates is that of dividing them into Anamniota and Amniota. In the former grouping one refers to a mode of reproduction in which eggs are laid in the water and the young develop in the water. In the latter grouping, comprised of reptiles, birds and certain mammals, a shelled egg is present. Although nearly all mammals bear their young alive and some reptiles do the same, the general pattern of embryonic development is similar. The term amniota is, of course, derived form the word amnion, one of the membranes surrounding the growing embryo in reptiles, birds, and mammals. The reptiles are divided into five orders: Chelonians (turtles and tortoises), crocodilians (crocodiles, alligators, and their relatives), saurians (lizards), serpentes (snakes), and rhynchocephalians (the tuatara).

Initial studies of sleep have been reported in all these orders except in the rhynchocephalian with its only extant species, the tuatara. It is in the reptilian class that one observes the striking diversity and specialization of adaptation, and it is in this class of vertebrates that most concerted efforts can be usefully directed at elucidating sleep behavior and sleep mechanism. The earliest polygraphic study of sleep was carried out on the margined tortoise (*Testudo marginata Schopfer*) (Herman, et al., 1964). Behavioral sleep was observed and electrographic studies revealed slow wave sleep, however, paradoxical (REM) sleep was not found. Following that earlier study many sleep researchers were inclined to suspect that paradoxical(REM) sleep was limited solely to mammals and birds, although in the latter class paradoxical sleep had been found to be of short duration and referred to as rudimentary. More recent studies of sleep in Chelonians have revealed results at variance with one another (Vasilescu, 1970 a, b; Flanigan, 1972).

Flanigan (1972) has correctly suggested that unanimity of observations has been difficult for many reasons, not the least of which could be limitations in methodological rigor. Later inquiries have profited from technical precision and greater familiarity with the animals under study. However, one cannot underestimate the effect of environmental conditions that can influence the outcome of any sleep study in lower vertebrates. Unfortunately, it is not always easy to pinpoint the specific role a particular external input may play in determining the ultimate results.

Vasilescu (1970 a, b) reported behavioral sleep and electrographic evidence of slow wave sleep and suggestive paradoxical sleep in the European pond turtle (*Emys orbicularis*). Of particular interest is the observation during wakefulness of a slight increase in frequency and amplitude of electrocortical activity associated with an arousal reaction. During slow wave sleep there was a slowing of the rhythm to approximately six cycles per second. During paradoxical sleep, marked reduction in the EMG associated with occasional phasic bursts, fast or slow eye movements either isolated or in bursts, and EEG activation was noted. The author stated that paradoxical sleep was observed in 15 percent of their animals (sample: 33 animals). Parenthetically, there is a similar American species, Blanding's turtle (*Emys Blanding*) (Schmidt and Inger, 1957), which is found primarily in the Great Lakes region of North America, illustrating a type of "disjunct distribution" which might permit a fruitful comparative study.

The eastern North American box turtle (*Terrapene carolina*) and the red-footed tortoise (*Geochelonia carbonaria*) from northern South America, were studied by Flanigan (1972). His decision to study Chelonians was based upon the recognition that this vertebrate order is phyletically quite separate from other reptilian orders. In his methodological approach, he defined sleep as a behavior requiring enumeration of particular criteria supporting that behavior. In brief, he mentioned 1) a stereotypic or species specific posture, 2) maintenance of physical quiescence, 3) an elevation of arousal threshold reflected in the intensity of an arousing stimulus and/or the frequency, latency or duration of an arousal response, and 4) state reversibility with stimulation. Since all these criteria were met, he indicated that behavioral sleep was present in these vertebrates. The EEG pattern during wakefulness and sleep varied only slightly. Thus cortical frequencies during arousal ranged from 4 to 26 Hz; the frequency range diminished to 2 to 21 Hz during quiescence. During arousal the amplitudes reached 19 μV and only reached 11 μV during quiescence. Sleep spindles, epochs of slow wave sleep and paradoxical sleep were not recorded in the turtle during behavioral sleep. Eye movements, both conjugate and nonconjugate, were present during wakefulness but were not recorded during quiescence. The author was impressed with the observation of large amplitude arrhythmic "spikes" in the turtle EEG recording. They occurred monophasically (30 to 50 msec duration) or polyphasically in a low- or high- voltage form (10 to 50 μV). These telencephalic spikes occurred at a rate of approximately one every 4 to 5 seconds and were highly correlated with behavioral quiescence. Spontaneous or induced arousal obliterated this spiking. During respiration high voltage spikes were present in the tectal derivations but were usually absent in the cortex. Since spiking has been observed in other reptilian species, in some amphibians, and many mammals, the author indicated that one might reasonably infer that ancient reptiles as well as those ancestral to birds and mammals may have exhibited a similar electrophysiological phenomenon. It would seem that these particular spikes represent one of the consistent electrophysiological findings throughout the vertebrate kingdom during sleep (Flanigan, 1972). Further studies will be required to clarify the significance of these spikes.

Studies of sleep in the crocodilians have been confined to *Caiman sclerops*

(Flanigan, et. al., in press) and *Caiman latirostris* (Peyrethon and Dusan-Peyrethon, 1969). The selection of the *Caiman sclerops* in Rechtschaffen's laboratory was determined by its being more closely related via ancient evolutionary lineages to birds and mammals than other living reptiles. As in the turtles, alterations in the EEG in the *Caiman* are minimal during behavioral sleep or quiescence) frequencies and amplitudes diminished only slightly. During wakefulness and arousal the frequency ranged from 5 to 26 Hz and the voltage reached 63 μV. During quiescence electrocortical activity ranged from 2 to 22 Hz with amplitudes up to 33 μV. Similar to the findings in the turtle there was an absence of spindles, slow wave sleep, and paradoxical sleep during behavioral sleep. No eye movements were recorded during behavioral quiescence and were rare during wakefulness. The telencephalic spikes observed in the *Caiman* ranged from 150 to 200 μV in amplitude and again spike frequency varied inversely with arousal, i.e., the greater the number of spikes noted the more prominent was behavioral quiescence.

Peyrethon and Dusan-Peyrethon (1967) also observed behavioral sleep in *Caiman latirostris*, reporting in addition the presence in their single specimen of mammalian-like paradoxical (active) sleep.

The first study of sleep behavior in lizards was carried out in two species of chameleons: *Chameleo jacksoni* and *Chameleo melleri* (Tauber, et. al., 1966). The choice of these species was determined by the fact of the lizard's being phylogenetically more advanced than the turtle. In addition, it was assumed that since the chameleon reveals a very highly developed visual-oculomotor organization with highly developed spontaneous voluntary eye movements during wakefulness, that this oculomotor patterning might be reflected during some stage of sleep. Evidence of behavioral quiescence and diminished response to arousal is striking in that the animal typically settles on a branch in the hours immediately prior to sunset, curls up his tail in watch spring fashion, and remains still; however, constant independent scanning eye movements of widely ranging angular travel persist. During this state prior to sleep, the lizard not only does not attack insects but ignores crickets which alight on his body. The head and belly come to rest on the branch and the clawed feet assume a loose straddling position in contrast to the tight grasping posture during wakefulness. The eyelids close in a circular manner and the eyeballs are slightly retracted. Unless disturbed, the animal will generally remain in this position throughout the night. During this behavioral sleep state, rapid eye movements can be clearly observed beneath the closed lids and occur in short bursts ranging from 1 to 7 minutes but are observed to last even up to 12 minutes duration. After several months of of direct observation, stainless steel wire electrodes were implanted on the forebrain surface for chronic recordings.

The EEG tracings in *C. melleri* revealed three different patterns correlated with three different behavioral states. During alert or vigilant behavior, frequency and amplitude were 10 to 12 Hz and 30 to 35 μV, respectively. When the animal appeared drowsy, there was a slowing to 7-9 Hz with roughly a 20 percent increase in voltage. Bursts of spikes at 4 to 6 Hz and of higher voltage emerged with behavioral sleep. The overall rhythmic activity then dropped slightly further, to 6-8 Hz alternating with lower voltage 13 to 18 Hz waves. The spikes appeared singly or in short clusters of 60 to 80 μV every 5 to 12 seconds. They completely disappeared with spontaneous or induced return to vigilance. EMG recording from neck and tail musculature revealed little change between that observed during wakefulness and behavioral sleep and at no time was there a sharp or sustained diminution of muscle tone. Heart rate averaged 18 to 22 beats per minute during alertness and 11 to 14 beats per minute during sleep. Quantitative estimations of arousal threshold were not determined nor was there evidence of a rapid state reversibility. Convincing criteria defining behavioral sleep and easily observable episodes of individual eye movements, as well as eye movement clusters during that state, led us to infer that the chameleon demonstrated a REM sleep state. Electrographic data failed to reveal even short epochs of mammalian-like slow waves so that the expected contrast in electrocortical recordings differentiating slow wave sleep from REM sleep observable in mammals was not present. In addition, the EMG recording was not sufficiently impressive to be comparable with respect to the hypotonia observed in the REM state in many mammals.

The behavioral criteria distinguishing wakefulness and sleep in the diurnal Mexican lizard (*Ctenosaura pectinata*) (Tauber et al., 1968b) presented no difficulties (23 adult specimens made up the sample for study). If in a state of relaxed wakefulness, the lizard was approached too closely, it would assume an attacking posture or would attempt to take flight. Voluntary independent eye movements in the presence or absence of head movements were easily observed. Alertness in the iguana, however, is in no way similar to what one familiarly observes in mammals, since its responses are so strikingly stimulus dependent. Behavioral sleep is characterized by complete flattening of the body and head upon the surface on which it is lying. The eyes are closed and in this condition one can touch and handle the animal gently, an action which would not otherwise be tolerated. Electrode implantation in the telencephalon (pyriform cortex and hippocampus) and midbrain tegmentum revealed predominant frequencies between 15 and 18 Hz and amplitudes between 15 and 50 μV during relaxed wakefulness. EMG amplitude was generally between 10 and 15 μV and the heart rate was 18 to 22 beats per minute. Different brain areas revealed voltage asymmetries. Spontaneous spikes were recorded irregularly from the forebrain and less often from the midbrain. These spikes were present during wakefulness and sleep and did not reveal correlation with the behavioral state. Of particular interest was the observation that habituation was very poorly developed in the iguana. Repeated entrance into the experimental room consistently evoked a behavioral and electrographic response. Eye movements were immediately increased in number as the experimenter was entering the room. This was followed immediately by the development of an attacking posture. The EEG arousal reaction consisted primarily of an amplitude augmentation even up to 200 μV with occasional frequency increases to 22 Hz. These electrographic responses were seen in forebrain and midbrain derivations but were not consistently symmetric. Of additional interest were the effects of sensory evoked stimulations resulting from visual-photic stimuli but the absence of evoked responses resulting from a variety of auditory stimuli. Sleep was characterized electrographically by an overall reduction of amplitude in forebrain and midbrain leads with the frequency ranging between 13 and 15 Hz. Arousal threshold increased progressively during the sleep period as tested by sensory stimulation as well as electrical stimulation of the midbrain reticular formation. The increase in arousal threshold plateaued at about midnight. During the first 2 or 3 hours after sleep onset, eye movements were not present, but thereafter single eye movements or a run of eye movements on either one or both sides, were recorded. The nighttime recording was done during darkness. The authors considered the eye movement findings as reliable since daytime recordings with eyes open or closed correlated with behavioral observations of eye movements. During sleep the heart rate slowed to 14 beats per minute from 18-22 beats per minute and occasional extra systoles were observed. The EMG showed only variable diminution throughout sleep.

In an unpublished communication M. Jeannerod, in respect to sleep studies in the skink, another lizard, wrote the following:

> I never published the skink material, for two reasons. First, I could record only one (the other two died). Second, I was never totally convinced that the "eye movements" I recorded were not artifacts: they always occurred when the animal was buried in the sand, and I could never observe them directly. The animal had fundamentally three stages of behavior. One was with motor activity such as crawling. Another was with behavior immobility, but with clear respiratory spindles at 5 to 10 per minute. The third one, with no respiratory spindles, low heart rate, and occasionally bursts of "eye movements" at a high frequency, and lasting for about 20 seconds or more. I would be personally very cautious in attributing these episodes to paradoxical sleep.

Peyrethon and Dusan-Peyrethon (1969) reported irregular cerebral activity with a frequency of 30 to 35 Hz and an average amplitude of 50 μV during wakefulness in an iguana (*Iguana iguana*). In addition, they noted the presence of diphasic waves lasting 250 msec and occurring approximately every 2 minutes. The amplitude of the waves was 100 μV. Respiratory rate was irregular at 20 breaths per minute. EMG activity was at a high level; nonconjugate eye movements were present. Cardiac rate was 17 to 20 beats per minute. Wakefulness averaged 25 percent of the total recording time, 50 percent of it during the day and 15 percent during the night. The iguana could be aroused from the beginnings of sleep by audio-visual stimuli and showed at that time orienting behavior — opening of the eyes and elevation of the head. During somnolence the cerebral tracing was identical with that of wakefulness but as soon as the eyes closed, frequency of the diphasic waves increased and there was some diminution in muscle tone. Respirations became slower. Once behavioral sleep occurred, eye movements ceased and auditory stimuli of great intensity were required to produce a change in state. There was progressive slowing of cerebral activity. The diphasic waves were still present while the EMG was almost totally abolished. At no time during behavioral sleep were eye movements observed. Unfortunately, the report was made on only one specimen and in addition, no information was given with respect to environmental temperatures, which frequently are critically correlated with different behavioral states.

As part of their report the authors studied one Caiman (*Caiman latirostris*). They observed in this species also irregular cerebral activity at 7-8 Hz with an amplitude of 20 μV. Superimposed on the background activity one could observe diphasic waves of 150 μV averaging 3 per minute. These waves correlated with the degree of attention, thus their frequency increased when the animal was stimulated by noise or light. They diminished on the other hand, with closure of the eyes. Cardiac rate was regular at 30 beats per minute. EMG recording was at a relatively high amplitude. Somnolence quickly followed wakefulness. The animal lay extended on the sand with its eyes closed with an occasional opening of one or the other lid. Electrographic activity showed slowing and there was progressive diminution of muscle tonus. This state was then followed by more evident behavioral sleep. The eyes were closed and there was no longer reaction to different auditory stimuli. With the reduction in EEG activity there was a concurrent diminution in muscle tone with amplitudes always less than 10 μV. Careful observation of the animal and of the polygraphic recording permitted one to observe during the course of behavioral sleep, short periods of 50 seconds duration characterized by rapid EEG activity, identical with that of wakefulness but the amplitude of which was the same as that observed during slow sleep. EMG was then consistently below 10 μV and rapid eye movements were recorded. There were also rapid small contractions of the digits of the forelimbs. Each period lasted an average of 50 seconds, the longest period being 64 seconds. Nine such periods per 24 hours, namely for 450 seconds, represented 1 percent of the total sleep time.

The third specimen in their study was an African python (*Python sebae*). In this species wakefulness was characterized by electrographic frequency of 20 to 22 Hz of low amplitude. EMG recording was prominent. Respiratory rhythm was irregular, 10 per minute, and cardiac rate was 35 per minute. The percentage of wakefulness was correlated with the state of alimentation. It comprised 35 percent of the circadian cycle when the animal was hungry and 15 percent during the phase of digestion. With respect to sleep, the satiated python coils himself up and is immobile for many hours without showing any movement. Respiration is slow, 3 to 4 respiratory movements per minute. The animal was essentially unresponsive to stimulation. Electrocortical activity slowed to 14 to 15 Hz and the amplitude increased. Diphasic waves of 100 μV at a frequency of approximately 20 per minute occurred (these waves disappeared during behavioral or electrographic wakefulness). There was considerable reduction in EMG recording and no eye movements were ever observed. Cardiac rhythm was regular at 30 beats per minute. This state of sleep occupied 85 percent of the recording during the period of digestion.

Since this was the sole report of a sleep study in one snake, it is of course impossible to draw any conclusions. One realizes, however, how necessary it will be to extend very considerably the inventory of reptilian studies. The python is an interesting choice of snake in that it is one of the most primitive members of the family of snakes. It is one of the well known large sized constrictors. From the standpoint of evolution, it is interesting to note that the Pythonidae and the Boidae are very closely related (Schmidt and Inger, 1957). The Pythonidae are egg laying and occupy Africa and Asia, while the Boidae, which give birth to living young, are found in the Western Hemisphere. The only important osteological distinction is the presence of the supraorbital bone (in the skull) of the Pythonidae. In view of the possible relationship of temperature regulation and sleep mechanisms it would be interesting to study the female python which is able to raise body temperature some 7 to 9 degrees above the ambient temperature when they are incubating their eggs. The increase of body temperature is allegedly associated with contractions of the body musculature. This phenomenon has been documented in the Indian python (*P. molurus*) but has not been reported in *P. sebae*. It would also be of interest to compare the recordings of the female python *P. molurus* with one of the other large pythons such as the reticulated python (*P. reticulatus*).

In regard to the predator/prey relationships and sleep patterns, a much greater familiarity with the habits and habitats of snakes would be necessary. Since snakes of every species, poisonous and non-poisonous, can be the object of predation either by other snakes or birds and some mammals, it is difficult to suggest a choice for study at present. By contrast, the marine iguana (*Amblyrhynchus christatus*) (Schmidt and Ingver, 1957), which inhabits the Galapagos Islands, is well protected from predation and has no significant enemies and could be expected to achieve undisturbed sleep.

Returning once more to the neuroanatomical substrates implicated in the sleep mechanisms reviewed by Broughton (1972), it is found that the groupings of reticular cells are much more pronounced in reptiles than in the vertebrate classes below reptiles. Thus, for example, the inferior reticular nucleus of the medulla reveals a distinct raphé grouping. There is also a separate lateral reticular nucleus contiguous with the nucleus of the vagus.

The nucleus magnocellularis is present and there are elements of the nucleus parvocellularis. There is evidence of a medial reticular nucleus composed of large cells close to the raphé. However, the preponderance of these cells are distributed laterally near the sixth nucleus. There is a division of the cells of the superior reticular nucleus into a dorsal and ventral group at the level of the fifth cranial nucleus with clustering of small cells in the raphé. These nuclei of the raphé are therefore separable into a superior and inferior part. The anlage of the locus coeruleus is said to exist at the angle of the lateral ventricle. The formation of the nucleus ruber has begun to emerge in the mesencephalon. The entire vestibular complex reveals definite evolutionary advancement over that noted in the higher fishes. Tangential, ventro-lateral (Deiter's) and the superior vestibular nuclei and a ventro-medial nuclear group, are present. Connections between these latter nuclei and the medial longitudinal fasciculus have been reported. The locus coeruleus can be found in all five orders of reptiles. In the Chelonians the beginnings of the neocortex emerge.

Studies of reptilian sleep have also emphasized additional neurophysiological issues which extend our understanding of sleep mechanisms. It was pointed out that animals with highly developed visual oculomotor systems might be expected to reveal more active eye movements during sleep in contrast to those species which were not strikingly eye-minded. This observation has generally held up in sleep studies of inframammalian vertebrates. Certain families in the reptile class, namely the diurnal lizards, in contrast to members of the other reptilian orders, possess foveate vision and excellent voluntary independent eye movements in the waking state. It is also known that the optomotor responses to monocular stimulation in animals with foveate vision are bidirectional while the response is unidirectional for the most part in animals lacking a fovea or area centralis (Tauber and Atkin, 1968). These observations indicate that the presence of homolateral tracts would not account for the bidirectional response since only in mammals are there both homolateral and contralateral visual pathways. In other words, the visual organization seemed to be the significant variable. The emphasis the reviewer attaches to visual-oculomotor organization is based on the well recognized observation that eye movements have been an unequivocal indicator of phasic activity during sleep and represent one of the indisputably reliable criteria of the REM state.

Of further informative value for a sleep researcher is a recent study (Glickstein et. al., 1972) of visual input to pontine nuclei in cats, in which it was revealed by anatomical and physiological evidence that a dense projection from cortical area 18 to the rostral pons is present. The authors indicated that "pontine cells respond best to moving targets in a preferred direction over a large receptive field, which usually includes the center of gaze. The results suggest a role for pontocerebellar pathways in visual control of movement." Visual inputs from the superior colliculus were also mentioned as additional connecting links with pontine nuclei. It would be reasonable to suspect that the pontine nuclei associated with triggering the REM state might eventually reveal important connections with the pontine nuclei in relaying inputs to the cerebellum. It would seem useful to explore the reptilian brain with respect to the possibility of there being visual inputs at least from the superior colliculus to the pontine nuclei.

The problem of interpreting the appearance of spikes during sleep in the reptilian class presents several difficulties. It is clear that spike activity seems to emerge in many instances during quiescence and sleep. It is also clear that in some of the material reported there is evidence of amplitude augmentation in the telencephalic derivations when the animal is exposed to increased vigilance. In the latter case, Hernández-Peón has suggested that inhibitory control in the central nervous system of lower vertebrates is poorly developed which might account for the patterned response (Tauber et. al, 1968). In the former case, it is conceivable that the spike activity during sleep might in some way be a precursor of slow wave activity (Rojas-Ramirez and Tauber, 1970). Whether these spikes are related to ponto-geniculo-striate spikes observed, for example, in the cat, cannot be evaluated at present.

Birds

The sleep researcher is able to more easily evaluate the problems of avian sleep since all species studied to date show evidence of paradoxical sleep and slow wave sleep. Although there are some qualifications to the above statement, nevertheless sleep in birds shows many similarities with that observed in mammals.

Before summarizing the behavioral and polygraphic studies of sleep in birds (aves), I would like to present some background information about the origin and radiation of birds. It is asserted, "of all vertebrate classes, the Aves are the easiest to define because of their very narrow monophyletic origin from reptiles and the extreme degree of uniformity in phenotypical features" (Bock, 1969b).

Despite the morphological similarity of all birds, their adaptive radiation is extensive and very complex. Most birds are diurnal and eye-minded like man. From the standpoint of origins, the separation betwen the phyletic lines within the reptiles from which birds and mammals arose is very ancient. Thus, it is believed that the split-off from the reptiles from which archosaurians (early birds) and synapsids (early mammals) occurred at least 250 million years ago (Middle Permian Period). It is generally believed that the split occurred as long ago as 300 million years, during the period of early reptilian evolution. Thus features shared in common with birds and mammals but which differ from those in reptiles could indicate either common ancestry or independent evolution in both groups. Birds may be traced back to the Thecodontia, the ancient reptilian stock of archosaurian radiation. The pseudosuchians, a suborder, have been regarded as the most probable reptilian ancestor, although this has not been unequivocaaly proved. The morphological changes reflecting the evolution of birds from reptiles occurred at different times and at different rates. The archeopterix, of which there are several specimens, was an animal dating back to the late Jurassic age and has provided us with the only evidence of avian evolution. In many ways it appeared reptilian; despite the evolution of forelimbs into wings, teeth were still present. Although the brain had early been described as typically reptilian, later studies revealed that the brain was actually avian in type. Modern birds had evolved presumably by the early Cretaceous period, although no fossil record of such evidence has been discovered. It is stated that avian evolution took place at a faster rate than mammalian evolution (Bock, 1969b).

There are several classifications of avian orders. However, various problems are presented by any of the classifications. The generally accepted classification of Wetmore contains 27 living orders of birds. The perching Passeriformes is the largest order and contains about 5100 of the 8600 species of living birds. This order alone is divided into approximately 75 families.

One large family of birds, namely the flightless birds (ostriches, rheas, emus, cassowaries, etc.) often referred to as ratites, should be of interest to the sleep researcher for comparison with carinates (keeled birds). Although flightless birds may not comprise an ancestral group of an early stage in avian evolution, their adaptation is so different from that of birds in general that they may offer some interesting findings. It is stated by Bock (1969b):

> that the ratites appear to be a monophyletic group of birds that evolved from a flying ancestor: hence, they are an advanced rather than a primitive group. Cobb and Edinger (1962) conclude that the brain of the emu is not primitive. Although we have no hints as to the nearest possible ancestor of the ratites this complex may be of interest to neurologists, permitting comparative study of the central nervous system in a group of large and morphologically diverse birds.

Bock also recommends the waterfowl, galliforms, pigeons, and parrots as ideal for comparative and neurophysiological studies because their behavior is well known.

The first polygraphic study of birds was carried out by Klein et. al. (1964) on three adult chickens, one adult pigeon, and 28 chicks, of which 24 were newly hatched. Electrode placement was in the hyperstriatum, neck muscles and around the orbits. Slow wave sleep similar to that reported in mammalian sleep studies was recorded with a frequency of 2-3 Hz and an amplitude of 100 μV. This sleep state was followed by a paradoxical stage consisting of low-voltage fast electrocortical activity, hypotonia but not complete loss of nuchal muscle tone, bursts of disconjugate rotatory eye movements, and bradycardia. The duration of this phase of sleep was quite short, averaging 6 to 8 seconds and never exceeding 15 seconds. The authors recorded paradoxical sleep in chicks as "a rudimentary" state, since in chicks it represented only 0.6 percent of total sleep time, while in adults it occupied only 0.3 percent of total sleep time.

Hishikawa et. al. (1969) in conducting their behavioral and electrographic study of young chickens housed them in individual cages. They recorded slow wave sleep and paradoxical sleep periods, the former periods lasting no longer than 6 minutes and the latter also lasting only 6-8 seconds. The total duration of paradoxical sleep comprised 7.3 $\pm$ 1.8 percent of the total sleep time. Three subsequent studies of sleep in the pigeon revealed unequivocal evidence of slow wave sleep and paradoxical sleep (Tradardi, 1966, Van Twyver and Allison, 1972; Walker and Berger, 1972). Of the three sleep studies, Tradardi (1966) did not report the percentage of paradoxical sleep in terms of total sleep time. However, Walker and Berger (1972) found that it occupied 7.3 percent, while Van Twyver and Allison (1972) reported it 6.9 percent of total sleep time. The overall observations indicated no disparity with respect to slow wave sleep patterns, for although of shorter duration than those observed in mammals, they were characteristically of low frequency and high amplitude. Electromyographic recordings in all instances revealed hypotonia during paradoxical sleep, but atonia such as observed in the cat during this stage of sleep was never recorded. There was uniform agreement with respect to the eye movement patterns observed during paradoxical sleep. They were clearly recordable although of short duration.

The sleep study of Van Twyver and Allison (1972) indicates the improved methods of conducting a sleep project in inframammalian vertebrates. They have consistently unmasked and pointed up the many challenging problems confronting the experimenter in dealing with the variables present in a sleep project. In contrast to other inframammalian sleep studies, they measured cardiorespiratory responses, brain temperature, and behavioral arousal thresholds with great care. They observed that the detection of slow wave activity during behavioral sleep depended upon the location of the recording electrodes. This was an important observation in that it might explain the problem that was not adequately answered by Rojas-Ramirez and Tauber (1970) in their study of the hawk and falcon. Although slow wave sleep and paradoxical sleep were found in the hawk (*Buteo jamaicensis borealis*) and the falcon (*Herpetotheres cachinnans chapmanni*), the slow waves rarely exceeded 45 μV in amplitude. Paradoxical sleep in these avian predators was characterized by clusters of 7-15 individual high amplitude asynchronous eye movement deflections, and they were not usually "yoked." The EEG activity revealed fast frequency and low amplitude. Myoclonic jerks similar to those observed in mammals were also present. Of particular interest was the observation that the EMG flattened out as soon as behavioral sleep was initiated. Thus EMG activity was essentially isoelectric during both phases of sleep. Paradoxical sleep in these two species of birds occupied 7-10 percent of total sleep time.

Two other observations in these birds of prey need to be mentioned: 1) occasional slow waves were present during states of alertness and 2) there were occasional small eye movement deflections during slow wave sleep. Since behavioral observations and electro-oculographic recordings were checked repeatedly during daytime observation, it was clear that the eye movement deflections were not artifacts.

Berger and Walker (1972) studied the sleep-wakefulness pattern in the burrowing owl (*Speotyto cunicularia hypugaea*). They described wakefulness as characterized by behavioral activity and a low-voltage high-frequency electroencephalogram and a high tonic neck electromyogram. Slow wave sleep revealed behavioral inactivity, high-voltage, slow wave patterns, and a reduction in muscle tone of the neck. Paradoxical sleep was characterized by a low-voltage high-frequency electroencephalogram. However, there was no further reduction in muscle tone of the neck. Furthermore, phasic eye muscle activity did not occur independently of eyelid movement. The mean duration of paradoxical sleep episodes was 11 seconds and equaled 5 percent of total sleep time.

To appraise and interpret the findings in the owl is a challenging task, for the owl has eyes which are immobile during wakefulness, as well as during behavioral sleep. Furthermore, it must be emphasized that the neck EMG during paradoxical sleep did not differ from that recorded slow wave sleep. The absence of eye movements and the lack of further reduction of EMG activity, make it difficult to assert unequivocally that paradoxical sleep is being reported. On the other hand, the authors indicate a suggestive distinction between the EEG activity during wakefulness in contrast with that recorded during paradoxical sleep, including a relatively elevated arousal threshold. However, no specific data were presented. Consequently, this reviewer is inclined to reserve judgment at this point. In addition to describing the sleep-wakefulness cycle in the burrowing owls, the authors hypothesize, "...that the evolution of REM sleep might be linked to that of binocularly coordinated eye movement, since the eyes of the owl are immobile." There is very little support for this hypothesis.

In summary, it does not strike this reviewer as important to focus attention on detailed distinctions between the findings with respect to sleep and wakefulness in birds. Thus, for example, the fact that hypotonia (neck EMG) is observable in the chicken and pigeon, while atonia is observed in the avian predators, does not seem to require a specific explanation. The striking fact is that behavioral sleep is unequivocally present and that the electrographic studies support and correlate with the behavioral findings.

Referring once more to Broughton's review of the neural substrates subserving sleep (Broughton, 1972), he indicates that the reticular elements in the brainstem of birds reveal a somewhat different organization from those observed in reptiles. The medial reticular nucleus and the superior reticular nucleus are very highly developed. Pontine reticular nuclei and brainstem raphe nuclei, structures that are analogous to those observed in mammals, are clearly present. Vestibular nuclei, including the descending and medial complex as well as the locus coeruleus, are also well developed in birds. Thus, it would appear that one could anticipate the presence of both types of sleep in the bird on the basis of their neuroanatomical brainstem structures, and indeed, the presence of these sleep states has been confirmed.

With a view to future sleep studies in birds, Bock (1969b) has pointed out which families of birds might be of importance by virtue of familiarity with their waking behavior. Stingelin and Senn (1969) have indicated that the evolution of the forebrain in birds has shown two different tendencies as reflected in parrots and owls. There are, of course, differences in the organization of the brain associated with the kind of sensory equipment necessary for their adaptation. Birds which have a large and specialized beak have a very large sensory trigeminal nucleus, whereas perching birds, among others, where beak touching is relatively less important, develop only a small touch center. An example is given of the snipe which has a nucleus for touch four times larger than that of a carrion crow, which is four times as heavy as the snipe.

For the sleep researcher several additional suggestions that could expand our understanding of sleep behavior in birds are the following: 1) recent studies of middle ear muscle activity during sleep revealed the presence of phasic muscle bursts during the paradoxical phase of sleep (Baust et. al, 1964; Dewson et. al., 1965; Pessah and Roffwarg, 1973). It would be of great interest to study middle ear muscle activity during sleep in the owl family (*Strigiformes*) where, as mentioned above, indicators of phasic activity, alleged to be present during paradoxical sleep, are ambiguous. 2) A comparison of bird species with regard to energy consumption and its correlation with sleep behavior might prove of value. Thus the hummingbirds (Order: Apodiformes; family Trochilidae) are known to fly at great speeds but are particularly famous for the rate of their wing beats which are alleged to reach 75 beats per second (Austin, 1961). They have tremendous flying muscles which are proportionately larger for their size and weight than in any other bird. The hummingbird, of course, is a small bird and one would expect that its metabolism would be extraordinarily high. It is claimed that the hummingbirds, however, can conserve their energy in several ways. Thus the body temperature of most diurnal birds drops about 5° to 10°at night, reaching a basal temperature of $100^{\circ}F$. In the hummingbird, the temperature may drop at night to $65^{\circ}F$. (Austin, 1961). Mountain species observed in the Andes enter a state of torpor during cold spells but become active immediately with sunrise and elevation of ambient temperature. The albatross (Order: Procellariiformes; family Diomedeidae) would present an interesting contrast to the hummingbird in that these birds utilize the wind primarily for loco-motion. They are a family of birds whose gliding flight is perhaps superior to that of any other bird. One might expect that their energy requirements would be relatively minimal despite their large size, because of their essentially exclusive use of the wing as an air foil. 3) A comparative analysis of eye movement densities during REM sleep in birds could be usefully explored. Active eye movements in the waking state are not only correlated with foveate vision but with beak configuration. It has been observed that birds with extremely long beaks are usually known to have voluntary independent eye movements, thus providing effective visual vigilance without the necessity for rapid head movements (Walls, 1963). The hornbills (Order: Coraciiformes; family Bucerotidae) are excellent representatives of such birds, as are also the pelicans (Order: Pelecaniformes) and the herons (Order: Ciconiiformes).

Certain investigators believe that the unequivocal demonstration of slow wave sleep and rapid eye movement sleep in both mammals and birds, and its existence or absence — to the degree thus demonstrated — in reptiles, amphibians, and fishes, have provided sufficient data to construct viable hypotheses concerning the origins of these two sleep states. Van Twyver and Allison (1972) from their studies of birds and primitive mammals (Echidna, *Tachyglossus aculeatus*), have indicated:

> that paradoxical sleep may have appeared late in mammalian evolution, well after the appearance of slow wave sleep. Because birds and mammals are independently derived from ancient reptilian stock, the presence or absence of paradoxical sleep in birds is of considerable interest . . . the presence of paradoxical sleep in both classes (marsupial and placental mammals, and birds) may be due to inheritance from a common ancestor (e.g., homology) or to parallel evolution. Because it is absent in the most primitive mammal (Echidna), we conclude that it has evolved independently in birds and therian mammals. Slow wave sleep (in birds) was also found to be similar to mammalian slow wave sleep. It was hypothesized on the basis of reptilian and mammalian studies that it too has evolved independently in birds and mammals.

However, this hypothesis does not do justice to the following facts. First, behavioral sleep is observable in certain families of teleostean fishes and in all members of the four orders of reptiles that have been studied to date. Second, no significant electrographic study of sleep-wakefulness has as yet been carried out in fishes. Third, behavioral and electrographic studies of amphibians do not suggest sleeping patterns if one applies mammalian criteria. Finally, the interpretation of electrographic information with respect to the reptilian class is still in many ways controversial, although it would seem to this reviewer that there is evidence of paradoxical sleep in certain diurnal lizards and, possibly, in the turtle.

Van Twyver and Allison have also suggested that homeothermy correlates convincingly with electrographic evidence of slow wave sleep in mammals and birds, but not in the lower vertebrate classes. However, in the latter groups the absence of the full complement of neuroanatomical substrates observed in mammals may not be essential to the mediation of sleeping behavior. In fact, mechanisms subserving sleep might be transmitted via different neural circuits. A further consideration is that if the correlation between homeothermy and slow wave sleep prevails, one would predict that warm-blooded fishes would reveal slow wave sleep.

Mammals

Early sleep studies of lower vertebrates reveal unexpected differences in polygraphic recordings from those reported for mammals. The absence of paradoxical sleep in the tortoise (Hermann et. al., 1964) and the presence of a "rudimentary" type of paradoxical sleep in the pigeon and chicken (Klein et. al., 1964) prompted researchers to recognize that knowledge of the evolution of sleep required an informed background in vertebrate evolution. The subsequent discovery of the absence of paradoxical sleep in the echidna (*Tachyglossus aculeatus*) (Allison and Goff, 1972; Allison and Van Twyver, 1972; Allison et. al., 1972), a monotreme, despite its presence in all placental and marsupial mammals studied to date, stimulated further interest in the ancestral lineages of mammals. What does it mean that slow wave sleep is present in therian (placental and marsupial) and nontherian (monotremes) mammals, while paradoxical sleep is present in all therian mammals but absent in the one nontherian representative?

Before addressing ourselves to the efforts made to solve this enigma, let me briefly review mammalian evolution. Romer (1963) reminds us that: "The reptilian stem from which mammals sprang was one of the first differentiated from the primitive reptile stock; and the first mammals themselves appeared nearly as early as the first of the dinosaurs." The pelycosaurs are the earliest representatives of the beginning differentiation of mammals from reptilian stock. Their fossil beds (late Carboniferous and Lower Permian) antedate the period when reptiles came to rule the globe. Their physical features reveal little departure from primitive reptilian stock. Therapsids, discovered in Africa, were mammal-like reptiles, believed to be descended from pelyco-saurs. They dated from the later Permian and Triassic. Many variants of mammal-like reptiles, some similar to the pelycosaurs but others fairly advanced in mammal-like characteristics, prevailed. It was in the early Triassic that the development of the ruling reptiles took place, leading to their senior occupancy of the globe. The archosaurs displaced these mammal-like reptiles. However, their mammalian descendants survived, if somewhat ingloriously, throughout the Mesozoic Era.

Subsequent evolution of mammalian forms indicates that nontherian and therian groups had a separate line of ancestry. The primitive monotremes retained their reptilian and egg-laying characteristics while other mammals which had oviparous ancestors achieved viviparity even during the Mesozoic period. It has been proposed that geographic isolation plus a life-style demanding minimal competition "preserved" them and saved them from extinction. The marsupials and placentals came to represent the two great living groups of mammals as evidenced by findings in the late Cretaceous beds. The marsupials flourished and attained great size in South America, a land mass that was cut off for over 150 million years until the Pleistocene. Thereafter, placental carnivores arrived once land connections were made and obliterated most of the marsupial stock with the exception of the opossums and a few other small pouched animals. Geographic isolation also played a significant role in Australia, permitting the marsupials to hold reign and paralleling the placentals in other areas of the globe until the arrival of man and the introduction of dogs and cats. In contrast to marsupials, placental mammals have made a much more successful adaptation by virtue of placentation. This reproductive mechanism has provided the opportunity for a lengthy period of development and maturation.

Despite the fact that monotremes are very poorly represented in the vertebrate kingdom today, they are, nevertheless, of particular interest to sleep researchers. They are representative of the very earliest mammals and their therapsid progenitors. Hopson (1969) states:

> The fossil evidence thus indicates that the ancestry of the mammals separated from the line that later gave rise to the living reptiles very soon after the origin of the class reptilia. This fact is significant in that it indicates that many of the features characteristic of living reptiles were never present in the early reptilian ancestors of mammals and therefore that modern reptiles cannot be considered to represent an evolutionary stage preceding mammals.

I have included this quotation because it clarifies a possible misconception that many of us have, namely, that mammals of all classes are direct descendants of living reptiles.

It is worthwhile to emphasize that: "The earliest therian mammals, the kuehneotheriids, were contemporaries of the eozostrodontids, indicating an extremely early separation of the stock leading to the living marsupials and placentals from that which gave rise to the monotremes" (Hopson, 1969). The monotremes have retained many features characteristic of the earliest mammals and are thus quite primitive. However, their mammalian status is undisputed.

In our search to acquire further evidence of brain patterns during sleep it is reassuring to discover ". . . the ear ossicles of monotremes do not differ in essentials from those of therian mammals (Doran, 1879). Yet, because these elements (i.e., malleus and incus) are still part of the jaw in the earliest known therians and nontherians, it follows that much of the morphological and functional similarity between the middle ears of modern therians and monotremes is the result of independent and parallel evolution.

> This example emphasizes the important point that natural selection acting upon similar structures inherited from a common ancestral stock can produce remarkably similar solutions to similar functional problems in long separated lineages. The possibility that some of the close resemblance between monotremes and therians may be *in part* the result of parallelism should be kept in mind in studies of other aspects of monotreme anatomy and physiology, including those on the central nervous system (Hobson, 1969)

There are two interesting inferences to the sleep researcher by virtue of the preceding quotation. 1) It seems quite clear that the monotremes and the therian mammals reveal parallelism along with their independent evolution from a common ancestral stock. Parallelism in the context in which it is used, refers to certain significant similarities shared by both lineages. It does not indicate, however, the extensiveness of these similarities. Thus, in terms of the Echidna (*Tachyglossus aculeatus*), there may have been paradoxical sleep at some time in its long history, since which it has disappeared for reasons we may never discover. On the other hand, it is also possible that the parallelism shared by monotremes and therian mammals did not include the sleep mechanisms associated with the state of brain activation. 2) The parallelism with respect to the ear ossicles present in both monotremes and therian mammals, suggests a profitable inquiry into the possible existence of phasic bursts of middle ear muscle activity during some stage of sleep. If the results are negative, this would add to the evidence that paradoxical sleep is absent in the monotreme. If on the other hand, the results are positive, this would indicate that REM sleep is present despite the absence of rapid eye movements.

As will be developed below, the Echidna shows remarkable similarity in body configuration and life style to several other representatives of different orders of mammals, illustrating convergent evolution. Paradoxical sleep has been demonstrated in some of these groups and will probably be found in all of them. Nevertheless, it has not been found in the Echidna. The Echidna (*Tachyglossus aculeatus*) has not changed very much or perhaps at all over millions of years. He is not a living fossil nor he is the ancestor of any living animal. Kurten (1969) has pointed out that the life style of the Echidna and his configuration are strikingly similar to three other mammalian species, none of which are monotremes. In addition, these three other species each belong to a different order of placental mammals (Affani, 1972): 1) The ant bear or anteater, *Myrmecophaga tridactyla* (Order: Edentata) which inhabits South America; 2) the pangolin, *manis* (Order: Pholidota) — four species inhabit Africa and three species inhabit south eastern Asia; 3) the aardvark, *Orycteropus afer* (Order: Tubulidentata) inhabits most of Africa south of the Sahara and Sudan. All four animals, though arising from different phyletic lines and occupying different areas of the glove, are predators which have come to resemble one another by adapting themselves to a similar lifestyle. They subsist essentially on termites and ants. Here we see a brilliant illustration of convergence.

From the standpoint of sleep research, there is conclusive evidence that two species of Edentates, the giant armadillo (*Priodontes giganteus*) and the common hairy armadillo (*Chaetophractus villosus*) reveal quiet sleep and paradoxical (active) sleep (Affani et. al., 1968; Affani, 1972). The daily mean percentages of wakefulness, quiet sleep, and paradoxical sleep were 24.5 percent, 50 percent, and 25.4 percent, respectively. During paradoxical sleep there were: a) the characteristic rapid eye movements; b) low-voltage fast EEG activity similar to that observed during wakefulness; c) muscle twitches; and d) an arousal threshold to subcutaneous electrical stimulation that was five times higher during paradoxical sleep than during quiet sleep. These two species of Edentates belong to the same order as the anteater or ant bear (*Myrmecophaga tridactyla*) whose sleep has so far not been studied. It is, of course, most probable that these latter Edentates will reveal both slow wave and paradoxical sleep. This would suggest that although convergence is striking in the Echidna and anteater, the degree of convergence might still not be complete enough for paradoxical sleep to be shared with the Echidna. Because the Echidna and the anteater show this convergence in life style and configuration, must we anticipate that their sleep patterns would, in general, be congruent? Perhaps the only answer is an empirical one based on devising additional tests to reveal phasic muscle activity and then determining whether evidence for paradoxical sleep can be demonstrated or excluded.

CONCLUSIONS

The preceding paragraphs dealing with the evidences of parallelism and convergence were emphasized in order to determine specific ways in which evolutionary studies might shed light on behavioral sleep and its electrographic correlates. The concepts of parallelism and convergence have their main importance in organizing morphological and physiological findings with respect to the various vertebrate groupings. However, the data reflecting the evidences of parallelism and convergence cannot specify precisely what morphological and physiological functions will be shared by the species under consideration. In other words, because the Echidna and the anteater reveal striking evidence of convergence, it does not follow that they will each share a fossorial way of living. Even if there are significantly similar features observable in two distantly related species, it would seem to me that the examination of a particular process has to be explored empirically. An inference with respect with respect to the prediction of a particular feature in a vertebrate, for example sleep patterning, is most reliably achieved by means of sleep studies. The fact that all therian sleep studies have revealed behavioral sleep with consistent evidence of a slow wave sleep phase and a paradoxical phase, (Snyder, 1966; Bert et. al., 1967; Jouvet, 1967; Tauber et. al., 1968a; Pegram et. al., 1969; Bert et. al., 1970a; Van Twyver and Allison, 1970; Affanni, 1972; Ruckebush, 1972) has permitted us to infer that the presence of similar findings in all subsequent therian sleep studies with a high degree of probability.

From what we have learned of the sleep patterns of the Echidna, *T. aculeatus*, it is reasonable to assume that slow wave sleep will be found in the remaining four species of Echidna and the single species of duck-billed platypus. Of the extant monotremes there are two families. One family of the spiny anteater consists of two genera, *Tachyglossus* and *Zaglossus*, comprising five species. The other family consists of a single genus, Ornithorhynchus. This genus contains one species (*Ornithorhynchus anatinus*) called the duck-billed platypus. A reliable guess as to whether paradoxical sleep will be found in any or all of these species is difficult to make. Noback and Allison (1972), in reporting on the brainstem reticular nuclei of the echidna, *T. aculeatus*, indicate that "at a gross cytoarchitectural level the neural structures thought to be actively involved in the generation of paradoxical sleep are present in the Echidna, and the lack of paradoxical sleep in this species is not explainable at this level of analysis." They suggest that histochemical studies, however, might disclose significant differences between the monotreme and therian brainstem.

While further research is being conducted to broaden the inventory of mammalian and inframammalian studies, it could be useful to borrow a leaf from the geneticist's book (Roe and Simpson, 1958; Dobzhansky, 1961) Simpson, 1961) by determining whether genetic analysis could shed light on some of the aspects of sleep patterns. One illustration of this approach has already appeared in the literature. Two strains of mice and their hybrids were studied. The authors state: "Our results clearly revealed both qualitative and quantitative differences in the EEG patterns during the states of sleep. No such differences were evident during waking . . . The circadian rhythm of the sleep-waking cycle was also different" (Valatx et al., 1972).

I would like to suggest a somewhat different type of a genetic experimental design utilizing the technique of backcrossing (Ehrman, personal communication). For example, let us assume that in a large sample of a particular species, one acquired quantitative estimations of sleep characteristics (quantity of REM sleep, slow wave sleep, cycle lengths, etc.) of that particular species. Let us then carry out a similar study in a subspecies. Let us assume that the results of these studies show a reliable difference in findings. If then mating of subspecies A and subspecies B took place, after which a further sleep analysis was carried out on the offspring, one might anticipate that: 1) the F_1 generation could reveal a strong dominance for either of the parent species. If this were the case, the question of dominance with respect to sleep could be noted. A more likely possibility of course would be 2) a result which would be intermediate between the parents. Of least likelihood would be 3) the finding that the sleep analysis of the F_1 generation would exceed or be seriously less than the sleep findings of either parent. For the purposes of the inquiry, let us assume that the results noted in the F_1 generation were to be intermediate with respect to either parent. One could then avail oneself of a classically powerful technique utilized by geneticists, namely backcrossing. That is, the offspring of the F_1 generation would be mated with the appropriate parent of subspecies A and B. Again, the generation F_2A and F_2B

would be exposed to quantitative sleep analysis in order to determine whether the sleep patterns are moving away or toward either of the original progenitors. It is also possible to continue further mating of subsequent generations, the sleep results of which could be usefully analyzed by genetic techniques, thereby revealing the direction of the sleep program. This type of experiment could be conducted with animals where hybridization occurs. Where hybrids are sterile, an experiment of this type would of course not be possible. However, in certain hybrid combinations, the female is fertile and the male is sterile. In this case, the female hybrid could be backcrossed with the male progenitor. One might then be able to determine whether the sleep patterns are sex-linked. If this type of genetic analysis were successful, one might anticipate that certain kinds of sleep patterns, including abnormalities such as insomnia, narcolepsy, sleep paralysis, and cataplexy are linked to genetic factors. This type of experimental program could be applied to mammals and inframammalian vertebrates alike.

REFERENCES

Affani, J.M., Observations on the sleep of some South American marsupials and Edentates. in, *The Sleeping Brain*, M. Chase, Ed., Brain Information Service, Los Angeles, Calif. 1972.

Affani, J.M., Samartino,G., and Morita, E., Observaciones sobre la actividad eléctrica del neocortex, paleocortex y bulbo olfatorio de Chaetophractus villosus. *Rev. Soc. Argent. Biol. 44*, 189-196 (1968).

Allison, T., and Van Twyver, H., The ecology of sleep, APSS, Santa Fe, New Mexico, 1970.

Allison, T. and Goff, W.R., Electrophysiological studies of the Echidna Tachyglossus aculeatus. III. Sensory and interhemispheric evoked responses, *Arch. Ital. Biol. 110*, 195-216 (1972).

Allison, T. and Van Twyver, H., Electrophysiological studies of the Echidna Tachyglossus aculeatus. II. Dormancy and Hibernation. *Arch. Ital. Biol. 110*, 185-194 (1972).

Allison, T., Van Twyver, H., and Goff, W.R., Electrophysiological studies of the Echidna Tachyglossus aculeatus. I. Waking and sleep. *Arch. Ital. Biol. 110,* 145-184 (1972).

Austin, O.L. Jr., *Birds of the World,* Golden Press, New York, 1961.

Baust, W., Berlucchi, G., and Moruzzi, G., Changes in the auditory input in wakefulness and during synchronized and desynchronized stages of sleep. *Arch. Ital. Biol. 102*, 657-674 (1964).

Berger, R.J., and Walker, J.M. Sleep in the burrowing owl (Speotyto Cunicularia Hypugaea). *Behav. Biol. 7,* 183-194 (1972).

Bert, J., and Collomb, H., L'electroencephalogramme du sommeil nocturne chez le Babuoin. Etude par telemetrie. *J. Physiol. (Paris) 58*, 285-301 (1966).

Bert, J., Collomb, H., Martino, A. L'electroencephalogramme d'un pro-simien. Sa place dans l'organisation du sommeil chez les primates. *Electroenceph. Clin. Neurophysiol. 23,* 342-350 (1967).

Bert, J., Kripke, D.F., and Rhodes, J. Electroencephalogram of the mature chimpanzee: Twenty-four hour recordings. *Electroenceph. Clin. Neurophysiol. 28*, 368-373 (1970a).

Bert, J., Pegram, V., Rhodes, J., Balzano, F., and Naquet, R. A comparative sleep study of two cercopithecinae. *Electroenceph. Clin. Neurophysiol. 28*, 32-40 (1970b).

Bock, Walter J., Discussion: The concept of homology. *Comparative and Evolutionary Aspects of the Vertebrate Central Nervous System, Annals of the New York Academy of Sciences 167* (Art. 1), 71-73 (1969a).

Bock, Walter J., The origin and radiation of birds. *Comparative and Evolutionary Aspects of the Vertebrate Central Nervous System, Annals of the New York Academy of Sciences 167*, 147-155 (1969b).

Broughton, R., Neurology and sleep research. *Can. Psychiat. Assoc. Journal 16*, 283-293 (1971).

Broughton, R., Phylogenetic evolution of sleep studies. in, *The Sleeping Brain*, M. Chase, Ed., Brain Information Service, Los Angeles, Calif. (1972).

Carey, F.G., Fishes with warm bodies. *Scientific American 228*, (No. 2), 36-44 (1973).

Dewson, J.H., III, Dement, W.C., and Simmons, F.B. Middle ear muscle activity in cats during sleep. *Exp. Neurol. 12*, 1-8 (1965).

Dobzhansky, T., *Genetics of the Evolutionary Process*, Columbia University Press, New York, 1961.

Dowling, H.J., American Museum of Natural History, New York, personal communication.

Ehrman, L., Department of Natural Sciences, State University of New York, Purchase, N.Y., personal communication.

Flanigan, W.F., Behavioral states and electroencephalograms of reptiles. in, *The Sleeping Brain*, M. Chase, Ed., Brain Information Service, Los Angeles, Calif., 1972.

Flanigan, W.F., Jr., Wilcox, R.H., and Rechtschaffen, A., The EEG and behavioral continuum of the crocodilian, Caiman sclerops. *Electroencephalography*, in press.

Gerard, R.W. and Young, J.Z. Electrical activity of the central nervous system of the frog. *Proc. Roy. Soc. B. 122*, 343-353 (1937).

Glickstein, M., Stein, J., and King, R.A. Visual input to the pontine nuclei. *Science 178*, 1110-1111 (1972).

Hermann, H., Jouvet, M., and Klein, M., Analyse polygraphique du sommeil de la tortue. *C.R. Acad. Science (Paris) 258*, 2175-2178 (1964).

Hishikawa, Y., Cramer, H., and Kuhlo, W. Natural and Melatonin induced sleep in young chickens. *Exp. Brain Res. 7*, 84-94 (1969).

Hobson, J.A. Electrographic correlates of behavior in the frog with special reference to sleep. *Electroenceph. Clin. Neurophysiol. 22*, 113-121 (1967).

Hobson, J.A., Goin, O.B., and Goin, C.J. Electroencephalographic correlates of behavior in tree-frogs. *Nature (London) 220*, 386-387 (1968).

Hopson, J.A. The origin and adaptive radiation of mammal-like reptiles and nontherian mammals. *Comparative and Evolutionary Aspects of the Vertebrate Central Nervous System, Annals of the New York Academy of Sciences 167*, (Art. 1), 199-216 (1969).

Jouvet, M. Biogenetic amines and states of sleep. *Science 163*, 32-41 (1969).

Jouvet, M. Neurophysiology of the states of sleep. *Physiol. Rev. 47*, 117-177 (1967a).

Jouvet, M. Neurophysiology of the states of sleep. in, *The Neurosciences*, G.C. Quarton, T. Melnechuk, and F.O. Schmitt, Eds. Rockefeller University Press, New York, 1967b, pp. 529-544.

Klein, M., Michel, F., and Jouvet, M. Etude polygraphique du sommeil chez les oiseaux. *C.R. Soc. Biol. (Paris) 158*, 99-103 (1964).

Kurten, B. Continental drift and evolution. in, *Continents Adrift (Readings from Scientific American)*, Vol. 12, 1969, pp. 114-123

McGinty, D. and Lucas, E.A. Sleep in amphibians. in, *The Sleeping Brain*, M. Chase, Ed., Brain Information Service, Los Angeles, Calif., 1972.

Nelson, G.J. Origin and Diversification of teleostean fishes. *Comparative and Evolutionary Aspects of the Vertebrate Central Nervous System, Annals of the New York Academy of Sciences 167* (Art. 1), 18-30, (1969).

Noback, C.R. and Allison, T. The brainstem reticular nuclei of the Echidna (Tachyglossus aculeatus). *Sleep Res. 1*, 90 (1972).

Pegram, V., Bert, J., Rhodes, J., and Naquet, R. Telemetry EEG of baboon sleep in the natural environment. *Psychophysiology 6*, 228 (1969).

Pessah, M.A. and Roffwarg, H.P. Spontaneous middle ear activity in man: A rapid eye movement sleep phenomenon. *Science 178*, 773-776 (1973).

Peyrethon, J. et Dusan-Peyrethon, D. Etude Polygraphique du cycle veille-sommeil d'un teleosteen (Tinca tinca). *C.R. Soc. Biol. (Paris) 161*, 2533-2537 (1967).

Peyrethon, J. and Dusan-Peyrethon, D. Etude Polygraphique du cycle veille-sommeil chez trois genres de reptiles. *C.R. Soc. Biol. (Paris) 163*, 181-186 (1969).

Roe, A. and Simpson, G.G., Eds., *Behavior and Evolution*, Yale University Press, New Haven, Conn., 1958.

Rojas-Ramirez, J.A. and Tauber, E.S. Paradoxical sleep in two species of avian predator (Falconiformes). *Science 167*, 1754-1755 (1970).

Romer, A.S. *Man and the Vertebrates*, Vol. I. Penguin Books, Baltimore, Maryland, 1963.

Romer, A.S. *The Vertebrate Body* W.B. Saunders Co., Philadelphia, Pa., 1970, 39 & 380.

Ruckebush, Y. Comparative aspects of sleep and wakefulness in farm animals. in, *The Sleeping Brain*, M. Chase, Ed., Brain Information Service, Los Angeles, Calif. 1972.

Schaeffer, B. Adaptive radiation of the fishes and the fish-amphibian transition. *Comparative and Evolutionary Aspects of the Vertebrate Central Nervous System, Annals of the New York Academy of Sciences., 167* (Art 1), 5-17 (1969).

Schmidt, K.P. and Inger, R.F. *Living Reptiles of the World*. Doubleday, Garden City, N.Y., 1957, 13-40.

Segura, E.T. and de Juan, A. Electroencephalographic studies in toads. *Electroenceph. Clin. Neurophysiol. 21*, 373-380 (1966).

Simpson, G. *Principles of Animal Taxonomy*, Columbia University Press, New York, 1961.

Snyder, F. Toward an evolutionary theory of dreaming. *Amer. J. Psychiat. 123*, 121-136 (1966).

Starck, W.A. and Davis, W.P. Night habits of fishes of Alligator Reef Florida. *Ichthyologia 38*, 313-356 (1966).

Stingelin, W. and Senn, D.G. Morphological studies on the brain of sauropsida. *Comparative and Evolutionary Aspects Vertebrate Central Nervous System, Annals of the New York Academy of Sciences 167* (Art. 1). 156-163 (1969).

Tauber, E.S., Roffwarg, H.P. and Weitzman, E.D. Eye movements and electroencephalogram activity during sleep in diurnal lizards. *Nature 212*, 1612-1613 (1966).

Tauber, E.S. and Atkin, A. Optomoter responses to monocular stimulation: Relation to visual system organization. *Science 160*, 1365-1367 (1968).

Tauber, E.S., Michel, F., and Roffwarg, H.P. Preliminary note on the sleep and waking cycle in the desert hedgehog (Paraechinus hypomelas). *Psychophysiology 5*, 201 (1968a).

Tauber, E.S., Rojas-Ramirez, J. and Hernandez-Peon, R. Electrophysiological and behavioral correlates of wakefulness and sleep in the lizard, (Ctenosaura pectinata). *Electroenceph. Clin. Neurophysiol. 24*, 424-443 (1968b).

Tauber, E.S. and Weitzman, E.D. Eye movements during behavioral inactivity in certain Bermuda reef fish. *Commun. Behav. Biol., Pt.A, 3*, 131-135 (1969).

Tradardi, V. Sleep in the pigeon. *Arch. Ital. Biol. 104*, 516-521 (1966).

Valatx, J.L., Bugat, R., and Jouvet, M. Genetic studies of sleep in mice. *Nature (London) 238* (5361), 226-227 (1972).

Van Twyver, H. and Allison, T. Sleep in the opossum (Didelphis marsupialis). *Electroenceph. Clin. Neurophysiol. 29*, 181-189 (1970).

Van Twyver, H. and Allison, T. A polygraphic and behavioral study of sleep in the pigeon (Columba livia). *Exper. Neurol.* 35 (No. 1), 138-153 (1972).

Vasilescu, E. Sleep and wakefulness in the tortoise (Emys orbicularis). *Rev. Roum. Biol.-Zool. (Bucharest) 15*, 177-179 (1970a).

Vasilescu, E. Isolated head of the tortoise (Emys orbicularis). *Rev. Roum. Biol.-Zool. (Bucharest) 15*, 273-276 (1970b).

Walker, E.P. *Mammals of the World*, Vols. I & II, John Hopkins Press, Baltimore, Maryland, 1964.

Walker, J.M. and Berger, R.J. Sleep in the domesticated pigeon (Columba livia). *Behav. Biol.* 7(2), 195-203 (1972).

Walls, G.L. *The Vertebrate Eye*, Hafner Publ. Co., New York, 1963.

Weber, E. Uber Ruhelagen von Fischen. *Z. Tierpsychol. 18*, 517-533 (1961).

Advances in Sleep Research, Vol. 1
© 1974, Spectrum Publications, Inc.

CHAPTER 3

Neuronal Unit Activity and
The Control of Sleep States

DENNIS J. McGINTY
RONALD M. HARPER
MARY K. FAIRBANKS

I. INTRODUCTION

The objective of this chapter is to reconsider the interpretations of studies of neuronal unit activity in relation to sleep. The study of changes in both spontaneous discharge and stimulus-evoked discharge of single neurons during wakefulness and sleep has been carried out in many laboratories for a variety of purposes. These purposes include the studies of general aspects of brain physiology during sleep, unit correlates of EEG slow waves, transmission in thalamic relay nuclei, control of motor outflow during sleep and, recently, the activity of cell groups which have been implicated in the active control of sleep behavior. Here these results will be summarized from the point of view of concepts which are central to the understanding of the mechanisms of the sleep process itself. We suggest ways in which the study of unit activity can provide definitive information about the physiological bases of sleep. Such a summary is premature, especially in the light of the fact that only a small fraction of the cell aggregates of the mammalian brain has been examined thus far, and because the smaller neurons within various groups are not easily sampled with contemporary procedures of unit recording in behaving animals. However, since we hope to stimulate the examination of theoretical issues, we have chosen an optimistic and speculative approach. Reviews of the studies of neuronal activity and sleep have been provided by Evarts (1967 a, b), Hobson and McCarley (1971), Hobson (1973), and Jacobs, McGinty, and Harper (1973).

Nearly all groups of neurons exhibit changes in characteristics of spontaneous discharge during sleep as compared to waking (W) and, generally, different changes within the two phases of sleep, slow wave sleep (SWS), and rapid eye movement sleep (REM). Since most of the cerebrum is not critically involved in the active neural control of the onset and maintenance of sleep behaviors (see Section II below), these ubiquitous changes in unit activity must reflect passive consequences of sleep, or at least the end-product of neural processes controlling sleep. These changes provide information about the state of the brain during sleep. They are reviewed in Section III.

The subsequent section (IV) is devoted to the discussion of cell aggregates which are thought to be directly involved in the neural control of sleep. On the basis of studies of the effects of localized lesions or of brain stimulation, certain regions of the brainstem and diencephalon have been suggested as sleep centers. The investigation of the unit activity of these regions has only recently begun, but the results are promising.

In Section V we take the opportunity to suggest some directions for future research and to discuss the usefulness of our own technical approach to unit recording.

Most studies have been concerned with the rate and pattern of "spontaneous" neuronal spike activity, that is, trains of spikes that occur in the absence of any obvious change in the environment or gross motor behavior. The interpretation of the significance of this spontaneous firing is not clear. Excitatory or inhibitory synaptic input modifying output, i.e., transfer across a neural relay, is characterized by temporal and spatial summation. An input consisting of slow spontaneous activity may not affect output because the threshold of depolarization in the target neuron may not be achieved. In neurons having primarily phasic functions, as in the case of phasic motor units or sensory neurons, slow background activity may not produce excitatory output in target neurons. On the other hand, in neurons with tonic functions, spontaneous activity represents the major output. Some neurons, such as visual pathway neurons, have both phasic (movement in visual field) and tonic (brightness) functions. Furthermore, in neurons with inhibitory influences on target neurons, the difficulty in interpreting the relative importance of discharge acceleration (inhibition) and deceleration (disinhibition) is especially obvious. Since our understanding of the behavioral or functional significance of synaptic output of most neurons in the brain is poor, the comprehension of the significance of spontaneous firing is also poor. The problem is especially acute in the study of neurons outside of well known sensory or motor pathways.

An Approach to the Relation of
Spontaneous Unit Activity to Sleep States

Given that the significance of spontaneous unit firing is obscure, what information can be obtained from studies of unit firing in relation to sleep? Sleep represents a widespread change in the function of the nervous system, a change in state. We feel that changes in spontaneous firing may be a reflection of nonspecific excitatory or inhibitory influences on cells. We speculate that these nonspecific influences are brought about by the action of specialized systems of neurons which have diffuse anatomical connections with virtually the entire brain. The existence of monoaminergic neurons having these anatomical properties has been documented. We suppose that nonspecific influences control the background level of resting polarization of the cell and, thus, the reactivity of the cell to discrete input. Changes in the level of excitability of cells may be the basis of the alternation of sleep and waking states. The neurons which control the diffuse changes in excitability can be considered to be primary elements of the control of sleep and wakefulness.

Several investigators have measured the reactivity of cells during different states directly. Thus it is possible to relate tonic spontaneous firing rate to neural excitability. The studies are reviewed below.

In summary, we assume that changes in neuronal unit activity during sleep in most brain sites represent consequences of the neural control of sleep, that is, either the result of withdrawal of influences which increase excitability, *or* the application of an influence which decreases excitability. On the other hand, certain groups of neurons should exhibit the state-specific changes in unit activity which are the sources of nonspecific excitatory or inhibitory influences. The data dealing with the neural control of sleep are considered from this point of view.

A goal of this review is to develop some testable hypotheses about the neural interactions underlying the cell groups which control sleep and other cell groups which reflect the consequence of sleep. We are concerned with the generation of experiments which may elucidate these mechanisms. For this reason, we speculate about interactions of hypothetical brain systems, whose definition is based on general anatomical and functional features rather than known physiological connections. The usefulness of our speculations will ultimately depend on the feasibility of the experimental assessment of our hypothesis, and rationality of our underlying model of neuronal function.

Slow Wave Sleep versus REM Sleep

Almost without exception, neuronal spike activity exhibits different characteristics in the two stages of sleep. Further, the great majority of neurons exhibit augmented firing rates during REM as compared with the quiet waking or SWS. In addition, a minority of neurons in most sites, as well as a majority of cells in certain limbic sites, exhibit autmented firing in SWS. There are two assumptions which may be derived from this general observation. First, we can assume, as originally emphasized by Evarts (1967 a, b), that sleep does not represent a condition of generalized inhibition or "rest" for the spike-generating process of cerebral neurons. It is possible that the spike-generating process of certain subsets of neurons may "rest" during particular phases of sleep. However, it is more likely that the basis of "fatigability," if such a phenomenon exists, will be found in some aspect of the synthesis, transport, or metabolism of transmitters, enzymes, or structural proteins rather than in the spike mechanism itself. Indeed, fatigability may reflect a more complex function of information processing in nerve nets that does not involve a deficit or excess of any element of the nervous system.

The second general assumption is that the characteristics of neural function in SWS and REM can be considered separately. It is true that there are common elements in the two sleep states, including the continuity of behavioral quiescence, and the interruption of recall of consciousness. It is an important challenge to find the substrate of this continuity. However, since the brain sites studied thus far do not show this continuity, it appears to be most useful to separate the discussion of the two states.

In order to make functional interpretations of data collected in unit activity studies, it is necessary to make additional assumptions.

Coding

Since our primary interest is the excitability of various systems, we feel that neural discharge rate is a useful functional parameter. However, it has been established empirically that spike train patterns are altered during sleep and must also be considered.

Sampling

In most regional unit studies a majority of units are found to share certain characteristics, while one or more "minority groups" exhibit different characteristics. In our discussions we are concerned with the characteristics of the majority. The largest cells within any brain region are undoubtedly sampled preferentially, partly as a result of the stage of development of our techniques (Towe and Harding, 1970). Thus, the "majority" corresponds to large cells. In this review we will speculate about the relationship among brain regions on the basis of the sampling of large cells. We believe that this is justified because these large cells are the primary output systems in many brain sites, as in the case of the pyramidal cells of the neocortex and hippocampus, and the Purkinje cells of the cerebellar cortex. Smaller cells may play a role in local interactions. Thus, the large cells provide information about the result of the integration carried out within a region. In most cases the minority groups may represent interneurons involved in local information processing.

II. BACKGROUND AND METHODS

Chronic Unit Recording Procedures

Most studies have been carried out in cats or in rhesus monkeys, while rabbits and rats have been occasional subjects. Thus far, studies of unit activity during sleep have been limited to extracellular recordings in unanesthetized animals. Paralyzed, unanesthetized animals have been employed to study changes in unit activity in relation to spontaneous alteration of EEG slow wave and fast wave activity assumed to mimic slow wave sleep and wakefulness.

The most frequently used procedure was developed by Hubel (1959) and by

Evarts (1966). Under surgical anethesia a section of skull is removed and a special stainless steel cylinder with an inside diameter of about 10 mm is cemented in place over the exposed dura and then capped to minimize infection. At the same time the animal is implanted with standard macroelectrodes (useful in sleep physiology) for recording EEG, EOG, and EMG. All electrodes and connectors, and rigid protruding posts are cemented securely to the skull. The posts are later attached to a frame in the recording enclosure or monkey chair in order to prevent head movement during recording sessions, while avoiding use of uncomfortable restraining devices applied directly to the animal's skin. After recovery from surgery, the animal is adapted to the movement restraining system. On each experimental day the cap is removed from the cylinder, and a matching cylinder is secured on top. The matching cylinder contains a piston under an oil-filled hydraulic chamber. A microelectrode protrudes under the piston. The piston can be advanced or withdrawn in small steps by a remote hydraulic drive system. In each experiment the microelectrode, sometimes within a protective guide cannula, penetrates the dura and makes a tract through the structures under study. The position of the tract can be varied within the cylinder. At the end of the day, the electrode and drive cylinder are removed. Typically, about 15 tracts are made through each cylinder. The electrodes themselves are usually stainless steel, a platinum iridium alloy, or tungsten, with the tip etched to a point with a diameter of about 1μ. The electrodes are insulated to within $10\text{-}20 \mu$ of the tip. Head restraint is usually required in order to avoid electrical artifacts caused by movement of the recording electrodes and cables.

We and a few others (Strumwasser, 1958; Olds, 1965; O'Keefe and Bouma, 1969; Jacobs and McGinty, 1971; Harper and McGinty, 1973) have used a different technique, in which the recording electrodes remain chronically within the brain. The electrodes consist of insulated 32-62 μ stainless steel or nichrome wires which are stereotaxically implanted during the initial surgical preparation. In our procedure a bundle of 6-10 microwires attached to a mechanical microdrive is lowered to a position just above the structure of interest. Appropriate connectors and macroelectrodes are implanted and cemented to the skull, as above, except that a restraint system is not required. During experimental session the electrode bundle is advanced slowly through the structure with the microdrive. One tract is made with each bundle. However, since the bundle contains six or more electrodes, and each animal is prepared with two or more bundles, the number of stable unit recordings obtained from each animal is comparable to that of the Hubel-Evarts procedure. Thus far, the microwire procedure has not been employed in neocortical structures.

The tips of the microwires are cut off bluntly and are much larger than tips of conventional microelectrodes, sometimes larger than the somata of the cells under study. Nevertheless, these electrodes yield adequate unit recordings while providing a number of distinct advantages over the conventional technique. These problems are discussed in detail in Section V. below.

An adequate unit recording experiment is characterized by the observation of a spike of constant amplitude exceeding background noise by a ratio of at least 2 to 1. The recording must be maintained through at least two of the three states. W, SWS, and REM. The microwire technique always yields recordings that are stable through a complete W, SWS, REM cycle.

The most common analytic procedures for unit data include visual inspection of simultaneously recorded polygraph and spike records, plots of electronic integrator output of neuronal rates over time, and counts of rates per unit time using electronic counting devices. To examine spike train pattern changes it is especially helpful to consider the distribution of the duration of intervals between spikes. This distribution is called the interval histogram.

Examination of the serial order of intervals is accomplished by means of the autocorrelation histogram. This procedure indicates both stability of successive intervals of a particular epoch and periodicity in the cell discharge. A variation of this technique, the cross-correlation histogram, examines relationships between two simultaneously recorded spike trains and will suggest the influence of one spike train upon another. Such statistics will find increasing use in the examination of how one neuron initiates activity in another neuron, and the functional connectivity of adjacent neurons during state changes.

Although it is useful to examine the activity of neurons in the time domain with statistics such as the interval, auto-, and cross-correlation histograms, it is sometimes more convenient to study the discharge of neurons in the frequency domain. By counting the number of discharges during successive short intervals, the variations in frequency over extended time periods can be examined. The spectral estimates on the frequency per unit time data provide another measure of periodicity (Sclabassi and Harper, in press). The example shown in Figure 1 illustrates a neuron firing in relation to the activity of hippocampal theta waves during SWS and REM. The application of the laboratory computer in carrying out these analytic procedures has been recently summarized (Harper and McGinty, 1973; Sclabassi and Harper, in press).

Neural Control of Sleep

Before considering these data relating unit activity to neural control of sleep and waking states, we wish to digress briefly to summarize the literature on the neural control of sleep.*

It has usually been assumed that sleep states, like other behavioral capacities (feeding, motor coordination, vision, etc.), are controlled by

---

*For comprehensive accounts of this literature, the reader should read the recent reviews of Moruzzi (1972), Jouvet (1972), and the papers of Villablanca (Villablanca and Marcus, 1972; Villablanca and Salinas-Zeballos, 1972).

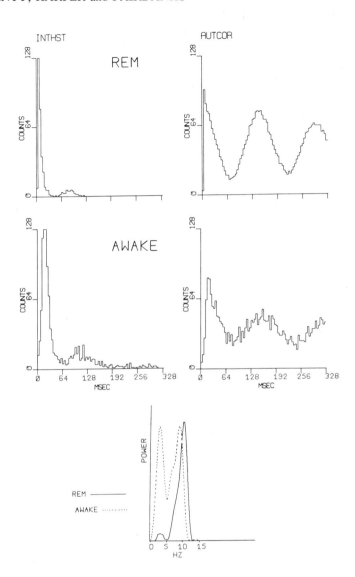

Fig. 1. An illustration of some analytic procedures useful in describing the patterns of spike firing. This hippocampal neuron from a rabbit discharged in a burst-pause pattern in synchrony with the EEG. During REM the frequency of this EEG rhythm increased and became more stable as compared to quiet W. The single cell firing paralleled this EEG activity. The two peaks in the interval histogram (left) correspond to the interspike intervals within the bursts and between the bursts. During REM the peaks are shifted to the left. The autocorrelations (right) show that the rhythmicity of the bursts is greater in REM. The spectral plot (bottom) illustrates the use of frequency domain techniques applied to spike train data. The plot with solid lines indicates the stability and high rate of repetition of spike bursts during REM, while the plot with dashed lines reflects the lowered frequency and increased variability of bursts during the alert state.

specialized cell groups ("centers") or systems of neurons. The localization of these cell groups has been studied primarily by the lesion method, i.e., determining the smallest lesion of a particular brain region required to selectively suppress sleep from the behavioral repertoire and the largest lesion of the brain which spares sleep. The latter (largest lesion) approach is epitomized by the study of sleep in animals with complete transections of the neuraxis.

With respect to REM sleep, the most basic result is the observation of Jouvet (1962) that most behavioral manifestations of REM sleep, i.e., periodic occurrence of discrete episodes of periods of atonia with rapid eye movements and phasic high amplitude waves in the pons, continue to occur after complete removal of the brain above the level of the rostral pons. Discrete lesion of the dorsolateral pontine reticular formation produces a partially selective abolition of REM sleep (Jouvet, 1962). There is general agreement that REM sleep is triggered by a lower brainstem mechanism. This concept is consistent with the biology of REM sleep. This state appears first in mammalian ontogeny, prior to the maturation of many neural elements of the forebrain. Further, REM sleep is a relatively stereotyped discrete behavioral state, reminiscent of other ontogenetically primitive physiological processes such as respiration or sucking. Such brain processes are primarily controlled by the brainstem.

The study of the locus of control of SWS has proven to be far more complex. In a chronic preparation with transection of the upper midbrain, a state with some properties of SWS is observed (Villablanca, 1966). Behavioral activity (generally restricted to continuous walking) is interrupted by periods of postural relaxation, behavioral quiescence, relaxation of the nictitating membrane and variable pupillary miosis. The variable miosis stage, to borrow the terminology of Villablanca (1966), is punctuated with episodes of REM sleep, as is normal adult SWS. The discrete quiescence state cannot be recognized in the animals with rostral pontine transections because the preparation is incapable of behavioral waking periods. Thus, discrimination of a discrete quiescent state is dependent on the upper brainstem. However, certain aspects of SWS are absent in decerebrate cats, especially the behavioral and postural preparations for sleep. Furthermore, there is strong evidence that forebrain mechanisms are also involved in SWS. Indeed, either total thalamectomy or total decortication (sparing only the thalamus, hypothalamus, and basal forebrain) produce nearly total suppression of SWS and REM sleep (Villablanca and Marcus, 1972; Villablanca and Salinas-Zeballos, 1972). Discrete lesions of the basal forebrain also produce a temporary suppression of sleep (McGinty and Sterman, 1968). In addition, the cyclic alteration of a wakeful condition and a SWS-like condition is observed even in the chronic isolated forebrain (chronic cerveau isolé) (Villablanca, 1965).

Since a quiescent state is present in high decerebrate preparations, and absent with the *addition* of diencephalon, or with the *addition* of forebrain, except thalamus, the abolition of sleep by forebrain lesion must result from a suppression of sleep mechanism, an imbalance in favor of behavioral activating processes. Thus, the forebrain modulates brainstem mechanisms in the normal occurrence of SWS. This concept is consistent with the fact that SWS appears both ontogenetically and phylogenetically (see Allison 1973) in relation to forebrain development. In addition, the lower brainstem plays a role in SWS by balancing the behavioral-activating mechanism of the upper brainstem (see Moruzzi [1964] for a review of the documentation of this influence).

In summary, the control of SWS appears to involve the integration of neural processes at several levels of the neuraxis. We believe that the neural control of SWS in mammals is most satisfactorily conceived by comparison with complex appetitive behaviors such as feeding, courtship and reproductive behavior, and agonistic behavior. Each of these behaviors is represented at the brainstem, diencephalon, and limbic systems. Generally, it is found that the complex instinctive or reflexive components of behavior, such as nutritional sucking, the lordosis reflex, sham rage, or REM sleep, are organized at the level of the brainstem. These reflexive components are modulated by processes originating in the forebrain. Diencephalic structures have been implicated in cyclic patterns in behavior, quantitative regulation of consumption, and coordination of behavioral and neuroendocrine processes of the pituitary. Limbic and neocortical systems control the selection of appropriate goal objects (edible vs. inedible foods, etc.), voluntary motor behaviors which prepare the organism for "consumption" (locomotion to appropriate sites, assumption of appropriate postures), learned adaptation to the environment, and perceptual controls over behavior. This point of view has been elaborated elsewhere (McGinty, 1971) and discussed in the scholarly and comprehensive review of Moruzzi (1972). We summarize the argument here because of its relevance to the interpretation of unit studies.

This conception does not preclude the possibility that specialized neuronal groups control SWS. However, such neurons must be reciprocally modulated by other cells at several brain sites, each of which controls certain elements of the complex behavioral process that corresponds to mammalian SWS.

III. CHARACTERISTICS OF CEREBRAL UNIT DISCHARGE DURING SLEEP

In this section we summarize results of studies of brain regions which are not primarily involved in the control of sleep. We will consider four types of data that characterize neuronal unit firing in SWS and REM, as contrasted with W: 1) changes in firing rate, including regional differences in rate data; 2) changes in responsiveness to afferent input of units in sensory pathways; 3) changes in firing patterns; and 4) changes in the temporal correlation in firing of neighboring cells. Table I summarizes the characteristics of unit activity in different brain sites during W, SWS, and REM. The table includes qualities of unit spike trains which, we feel, are most useful in distinguishing functional changes during sleep. These qualities are the profile of rate changes across sleep-waking states, and the temporal patterns of firing.

Table I illustrates several points. The various regions of the brain exhibit distinctive types of changes in firing during SWS. However, some sites appear to share certain properties. The majority of cells in the thalamic relay nuclei and cortex exhibit both similar rate change profiles and patterns during SWS. Certain cell groups in the limbic system exhibit a common

TABLE I

A summary of Neuronal Discharge Rate and Pattern during the Sleep-Waking Cycle. The profile shows how discharge rates changed during the sleep-waking cycle. Representative studies were selected to emphasize the existence of three systems, thalamocortical, limbic-hypothalamic, and monoaminergic. The information provided for each study is indicated by the format shown on the right. The discharge rates in the diagram are given as percentages of the SWS rate which is provided in the second column. The discharge patterns in SWS are described as burst-pause (B-P) (see text), regular (R), indicating a tendency for equal interspike invervals, or irregular (I), indicating a tendency for a random distribution of interspike intervals. Abbreviations: C: cat; M: monkey; R: rat; Ra; rabbit. In some cases rate data for the majority or plurality type of cell were not available (N.A.), and the rate change profile was estimated by the authors.

CORTEX - THALAMUS			LIMBIC-HYPOTHALAMIC			BRAIN STEM		
Vis. Cx.[b] M	7 B-P		Ant. Hyp.[j] RA	N.A.		D. Raphé[o] C	1.4 R	
Mot. Cx.[c] M	8 B-P		Misc.[j] RA	N.A.		Sub. Coer.[p] C	1.1 R	
Assoc Cx.[d] C	11 B-P		Amyg.[k] C.	0.6 I		L. Coer.[q] C	4.2 R	
Assoc Cx.[e] M	4 I		VMH.[l] C	3-10		MRF[r] C	16 R	
Vis. Cx.[f] C	4 B-P		Hippo.[m] R	N.A.		MRF[s] C	8 B-P	
LGN[g] C	13 B-P		Hippo.[n] C	N.A. B-P		FTG[t] C	5 I	
LGN[h] C	17 B-P							
n. ret. thal[i] C	19 B-P							

FORMAT:

Site[Ref]   SWS Rate (Profile)
Species   Pattern

b. Evarts (1962).
c. Evarts (1964).
d. Noda and Adey (1970).
e. Desiraju (1972).
f. Hobson and McCarley (1971b).
g. Sakakura (1968).
h. Mukhametov et al. (1970a).
i. Mukhametov et al. (1970b).
j. Findlay and Hayward (1969).
k. Jacobs and McGinty (1971).
l. Oomura et al. (1969).
m. Mink et al. (1967).
n. Noda et al. (1969).
o. McGinty et al. (1973).
p. McGinty and Sakai (in press).
q. Chu and Bloom (1973).
r. Kasamatsu (1970).
s. Huttenlocher (1961).
t. McCarley and Hobson (1971).

profile which is reciprocal to the thalamocortical profile. The activity of samples of cells found in studies of the midbrain reticular formation and hypothalamic sites is heterogenous, that is, lacking a homogenous majority or plurality. However, two groups of brainstem cells exhibit a unique profile which is distinct from that of forebrain units. These two groups are thought to represent the 5HT-containing cells of the raphé system and the NA-containing cells of the subcoeruleus region of the pons.

Our discussion will emphasize three functional groups which are defined by common profiles of rate changes in sleep, the thalamocortical system, part of the limbic-hypothalamic pathway, and the monoaminergic cell groups. We speculate that these three groups provide models of functional systems in the brain.

Unit Activity and SWS

Thalamocortical System

The majority of units recorded in the thalamic relay nuclei and the cortex exhibit reduced spike rates in SWS compared with W. The reduction typically ranges from 20-50%, but substantial firing rates are maintained in SWS. The more striking change during SWS is the transformation of the temporal pattern of the spike train. The relatively "well-spaced" spikes of wakefulness are replaced by a burst-pause pattern. The bursts consist of groups of 2-10 repetitive spikes attaining transient rates reaching several hundred spikes/sec. These bursts are separated by long pauses in firing. An example is shown in Figure 2. As indicated in Table I this pattern is pervasive during SWS. The mechanism of this phenomenon has been the subject of extensive investigation in acute animals (Purpura and Shofer, 1963; Anderson et al., 1964; Anderson and Andersson, 1968; Purpura, 1970), but it is beyond the scope of this paper.

Mukhametov and Rizzolatti, (1970) reported an interesting observation that may elucidate the origin of the burst-pause pattern. These workers analyzed the evoked unit changes in the lateral geniculate nucleus (LGN) produced by flashes of light in each stage of the sleep-waking cycle. The flashes were produced by a miniature lamp fixed to a glass contact lens. LGN units typically respond to retinal stimulation by transient rate increases ("on" response) or decreases ("off" response) (Hubel and Wiesel, 1961). These typical evoked excitatory "on" responses, as well as inhibitory "off" responses, were examined for changes in firing patterns as well as firing rate. Mukhametov and Rizzolatti (1970) found that an inhibitory transient (off response) during a quiet-waking state could produce the burst-pause pattern normally found in sleep. The same stimulus during sleep could greatly exaggerate the ongoing burst-pause pattern, that is, produce maximum bursts followed by maximum pauses. Conversely, the excitatory transient during SWS could restore the spaced firing pattern of W. These observations indicate that the firing patterns of cells can be altered by direct retinal influences on the excitability of the LGN neurons. However, LGN firing exhibits discharge variations during sleep under experimental conditions in which optic tract discharge is constant. Thus, the burst-pause pattern may result from direct afferent input reduction (off response) or from an impinging influence other than that in the optic tract. This nonvisual input may be either inhibition or withdrawal of facilitation. Conversely, increases in unit firing and the appearance of spaced spikes may result from optic or nonoptic excitatory input to the LGN. The burst-pause pattern appears to result from reduction of excitation.

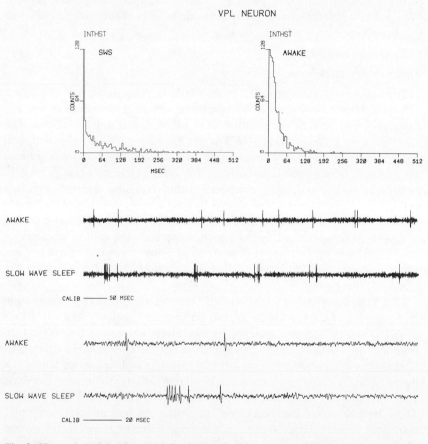

Fig. 2. Illustration of the characteristic changes in firing pattern of thalamic neurons during SWS and W (awake). During W the firing pattern is characterized by isolated cell discharges with very few high frequency bursts (traces 1 and 3). During SWS, however, the discharges occur mainly in short high frequency bursts separated by longer pauses (traces 2 and 4). The interval histograms (top) indicate the preponderance of very short intervals during SWS compared to the alert state. The SWS histograms also reveal a wider distribution of long intervals than seen in the alert state, reflecting the increased variability of intervals between successive discharges during SWS.

As suggested in the introduction, the change in spontaneous firing rate may reflect changes in a level of tonic excitability of neurons. This possibility has been examined directly in two ways. Sakakura (1968) was able to observe spontaneous EPSP's in some recordings in the LGN. He noted the number of EPSP's resulting in spikes, as well as those failing to do so, in each stage of sleep and wakefulness. In this way he could estimate the fraction of EPSP's which generated a spike. His data are compared with the spontaneous rate of firing in the same unit, as shown in Figure 3. The data show that the spontaneous firing rate and the probability of spike generation by an EPSP are closely parallel.

A second procedure is to measure the probability of evoking a spike with an afferent stimulus. This approach was also employed by Sakakura (1968), by stimulation of the optic tract, and by Mukhametov and Rizzolatti (1970), with flashes from a minature lamp fixed to a glass contact lens, as mentioned above. The results of these studies are like those derived from the study of spontaneous EPSP's. The responsiveness of the LGN to afferent stimulation is proportional to the spontaneous firing rate.

These data suggest that the excitability of LGN neurons to optic tract input

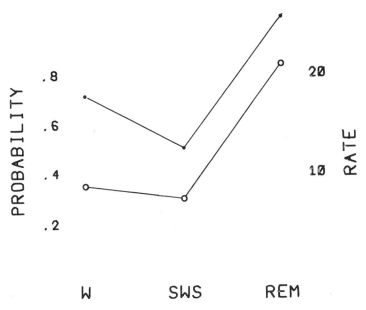

Fig. 3. Comparison of the rate of spontaneous unit discharge (connected dots) with the probability of spike elicitation by EPSP's (connected circles) in an LGN cell during waking (W), slow wave sleep (SWS), and rapid eye movement sleep (REM). The data show that the relative rate of spontaneous firing during the sleep-waking cycle is generally proportional to the excitability of the cell as measured by the EPSP method (see text) or by studies of response to afferent input. Similar results have been obtained in studies of midbrain reticular units. These data were taken from the report of Sakakura. .

is modulated by input from nonvisual influences. The spontaneous firing of LGN neurons is a measure of this background excitability. The source of this change in background excitability is responsible for changes in sensory transmission in sleep.

The change in unit firing pattern in SWS is paralleled by another process, the correlation of spike activity of neighboring units. This phenomenon has been carefully documented in neocortical and hippocampal sites by Noda and Adey (1970). The results were based on a series of recordings from single electrodes in which two discriminable spike trains could be observed. These two trains were separated on the basis of amplitude. The temporal association in the two spike trains was analyzed by digital computer. The analysis showed that the second neuron of each pair was sometimes active with a higher probability at the time of occurrence of the discharge of the first neuron. This temporal association in discharge was pronounced during SWS but was reduced during W and absent in the majority of units during REM. These data indicate that the occurrence of the burst-pause pattern in SWS is associated with synchronized firing in adjacent units.

The burst-pause pattern in thalamocortical cells is not a specific correlate of behavioral sleep. This phenomenon may be observed during slow wave EEG activity in the absence of sleep behavior. There are certain conditions under which it is possible to dissociate the usual EEG correlates of sleep and waking. For example, large doses of atropine administered to alert rabbits will synchronize the EEG with large slow waves which bear some semblance to those seen during quiet sleep. Under these conditions many neurons in thalamic and limbic structures discharge as if the animal were asleep with slow waves, even though behaviorally the animal is not sleeping (Harper, 1973). This result is illustrated in Figure 4. This experiment is not intended to show a resemblance between the atropine condition and quiet sleep. Rather, it demonstrates that the burst-pause pattern is a passive consequence of sleep behavior that may, in fact, be simulated in a waking animal.

Cell groups thought to be directly involved in regulation of motor function, such as the red nucleus and cerebellar Purkinje cells, are distinct in their alternation of firing pattern during the sleep-waking cycle. During SWS, red nucleus (RN) neurons become more variable but do not adopt the short high frequency burst characteristic of the thalamocortical cells. In REM these neurons can fire in high frequency bursts but the bursts are irregular and are not necessarily followed by long pauses. It should be made clear that, in describing the burst-paust activity of neurons, we distinguish between short high frequency bursts that characterize thalamocortical neurons during quiet sleep and long sustained bursts of activity that characterize, for example, red nucleus neurons in REM. This activity is perhaps best described by the histograms of the distribution of intervals between spikes given in Figure 5. Clearly, there is no abundance of very short intervals during quiet sleep, as is the case with thalamic neurons. In a thorough study of cerebellar Purkinje cells, McCarley and Hobson (1972) have demonstrated that the variance, third and fourth moments, and the percentage of intervals in the first order interval histogram are functions of mean discharge rate. These properties could not be characteristic of cells which discharge in a burst-pause pattern, like thalamic neurons.

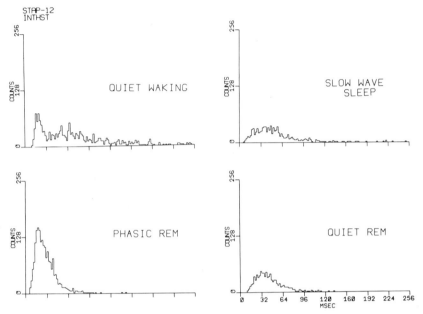

Fig. 4. These plots represent the distribution of intervals between spike discharges from the hippocampus of a rabbit during states of waking, quiet sleep, and waking after administration of 5 mg/kg atropine sulfate. Atropine administration cuases large slow waves to develop in various brain structures of the waking animal. The interval histograms are very similar for the atropine and quiet sleep states, while the shape of the histogram during the alert state is different from these two conditions. The difference arises from the preponderance of short intervals, reflected in the recordings as a change to a burst-pause pattern of discharge. These plots demonstrate a dissociation of phenomena which characterize a state: slow waves appear during quiet sleep and also in the waking state under atropine. The single neurons are discharging in a pattern that corresponds to the EEG activity rather than to the behavior.

Behavioral Functions and Sleep

The studies reviewed above dealt primarily with thalamic relay nuclei and sensory cortex where anatomical and functional properties of large cells are partially understood. Analysis of unit firing outside of known sensory and motor systems is more difficult to interpret. A majority of units recorded in many hippocampal and hypothalamic sites decrease their discharge rates in SWS as do thalamic and neocortical cells. However, certain limbic subgroups exhibit increased discharge in SWS. The majority of units of the basolateral amygdala (Jacobs and McGinty, 1971) and the ventromedial hypothalamus

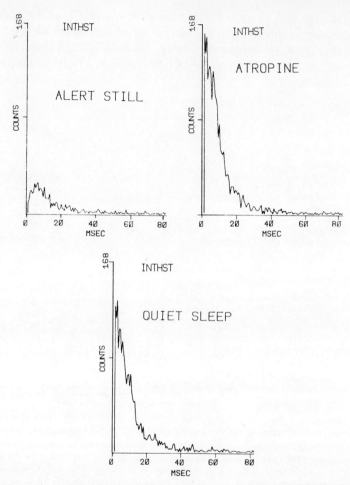

Fig. 5. Plots of interval histograms for a cat red nucleus neuron during four states. Note that there are few very short intervals during SWS. This histogram for SWS should be compared to the histogram for the thalamic neuron in Fig. 2. The distribution of intervals during phasic REM reflects the bursts of increased spike discharge during that state. These bursts, however, are not simply more enhanced versions of the type of burst-pause patterns seen in thalamic neurons during SWS; the phasic REM discharges are characterized by more sustained periods of firing, and the extremely short intervals characteristic of thalamic burst-pause patterns are missing.

(Oomura et al., 1969) of the cat, and a plurality of units of the anterior hypothalamus of the rabbit (Findlay and Hayward, 1969) exhibit an increase in rate in SWS. These sites are anatomically interrelated and functionally involved in "behavioral inhibition." That is, these sites function in the limitation or regulation of behaviors such as feeding, exploration, or reactivity to specific sensory stimuli. Following lesions of these sites, these normal behaviors occur with an exaggerated frequency.

However, the extrapolation of behavioral concepts to cellular functions is not readily achieved. The anatomical and functional relationships of most cells in limbic, hypothalamic, and brainstem sites are virtually unknown. Lesion and stimulation of these sites almost invariably produce multiple behavioral effects, reflecting the fact that most of these sites contain not only mixtures of cell types, but also major ascending and descending fiber pathways. The increase or decrease of unit discharge during sleep, observed in a randomly encountered limbic or brainstem neuron, has little meaning unless the functional correlates of these changes are known. For this reason we have proposed a method of analysis of such cells based on a comparison of behavioral correlates of unit discharge during wakefulness and changes during sleep.

This procedure involves the study of each unit in a series of behavioral conditions, chosen on the basis of probable functional relation. For example, discharge of cells in a given region may be studied for specific correlations with movement, sensory input, autonomic functions, drive states, EEG correlations, or complex behavioral functions. This approach can provide three important benefits: 1) the establishment of criteria for identification of cell types in heterogeneous regions; 2) the discovery of powerful influences on unit discharge; and 3) the initial steps in the study of the integrative action of the cells under study. These benefits are illustrated in the study of basolateral amygdala unit discharge. This complex experimental program, which is summarized briefly below, has been described in detail elsewhere (Jacobs and McGinty, 1971, 1972; Jacobs, 1973).

The first step in this analysis was the investigation of the behavior of each unit during the sleep-waking cycle. On the basis of this analysis, basal amygdala units could be divided into two discrete groups. Approximately 60% of the encountered units significantly increased their rate of firing during SWS as compared to W or REM. The cells which discharged fastest in SWS were characterized by slower firing rates overall (median rate = 0.5 spikes/sec in SWS compared with 1.8 spikes/sec in SWS for the remaining cells). The difference in rate between the two groups was greater in W and REM.

Following the sleep study, the units were studied during conditioning experiments or during sensory stimulation tests. The conditioning experiments were chosen on the basis of previous studies indicating that the amygdala played a role in behavioral inhibition. Two types of conditioned inhibition experiments were carried out. In the first experiment a specific EEG rhythm, the sensorimotor rhythm (SMR), was reinforced in an operant paradigm. This conditioning procedure was chosen because previous studies had shown that SMR was associated with inhibition of phasic motor behavior. Spontaneous occurrences of the SMR recorded over the sensorimotor cortex and detected by a frequency analyzer (tuned to respond to 13.5 Hz) were followed by the delivery of hypothalamic brain stimulation previously found to provide positive reinforcement. The conditioning procedure increased both the frequency and duration of the trains of SMR. The rates of unit discharge in intervals containing the SMR were compared with contiguous equal intervals without SMR. The response of the units to hypothalamic stimulation was also assessed.

The second conditioning experiment was a variant of the conditioned emotional response paradigm. In the first stage of the experiment, food deprived cats were presented with 30 trials consisting of a 10 sec 1 kHz tone followed by a 0.5 sec strong aversive air puff. The air puff caused the cats to withdraw to a corner of the chamber. In the testing phase of the study, the tone was presented alone during free feeding from a bowl. During the tone feeding was suppressed, indicating successful aversive conditioning. Neuronal discharge rates were measured during the suppression of feeding and compared with rates in the preceding 10 sec periods.

The sensory stimulation tests consisted of presentation of both simple stimuli (tone, clicks, changes in illumination, flashes, white noise) and complex stimuli (meows, cat howls, olfactory stimuli such as smoke, a rat in the chamber, hand threats, rustling of shavings, etc.). The latter tests were based on a previous report that basal amygdala units may respond to specific complex stimuli. We were able to replicate this result; basal amygdala units may respond exclusively to one or two unique complex stimuli, and be absolutely unresponsive or suppressed by all other stimuli.

The results of all of these experiments are summarized in Table II. The initial classification of cells on the basis of the sleep-waking state rate profile

TABLE II

	Classification: SWS	Fastest Rate W or REM
Median rate (spikes/sec) SWS	0.5	1.8
1. Increased discharge during SMR [a]	8/10	0/7
2. Decreased discharge following hypothal. stimulation [a]	6/10	1/7
3. Decreased discharge during conditioned suppression [a]	5/8	1/5
4. Acceleration to complex stimuli [a]	9/36	0/36

[a] Proportion of cells exhibiting statistically significant discharge rate changes.

could be used to predict differences in various behavioral situations. Thus, 80% of the SWS-fastest cells increased their discharge rate during SMR conditioning, while none of the other cells did so. Similarly, SWS-fastest cells discharge was inhibited during conditioned suppression and by hypothalamic stimulation. In addition, only SWS-fastest cells were found to respond to complex sensory stimuli. Only nine complex stimuli were found to be effective, probably because of the impossibility of testing the wide range of complex stimuli that could be relevant to the cat. The differences in the response of the two populations were statistically significant in the case of each procedure.

We hypothesized that discharge of one class of amygdala unit is instrumental in a certain type of behavioral inhibition involving phasic motor inhibition (SMR conditioning). These same units respond to specific complex stimuli. Since lesion studies had indicated that this brain site suppressed behavioral approach to inappropriate stimulus objects (inedible foods, irrelevant stimuli), we suggested that these units may mediate inhibition of motor behavioral responses to specific complex stimuli.

On the basis of this analysis, the increase in firing in SWS may be understood. During W, a small fraction of these amygdala units are active at any instant, because their activity is dependent on highly specific stimuli. During sleep all the members of this class are active simultaneously. This mass action of units that appear to be involved in motor inhibition may play an active role in the modulation of sleep by the forebrain. Units of this class in the amygdala, and possibly in other limbic sites as well, may explain the suppression of sleep after forebrain lesions (McGinty and Sterman, 1968; Villablanca and Marcus, 1972; Villablanca and Salinas-Zeballos, 1972). That is, removal of the inhibitory influence of these cells may prevent SWS.

Ben-Ari and LaSalle (1971) have also found it useful to divide basal amygdala units into two classes, based on discharge rate. Slow firing units were found to exhibit habituation to stimuli. Because of the similarity in the classification procedure, we can compare our results directly with theirs, and thereby expand our understanding. Interlaboratory comparison of data obtained from heterogeneous structures is impossible in the absence of some method of classification.

REM Sleep

The majority of neurons of most regions of the brain exhibit augmented discharge during REM sleep. Firing rates exceeding those of SWS and quiet W are found in the thalamus, cortex, and many limbic and hypothalamic-brainstem sites. Further analysis of the increased firing in REM has compared the rate changes in relation to tonic and phasic periods within REM sleep and in relation to active W compared with quiet W. In both cases the objective has been to distinguish periods with movements or behavioral arousal from quiescent periods. For example, it has been reported that visual cortex units exhibit comparable rates in REM and *alert* W. LGN unit discharge was found to be faster in REM than in quiet waking only during periods containing PGO waves (Mukhametov et al., 1970a). It appears likely that in many structures discharge rates in quiet W are comparable to rates in REM without phasic events, while discharge rates in active W are comparable to phasic REM rates. Because of the difficulty in collecting artifact-free records in alert, active W states, this issue has not been completely resolved.

Investigators of unit discharge cannot help being impressed with the widespread augmentation of unit firing in animals who are behaviorally asleep. Since release of neuronal discharge during REM is accompanied by tonic inhibition of motoneurons (Pompeiano, 1967), it may be suggested that the behavioral expression of the activation of the brain is prevented at the motoneuron level. However, it must be remembered that the acceleration of unit discharge in REM does not necessarily reflect the same excitatory process as that which is manifest in wakefulness. There are striking functional differences between these two states, including the lack of high levels of sensory (including proprioceptive) input during REM. It is plausible that accelerated unit discharge during W, especially in thalamic sites, is more dependent on sensory excitation, while the same acceleration in REM may reflect nonsensory input. On the other hand, the magnitude of the influence during W of nonsensory input to the thalamus is not well known. Processes such as corollary discharge associated with eye movements and other motor events may provide strong excitatory inputs. Acceleration of unit discharge in a given cell may reflect a variety of influences.

PGO Waves

Among the most fascinating aspects of REM sleep is the occurrence of high amplitude slow waves, either single waves or as bursts of 2-5 waves. These waves are found in the *pontine* reticular formation, lateral *geniculate* nucleus, and *occipital* cortex, hence the name PGO waves. These waves are coincident with rapid eye movements, or lateral EMG activity, and normally occur only during REM, and during SWS for an approximately 1 minute period preceding REM. Smaller amplitude slow waves *following* eye movements may be seen in the same structures during W. These PGO waves are of interest because they are the most readily studied example of the phasic elements of REM sleep. In addition, Dement (1969) and his associates have suggested, on the basis of a variety of studies, that PGO waves may be an important manifestation of the biological function of REM sleep.

The unit activity of LGN neurons and optic tract terminals has been carefully studied in relation to local PGO waves. With respect to LGN units, bursts of firing have been correlated with the falling phase of PGO waves, while the initial rising phase is correlated with a slight suppression of firing. Optic tract discharge itself does not vary. Both Bizzi (1966) and Sakakura and Iwama (1967) have demonstrated that the optic tract terminals are depolarized coincident with the rising phase of the PGO waves, an apparent example of presynaptic inhibition.

FTG Neurons

The gigantocellular tegmental field (FTG) of the pons has been proposed by McCarley and Hobson (1971) as a control center for the manifestation of REM (see also Chapter 4, this volume). Unit recordings in restrained cats had shown that during W and SWS there is very little neuronal discharge from this area. The firing rate of these cells increased dramatically with the onset of REM. The highly specific change in rate, often exceeding a tenfold increase, has been interpreted as supporting the hypothesis that these neurons are instrumental in the triggering of REM. We are presently recording extracellular single units from unrestrained cats in an attempt to verify this hypothesis.

We have studied 30 units in the medial pontine tegmentum, of which 13 appear to correspond to the cell type described by McCarley and Hobson (1971). These units were recorded from the medial gigantocellular field (L1-L2) of the pons. This type of cell discharged at a very low rate, with silent periods, during quiet W and SWS. During SWS the discharge rates increased when PGO waves appeared. During REM these cells became tonically and phasically active with at least a tenfold increase in rate (see Fig. 6). An integrator record of a typical unit is shown in Figure 7. The augmentation of firing preceding and during REM is striking.

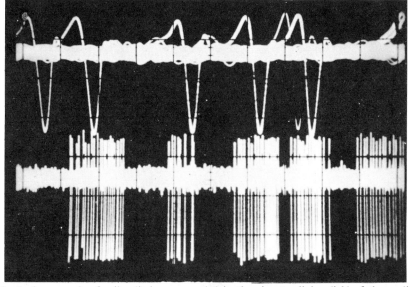

Fig. 6. An example of spike discharge recorded in the gigantocellular field of the medial pontine tegmentum. Short bursts of activity (upper trace) were during rhythmic grooming movements during W.

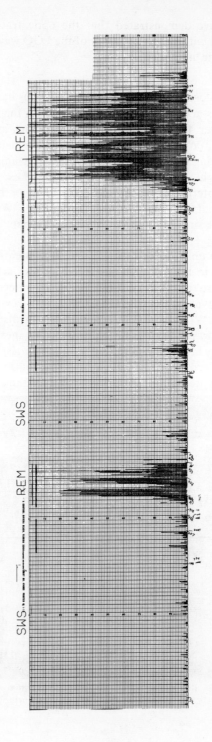

Fig. 7. The rate of a pontine tegmental neuron during an 80 min. record of sleep, including two REM periods. Each vertical line represents the number of spikes in 5 sec.; a full scale vertical deflection corresponds to a rate of 100 spikes/sec. The rate of firing of the cell was low during SWS, but increased markedly during REM (indicated by double horizontal line at the top of the figure). The discharge rate also increased during PGO waves during SWS (single horizontal line).

A specificity criterion for a REM control center would dictate that discharge rate changes occur uniquely in REM. This was not true for these units. During active W these cells exhibited bursts of firing which were correlated with movements of the head or neck region. These movements were frequently specific, i.e., turning the head to follow an object going across the visual field from left to right, or twitching the right ear when it was touched. An example is shown in Figure 8. Initial tests with head restraint during W produced a nearly total suppression of unit activity, even during eye movements or mild struggling. This experiment is illustrated in Figure 9. Thus, discharge rates of these cells are low during quiet W or during head restraint because of the absence of head movement.

This cell type appears to correspond to proposed REM control center neurons observed in the restrained cat. These units have the same pontine localization, augmented discharge prior to REM, tonic increase during REM, and relatively low rates during quiet W and SWS. However, correlations observed between W movements and unit discharge in freely moving cats suggest that other possible functions for these neurons should be considered. This cell seems to be involved in some aspect of motor function such as the coordination of head and eye movements. A behavioral analysis, like that applied to the amygdala neurons, is needed.

Discussion

We have reviewed studies of neurons which lie outside of brain regions which have been specifically implicated in the neural control of sleep. We have considered these results from the point of view of the question of how the control of sleep may be implemented. A strategy for the investigation of this question has been suggested. The following tentative conclusions can be offered.

1) The burst-pause pattern of most thalamic and cortical neurons during SWS results from withdrawal of a diffuse excitatory process. The burst-pause pattern is not a specific correlate of SWS.

2) Neurons having inhibitory functions in W may exhibit increased firing in SWS. This was suggested on the basis of a detailed study of amygdala neurons and the similarity of unit changes during sleep between these neurons and other limbic sites thought to have behavioral inhibitory functions. Evarts (1967a, b) has suggested that neurons which have slow discharge rates in W accelerate in SWS, while fast cells decelerate. That is, differentiation of function is reduced in SWS. Further studies are required to assess these two hypotheses.

3) During REM most neurons exhibit firing patterns like those seen in W. This result is particularly obvious in the case of neurons involved in motor control. The source of the excitatory influences in W and REM are not known.

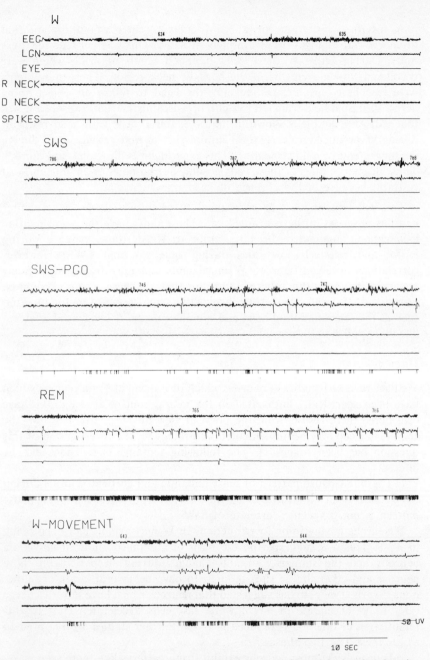

Fig. 8. Polygraph record including pontine neuronal discharge (from Schmitt trigger) during sleep states and waking. Discharge was slow during quiet W and SWS, but increased during SWS with PGO waves and was characterized by high frequency bursts during REM. The same cell is active during W with head movement.

HEAD RESTRAINED

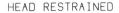

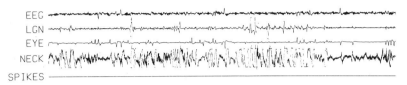

NO RESTRAINT

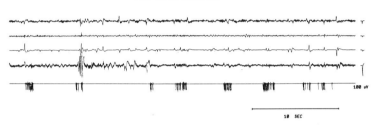

Fig. 9. A pontine neuron that normally fires slowly except during REM and during head movements. This cell normally discharges during head movements to the left. During W the discharge does not occur if head movements are prevented by restraint, even if the cat was struggling and moving his eyes.

IV. NEURAL CONTROL OF SLEEP

Thus far, we have considered studies of brain loci which have not been found to directly control sleep, but rather appear to play secondary or passive roles. As noted in the introduction, the primary control of REM sleep appears to be carried out in the pontine tegmentum. SWS has a more diffuse basis but the simple alternation of behavioral activity and behavioral quiescence requires midbrain structures. Cyclic and appetitive behavioral characteristics of SWS appear to be diencephalic and telencephalic functions. Thus, attempts to study neurons involved in REM have logically explored pontine sites, while midbrain sites may be studied in connection with behavioral activation and quiescence. The pioneering work of Jouvet (1967, 1969) has lead neurophysiologists to study the locus coeruleus and n. ret. pontis oralis and caudalis of the pons and the raphé system of the midbrain and pons. Jouvet (1967, 1969) has particularly emphasized the NA-containing cells of the pons and 5HT-containing cells localized in midline nuclei of the midbrain, pons, and medulla. This work has been begun only within the last two or three years and most findings are tentative. However, the results are promising and provocative.

Monoaminergic Functions

The study of monoaminergic function was greatly stimulated by the now well known work of the Swedish group (Dahlstrom and Fuxe, 1965; Anden et al., 1966a), which developed the histo-fluorescent technique for the anatomical localization of monoamines in the brain. It is now widely accepted that cerebral monoamines are localized exclusively within specialized systems of neurons whose perikarya are localized within nuclei in the brainstem except for a group of dopamine-containing cells in the infundibular region of the hypothalamus. These cells give rise to long axons which project to terminal regions in the forebrain, brainstem, and spinal cord. Certain aspects of the model have been clarified by recent studies. Moore (1970) had suggested that some forebrain monoamines might be contained in cells of forebrain origin because, following lesions of the ascending pathway and presumed degeneration of terminal areas, substantial quantities of forebrain monoamines are still found. This finding may have resulted from the fact that ascending pathways are more diffuse than had been originally thought. At any rate, complete lesions of the brainstem midline groups result in nearly complete loss of forebrain 5HT and a parallel loss of tryptophane hydroxylase (Kuhar et al., 1971). The early difficulty in visualizing fluorescent terminals in neocortical sites, where substantial quantities of CA were detected neurochemically, has been remedied by improvements in the histofluorescent techniques (Nystrom et al., 1972).

The release of monoamines appears to be under the control of a feedback mechanism. This mechanism has been elucidated by Aghajanian et al. (Aghajanian et al., 1970a, b; Aghajanian, 1972). They have shown that a variety of pharmacological treatments which increase 5HT levels in the brain cause the suppression of unit discharge of raphé neurons. Among the drugs which produce suppression of unit activity are monoamine oxidase inhibitors (Aghajanian et al., 1970a), tricyclic antidepressants (Aghajanian et al., 1970b), and L-tryptophane (Aghajanian, 1972)—the precursor of 5HT. These results are interpreted to indicate that increased stimulation of receptors for 5HT by elevation of available 5HT causes a feedback suppression of 5HT-neuronal discharge.

Graham and Aghajanian (1971) have also studied feedback control of the norepinephrine-containing neurons of the locus coeruleus of the rat. In this case, administration of amphetamine, a powerful sympathomimetic agent which is thought to release norepinephrine from nerve terminals suppressed locus coeruleus unit discharge. This feedback control system has also been studied indirectly by the Swedish group (Anden et al., 1969). They have shown that a variety of drugs which *block* catecholamine receptors *increase* release of catecholamine, while receptor stimulants decrease release. In the latter experiments, release was measured indirectly by examining rates of decrease in terminal catecholamine levels after synthesis inhibition.

This feedback control system complicates the interpretation of pharmacological treatments which are thought to augment or decrease receptor stimulation by augmenting or decreasing monoamine levels. Feedback compensation will tend to minimize changes in receptor stimulation. Indeed, it is plausible that exogenous sources of monoamines may be distributed to terminal areas in a nonuniform manner and cause an increase in stimulation of some receptor sites and, through feedback inhibition, a decrease in stimulation at others.

Although the Swedish group has studied the monoaminergic system primarily in the rat, the distribution of cell bodies and pathways in the cat has been described as well (Pin et al., 1968). There are slight difference in the two species. For example, in the cat, scattered cells containing 5HT have been found in the red nucleus. The catecholaminergic cells of the dorsal pons are densely packed in the rat, but in the cat they are more diffuse, being found in the locus coeruleus, subcoeruleus, n. parabrachialis medialis, and lateralis. The cells of the principal nucleus of the locus coeruleus are generally oval, while the cells of the subcoeruleus complex are frequently larger and multipolar.

The hypothesis that monoamines play some role in the modulation of the sleep-waking process has been generally supported by a variety of experimental approaches, including lesion studies, pharmacological studies, and biochemical studies. That is, almost any experimental treatment that affects monoamines will affect sleep, while experimental manipulation of sleep may affect monoamines. However, no consistent set of results has emerged. The specific theory of Jouvet (1967, 1969) that the action of 5HT is required for the occurrence of SWS and that the action of NA, specifically in neurons originating in the locus coeruleus of the pons, is required for REM is only partially supported by the data. For example, depletion of brain 5HT by synthesis inhibition with single doses of parachlorophenylalanine (PCPA) suppresses sleep in the cat. However, during chronic administration of PCPA sleep returns to normal (Dement et al., 1972). Single doses of PCPA produce inconsistent or partial effects in rats. In man, PCPA affects REM rather than SWS.

In the case of the function of norepinephrine, electrolytic lesions of the locus coeruleus and subcoeruleus suppress REM in the cat (Mouret and Delorme, 1967). The depletion of NA by synthesis inhibition with α-methyltryosine may augment rather than suppress REM (Iskander and Kaelbling, 1970; King and Jewett, 1971).

Monoamines have been implicated in the regulation of a variety of functional processes in addition to sleep, including general arousal and exploration, temperature regulation, feeding, pain perception, sexual behavior, aggression, "reward" mechanisms, and conditioned behaviors (see Barkas and Usden (1973) for a review). Since treatments that alter monoamine (MA) function may affect all of these behaviors, it is difficult to ascribe a change in sleep patterns to be solely the result of a specific effect on sleep mechanisms.

Unit Recording of Monoamine Systems

Measurement of the time of release of monoamines in relation to behavioral activities or events can best be accomplished by direct recording of the neuronal discharge of monoamine-containing neurons. There is substantial evidence that monoamines in cerebral neurons are released by the depolarization of axon terminals by nerve impulses, just as ACH is released by motoneurons. This evidence comes from three sources: stimulation experiments, lesion experiments, and pharmacological experiments.

The experimental problem is to determine the relationship between the release of monoamines in terminal regions such as the forebrain or spinal cord, and the occurrence of nerve impulses in the brainstem perikarya. This can be accomplished by measuring increases or decreases in transmitter concentration in terminals, or decreases or increases in monoamine metabolites such as 5-hydroxyindoleacetic acid (5HIAA) following, respectively, decreased or increased neuronal activity.

Changes in monoamine concentration are more predictable under conditions of synthesis inhibition. The approach was used by Anden et al. (1969) in the study of spinal norepinephrine and 5HT levels. Normally, after synthesis inhibition, monoamine levels gradually decline, as a result of gradual release and metabolism of pre-existing monoamine stores. Caudal to a spinal transection, before nerve degeneration, the same decline of monoamine levels is greatly diminished (Anden et al., 1966b). The authors' conclusion was that decline of monoamine levels after synthesis inhibition did not occur caudal to the transection because nerve impulses no longer reached terminals to release monoamine stores.

Control experiments indicated that the failure of release was not the result of metabolic changes after transection. This study suggests that release of monoamines requires nerve impulse flow. This interpretation was supported by additional studies showing that stimulation of bulbar 5HT- or norepinephrine-containing neurons after synthesis inhibition would *accelerate* the respective decline of 5HT and NA levels (Dahlstrom et al., 1964).

Several groups have replicated the observation that stimulation of the 5HT-containing neurons of the midbrain resulted in decreased forebrain 5HT levels and increases in 5HIAA levels (Aghajanian et al., 1967; Eccleston et al., 1969; Kostowski et al., 1969; Gumulka et al., 1971). Thus, within ascending 5HT systems, as in bulbospinal systems, 5HT is released by neural discharge. Pharmacological studies also support this result. LSD suppresses the neuronal discharge of midbrain raphé neurons (Aghajanian et al., 1968). This drug has also been found to raise forebrain 5HT levels and reduce 5HIAA levels (Freedman, 1961).

The ascending NA-containing neurons with perikarya in the locus coeruleus of the pons also share this property. Arbuthnott et al. (1970) have shown that electrical stimulation of the dorsal pathway arising from the locus coeruleus causes disappearance of NA in hippocampal and dorsal neocortex, ipsilateral to the site of stimulation.

In summary, a variety of studies support the concept that the occasions of release of monoamines from nerve terminals can be determined by observation of the neural discharge of the perikarya in the brainstem.

5HT-Containing Neurons

Our investigations of the unit activity of 5HT-containing neurons (McGinty, 1973; McGinty et al., 1973) have thus far been restricted to the dorsal raphé nucleus of the caudal midbrain. This nucleus lies in the ventromedial portion of the central gray, under the aqueduct of Sylvius, dorsal and medial to the medial longitudinal fasciculus. The anterior portion is medial to the nucleus of IV and caudal to III. The posterior portion is medial to the dorsal tegmental nucleus. This nucleus was chosen for our initial studies because it is the only cluster of cells that consists nearly entirely of 5HT-containing neurons. Other nuclei generally consist of scattered cells or pairs of cells in the midline, adjacent to other cell types. Thus, in the dorsal raphe nucleus alone, it is possible to be relatively certain that a histologically localized electrode placement is among 5HT-containing cells.

We have recorded the unit discharge of 43 cells from electrodes which were placed in the region of the dorsal raphé nucleus, within 0.5 mm of the midline, excluding occulomotor neurons of n. IV. Of this sample, 34 (81%) exhibited a homogeneous pattern of activity. These cells exhibited a slow regular pattern of firing during W at rates between 0.5 and 5.0 spikes/sec. We operationally defined a class of cells as those with W rates within this range. The following discussion is concerned with this class of neurons.

The assumption that we recorded from 5HT-containing neurons is based on the histological data (see Fig. 10), the homogeneity of the characteristics of the neurons as could be expected from a homogeneous cellular group, the similarity of our results and those of Aghajanian and his associates (Aghajanian et al., 1970a, b), who have studied this nucleus in the anesthetized rat, and the consistency of the behavior of the cells with facts relating 5HT and PGO waves (discussed below).

The changes in firing rate in relation to the sleep-waking cycle are shown in Figure 11. There are two principal findings. First, the rate of firing in SWS compared with W is reduced by about 50%. Second, the firing rate in REM is reduced 90% compared with W. The reduction in firing in SWS compared with W was significant for 27 of the 34 individual neurons, while the reduction in REM compared with SWS was significant in 29 of 34 (2-tailed "t" test, $p = 0.01$).

The reduction of raphé unit firing in SWS implies, as argued above, that the release of 5HT is reduced in SWS. This result is inconsistent with the theory of Jouvet that 5HT is directly involved in the maintenance of SWS. However, it can be argued that our results are not conclusive because 1) our recordings were restricted to only one raphé nucleus, 2) our recordings may have selectively sampled a subset of large cells which behave differently than small cells, and 3) the sleep-enchancing role of 5HT may be carried out during W through the suppression of behaviors which interfere with sleep.

With respect to the first objection, it must be pointed out that lesions of the dorsal raphé nucleus are sufficient to produce the suppression of sleep that

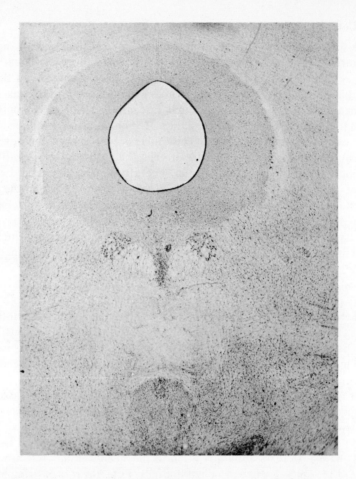

Fig. 10. A small lesion marking the tip of an electrode in the dorsal raphé nudens at the level of the n.iv. Raphé units which exhibit suppression of discharge during REM are invariably detected near the midline, but not by electrode placements more than 0.5mm laterally.

was observed by Jouvet after more extensive lesions (Morgane and Stern, 1973). Second, preliminary reports of recordings from pontine raphé nuclei also indicate a reduction of unit discharge in SWS (Sheu et al., 1971). With respect to the objection based on sampling of large cells, we reiterate that the pattern of firing which we observed was identical to that obtained with small tipped microelectrodes in the rat, and that in the cat we do not find any minority group that would suggest the presence of small cells which increase firing in SWS. More importantly, we feel that the third explanation, that 5HT may facilitate sleep through a role during wakefulness, is a plausible explanation which incorporates a wide variety of observations. Before considering this hypothesis in detail, we wish to discuss the results obtained in REM sleep.

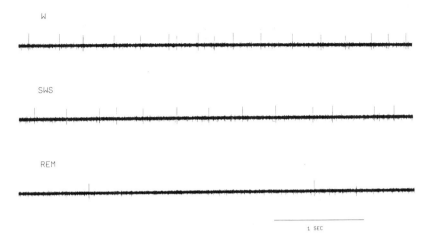

Fig. 11. Raphé unit spike activity during W, SWS, and REM. Spike activity is slow and regular during W. The rate of firing is reduced during SWS, but the regularity of discharge is maintained. During REM discharge is markedly reduced. The amplified signal was digitized 33 K Hz, and plotted by a laboratory computer.

5HT and REM Sleep

The depression of raphé unit firing during REM is the most striking aspect of this experiment. With the exception of the neurons of the subcoeruleus region of the pons, described below, and motoneurons, this is the only known example of a state-specific change in unit firing of a large class of neurons.

Certain details of this phenomenon require detailed description. The depression of dorsal raphé unit discharge anticipates the onset of the tonic aspect of REM, as suggested in Figure 12. Raphe units appeared to pause before the SWS-PGO waves that precede REM. These units may also resume firing within a REM period during interruptions in the train of PGO waves. Thus, the depression of raphé unit discharge appears to be specifically related to the phasic rather than the tonic aspect of REM.

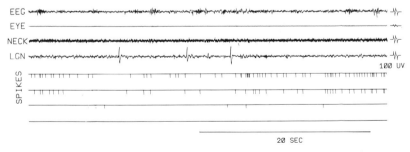

Fig. 12. Polygraph record during SWS with isolated PGO waves. Two typical raphé units were recorded simultaneously. The spike activity of the raphé neurons tends to slow before SWS-PGO waves in most dorsal raphé cells.

A more detailed analysis of the relationship of raphé unit discharge and PGO waves in 10 typical units is shown in Figure 13. The intervals between six successive raphé unit spikes preceding isolated PGO waves were measured for each of 15 PGO waves in each of the 10 cells. The mean duration of the 15 observations was increased significantly in the intervals immediately preceding PGO waves in 8 of the 10 units. Thus, we conclude that the release of 5HT is interrupted prior to the occurrence of PGO waves. This observation supports the concept that 5HT tonically inhibits the release of PGO waves.

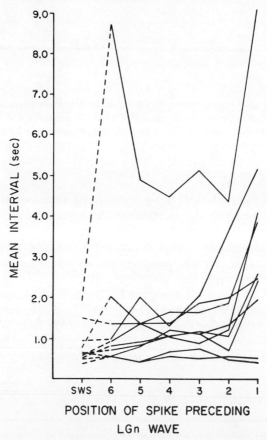

Fig. 13 The mean intervals between raphé unit spikes were measured during SWS and preceding PGO waves for 10 different cells. The last interval before the PGO wave is on the right (#1), the preceding is #2, etc. The last interval before the PGO wave was increased significantly in 8 of the 10 units. In 6 out of 10 units, two or more intervals were increased. Each point is the mean of 15 measurements.

This concept is completely consistent with a variety of well documented studies. First, PGO waves which are normally confined to REM and pre-REM periods are released in W and SWS after depletion of brain 5HT with the synthesis inhibitor, PCPA (Delorme et al., 1966). The release of PGO waves outside of REM has also been observed after treatment with reserpine, which depletes brain 5HT by a different mechanism (Delorme et al., 1965). Finally, electrical stimulation of the dorsal raphé nucleus during REM blocks the occurrence of PGO waves. This experiment is shown in Figure 14. As first proposed by Dement (1969), this insomnia seems to result from the disruption of sleep onset by the intrusion of PGO waves. Waking PGO waves are correlated with behavioral activation.

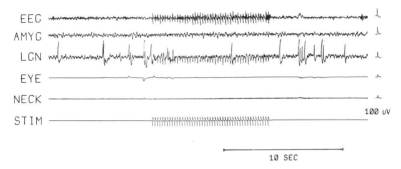

Fig. 14. Electrical stimulation of the dorsal raphé nucleus suppressed the ongoing train of PGO waves during REM. In an analysis of 20 trials, significant PGO suppression was found during the last 8 sec of the 10 sec stimulation period, and for 1 sec following the end of the period. The stimulus consisted of 0.5 msec square waves, 5.0 volts, 5 pulse/sec with 10 sec trains repeated at 20 sec intervals.

The consistency between the pharmacological and physiological data relating levels of brain 5HT to inhibition of release of PGO waves, and the temporal relation between pauses in raphé unit discharge and PGO waves would appear to confirm the concept that sustained raphé unit discharge "gates" the release of PGO waves. This consistency also reinforces our view that our recordings of dorsal raphé units are representative of an important class of 5HT-containing neurons.

The concept that 5HT normally inhibits PGO waves during wakefulness provides an interpretation to account for the insomnia after PCPA treatment and raphé lesions. The phasic events represented by PGO waves that are normally gated during W may disrupt sleep. The onset of insomnia after PCPA first occurs when PGO waves appear in W (Dement et al., 1972). During chronic PCPA treatment in the cat the amount of sleep returns to normal levels (Dement et al., 1972). This may be explained as the result of the cat's habituation to the arousing influence of intruding PGO waves, or to other adaptations in the arousal process. In addition, PCPA produces only an inconsistent and partial suppression of sleep in the rat. This species lacks PGO waves, so sleeping may be less dependent on suppression of the phasic events.

Norepinephrine-Containing Neurons

Our initial studies of the dorsal pontine system (McGinty and Sakai, in press) were concentrated on the medial portion of the subcoeruleus region, adjacent and ventral to the tract of the mesencephalic n. of V and medial to the brachium conjunctivum. This location contains a relatively high density of large NA-containing cells, the largest cells of the region. Thus, the majority of cells sampled by microelectrodes in this region are likely to be representative of the norepinephrine-containing group.

Among 51 units that have been studied thus far, 23 (45%) exhibited several common properties, while the remaining cells appeared to belong to small populations representing several different cell types. The large homogeneous group of units was characterized by slow regular firing during W (1.0 - 3.5 spikes/sec), slight reduction in firing during SWS (0.5 - 2 spikes/sec), and a more striking reduction or *total abolition* of firing in REM sleep. In most units firing was reduced at least 90% in REM relative to W. Silent periods lasting at least 10 sec were observed in all cells of this type. Slowing of unit firing usually preceded PGO waves occuring during SWS prior to REM. This result is shown in Figure 15.

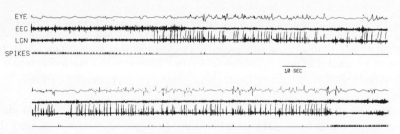

Fig. 15. Polygraph record shoing spike activity of a neuron from the subcoeruleus region of the dorsolateral pontine tegmentum of the cat. This cell type exhibits slow regular discharge during W and SWS, similar to that of dorsal raphé neurons. As shown in the figure, spike discharge slows markedly during REM, and prior to PGO waves in the LGN preceding REM. We believe these cells represent a class of norepinephrine-containing cells and that the release of norepinephrine is interrupted during REM.

Our conviction that we have sampled NA-containing neurons is based on the homogeneity of the sample obtained in a region where the largest cells contain NA. It should be noted that similar results have been obtained by Hobson (1973b) in recording from this region. Chu and Bloom (1973) have reported somewhat different results from recordings in the principal nucleus of the locus coeruleus. The medial cells exhibited grouped discharge in REM, apparently correlated with PGO waves. Similar rates of firing were observed in REM and alert waking. As noted above, the NA-containing cells of the principal nucleus have a different cytoarchitecture than the subcoeruleus cells, and it is reasonable to expect that they would exhibit different functional properties.

The depression of unit firing in subcoeruleus neurons is contradictory to the theory of Jouvet that NA-containing cells of this region directly facilitate REM. However, this result is not at variance with many basic experimental facts. The suppression of REM after lesions of this region could be the result of removal of a system which facilitates REM by cessation of activity rather than augmention of activity. Pharmacological depletion of NA by synthesis inhibition with α-methyl-tyrosine augments sleep. The latter result is consistent with the idea that NA normally suppresses REM.

Speculations on Monoamines and Sleep

In Section II above we reviewed lesion studies showing that REM sleep was organized in the dorsal pons and that the most basic aspect of SWS, the alternation of tonic wakefulness and tonic quiescence, is dependent on the midbrain. Subsequently, we argued that the neural control of SWS may be accomplished by nonspecific influences on the excitability of thalamic and cortical neurons, while the essence of REM was the activation of the brain while motor expression was blocked. We noted that the 5HT-containing neurons of the midbrain and the NA-containing neurons of the pons have diffuse and widespread neural connections and are, thus, physiologically suited to modulate SWS and REM. Our unit recording data support this conception of monoaminergic neurons. These cells exhibit slow, relatively stable discharge that may mediate slowly changing functions such as drive, arousal, or state. We feel that it is useful to speculate about the role of monoamines in sleep control. Our emphasis on the role of 5HT and NA closely parallels the approach of Jouvet (1972), whose theory encouraged our own investigation of these systems. However, our conception differs from that of Jouvet in critical details.

1) The rate of activity of the 5HT- and norepinephrine-containing neurons is compared in Figure 16. The two monoamine systems exhibit a close interaction, with both systems maximally active in wakefulness and minimally active in REM. The level of behavioral facilitation may be a positive function of the joint action of the two systems. Direct electrical stimulation of either system produces arousal (Crow et al., 1972). We speculate that these systems facilitate the integration of coupling *between* various brain systems that is required for coordinated behavioral expression. That is, monoamines may facilitate connectivity between different "functional groups" in the brain. This point of view implies that the characteristic of brain function in REM is the uncoupling of systems. The definition of functional groups cannot be specified with precision, but we wish to emphasize the poor interaction between sensory input, cognition, premotor systems, and motor expression. Except for the motoneurons, each of these systems seems to exhibit similar activity in W and REM, but during REM, integration is absent.

2) The pattern of unit discharge of brain systems, as reflected in neuronal discharge rates, may be a reflection of an antagonistic interaction of the two

systems. Specifically, we speculate that the ratio of activity in norepinephrine
and 5HT cells may determine this aspect of neural activity. This ratio is
shown in Figure 16. The shape of this function is reciprocal to that in the
thalamocortical system and the same as that in the limbic inhititory sites. In
this model norepinephrine acts to reduce the excitability of the
thalamocortical system. Note that, during the orienting response to a novel
stimulus, the activity of NA-containing neurons is suppressed (Fig. 17).

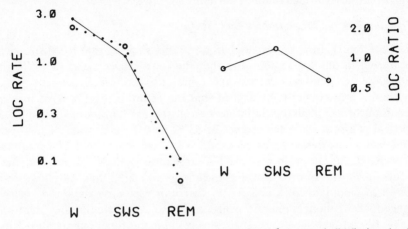

Fig. 16. Left: Median rates of unit discharge of dorsal raphé neurons (solid line) and subcoeruleus neurons (dotted line) during W, SWS, and REM. Note that rate is plotted on a log
scale. These two classes of neurons exhibit a unique pattern and closely related rate changes in
the sleep-waking cycle. We believe that these functions indicate the rate of release of 5HT and
norepinephrine (NA), respectively, in the forebrain. Right: NA/5HT units during SWS. We
speculate that the behavioral facilitation is produced by the joint activity of these two systems,
while the excitability of specific neuron systems may be determined by the ratio or some other
measure of differential between the systems.

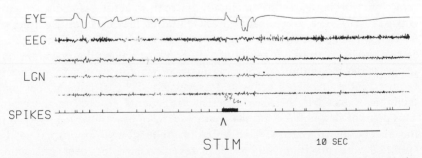

Fig. 17. Polygraph record including indication of spike activity in a subcoeruleus neuron during
W. Any stimulus that elicits an orienting response produced a transient suppression of spike
activity in these cells. In this case a brief train of high frequency electrical stimulation of the
midbrain reticular formation produced the response. The slow fairly regular discharge was
typical of subcoeruleus neurons. The three lower polygraph traces are all derived from LGN
electrodes.

3) Mammalian sleep states must be regarded as the resulants to coordinated processes in many systems. SWS reflects the changes in the brain that are *permitted* by the reduced levels of release of monoamies, including the expression of appropriate behavioral activities by the forebrain. REM sleep reflects changes in the brain permitted by further reduction in monoamine release. The gradual reduction in monoaminergic unit discharge may be possible only during SWS, while selective depression of either system may disrupt sleep.

V. PROPOSED STUDIES

The unraveling of the problem of the control of sleep will require many types of experimental approaches, but a major contribution must come from unit recording studies. We believe that our studies of monoaminergic neurons, reviewed above, offer proof of the value of unit recording studies in the evolution of theoretical concepts. However, the simple correlational unit study that has been employed by us and others can yield little more than interesting speculations. We wish to suggest ways in which the present level of analysis can be extended so that more definitive answers can be obtained.

1) Behavioral classification and behavioral control. The rationale underlying the extensive testing of behavioral influence on neuronal discharge was outlined above in Section III. This approach provides classification of neuronal types, identification of important correlates of cell discharge, and initial information about integrative action of the cells. By thus defining the physiological function of each cell type, the changes that occur during sleep can be understood. In addition, behavioral testing should exclude trivial explanation for changes observed during sleep, such as altered posture, or autonomic changes.

2) Cyclic properties of sleep. The alternation of sleep and waking and of SWS and REM are rhythmic processes. This rhythmicity may proceed in the absence of overt sleep-waking behaviors. Neurons directly involved in sleep must exhibit stable changes in relation to these cyclic processes. The phase relations between cyclic changes in various systems should reveal the sequential events in the sleep cycle.

3) Cellular interactions. We have suggested that the changes in some brain sites underlying sleep involve altered excitability to afferent imputs. These changes have been measured directly in the case of LGN neurons using nonphysiological stimuli. Excitability studies must be extended to a variety of brain sites. This paradigm can also be used to study the coupling among "functional groups" such as thalamocortical systems, premotor systems, and limbic systems. The study of excitability changes in sleep would be improved by the difficult experiment of stimultaneous recording of pairs of cells with demonstrable connections. The excitatory or inhibitory influence of spike discharge of one cell on the other could be measured statistically during the states of sleep and wakefulness. This type of study would avoid the use of

stimulus evoked bombardment which may not mimic normal input. In all studies, excitability changes must be related to spontaneous firing rate.

4) Monoaminergic influences. We have speculated that monoamines are the causal agents of diffuse changes in altered excitability during sleep. This concept can be tested by measuring excitability changes in thalamic, cortical, or limbic sites, following stimulus-evoked release or spontaneous release (determined by unit recording techniques) of 5HT or norepinephrine. These systems should also be studied during drug treatments which alter sleep patterns. For example, treatment with 5HTP appears to augment SWS, but it is possible that net changes in brain excitability produced by this drug are the opposite of that seen after increase in neurally released 5HT. This paradoxical effect could result from overcompensation for exogeneous 5HTP by negative feedback or antagonistic systems. Finally, the interactions between the monoaminergic systems must be studied directly.

The technical requirements for the studies listed above include the maintenance of stable unit recordings through extended periods and, in some cases, the stimultaneous recordings from two or more non-adjacent cells. The pursuit of these studies has awaited the required technological developments. We believe that the microwire unit recording technique fulfills these requirements. (Harper and McGinty, 1973). This technique makes it possible

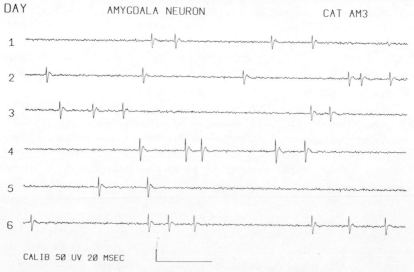

Fig. 18. This figure documents the ability to record from a single neuron for very long periods of time. In these traces, amygdala single neuron discharges recorded from a fine wire microelectrode are plotted for 6 consecutive days. The waveforms of the neuron retain their basic shape over the 6 day period. The size of the waveform grew appreciably larger on day 4, reflecting perhaps movement of the electrode closer to the neuron. Plots of these waveforms, together with continuous measures of characteristics of the waveshape, provide strong evidence that very long-term recordings of single neurons are possible with the fine wire technique.

to record from single neurons for several days. A recording from a single amygdala neuron extending over a five day period is seen in Figure 18. These long-term recordings allow time for extensive behavioral testing, pharmacological treatments, or cyclicity studies. These studies are also facilitated by the lack of the requirement for physical restraint of the subjects and the use of relatively simple electronic apparatus. The simultaneous recording of two or more cells from separate electrodes is straightforward. The development of analytical procedures for examination of multineuronal interactions is in progress. The quality of the recordings obtained with the microwire technique is equal to that obtained with conventional microelectrodes in unanesthetized animals, as attested by the examples presented in this paper.

An objection to this technique is based on the skepticism that a recording tip that is equal to or larger than the perikarya cannot record spike activity. We believe that this skepticism is founded on a misconception. The success obtained with "large" microelectrodes may be explained by the fact that the spike field around the perikarya is apparently quite extensive. This fact is well known to investigators with experience in structures such as the LGN where cell packing is high. It is usual to observe more than one spike train from electorde tracts in such structures; only careful movements of the electrode position are sufficient to produce well isolated spike trains. Our interpretation is supported by the observation that microelectrode movements of 100-400 μ may be required to move an electrode past the field of a single neuron.

Summary

We have attempted to relate the study of neuronal unit dicharge in the brain to current conceptions of the neural control of sleep. We have speculated freely and suggested experimental strategies with the hope of stimulating research on this complex problem. We hope that the usefulness of these strategies will compensate for the errors in our speculations.

This work was supported by the Veterans Administration, and USPHS Grants MH 10083 and NS 02501.

REFERENCES

Aghajanian, G.K. Influence of drugs on the firing of serotonin-containing neurons in brain. *Fed. Proc. 31;* 91-96, (1972).

Aghajanian, G.K., Rosecrans, J.A. and Sheard, M.H. Serotonin: Release in the forebrain by stimulation of midbrain raphé. *Science 156;* 402-403, (1967).

Aghajanian, G.K., Foote, W.E. and Sheard, M.H. Lysergic acid diethylamide: Sensitive neuronal units in the midbrain raphé. *Science 161;* 706-708, (1968).

Aghajanian, G.K., Graham, A.W. and Sheard, M.H. Serotonin-containing neurons in the brain: Depression of firing by monoamine oxidase inhibitors. *Science 169;* 1100-1102, (1970a).

Aghajanian, G.K., Foote, W.E. and Sheard, M.H. Action of psychotogenic drugs on single midbrain raphé neurons. *J. Pharmacol. Exp. Therap 171* 178-187, (1970b).

Allison, T. Comparative and evolutionary aspects of sleep. *The Sleeping Brain,* in M.H.Chase, Ed., UCLA Brain Information Service, Los Angeles, 1973, pp. 1-57.

Anden, N.E., Dahlstrom, A, Fuxe, K., Larsson, K. Olson, L., and Ungerstedt, U. Ascending monoamine neurons to the telencephalon and diencephalon. *Acta Physiol. Scand. 67;* 313-326, (1966a).

Anden, N.E., Fuxe, K. and Hokfelt, T., The importance of the nervous impulse flow for the depletion of the monoamines from central neurons by some drugs. *J. Pharm. Pharmacol. 18;* 630-632, (1966b).

Anden, N.E., Corrodi, H., and Fuxe. K., Turnover studies using synthesis inhibition. *Metabolism of Amines in the Brain,* in, G. Hooper, Ed., MacMillan, Edinburgh, 1969, pp. 38-47.

Andersen, P., Eccles, J.C. and Sears, T.A. The ventrobasal complex of the thalamus: Types of cells, their responses and their functional organization. *J. Physiol. 174;* 370-399, (1964).

Andersen, P. and Andersson, S.A. *Physiological Basis of the Alpha Rhythm,* Appleton-Century-Crofts, 1968.

Arbuthnott, G.W., Crow T.J., Fuxe, K., Olson, L., and Ungerstedt, U., Depletion of catecholamines in vitro induced by electrical stimulation of central monoamine pathways. *Brain Res. 24:* 471-483, (1970).

Barkas, J. and Usden, E. Eds., *Serotonin and Behavior,* Academic Press, New York, 1973.

Ben-Ari, Y., and Le Gal LaSalle, G. Relationship between spontaneous and evoked unit activity in the amygdala of the cat. *Brain Res. 32;* 474-478, (1971).

Bizzi, E. Changes in the orthodromic and antidromic response of optic tract during the eye movements of sleep. *J. Neurophysiol. 29;* 861-870, (1966).

Chu, N. and Bloom, F.E. Norepinephrine-containing neurons: Changes in spontaneous discharge patterns during sleeping and waking. *Science 179;* 908-910, (1973).

Crow, T.J., Spear, P.J. and Arbuthnott, G.W. Intracranial self-stimulation with electrodes in the region of the locus coeruleus. *Brain Res. 36;* 275-287, (1972).

Dahlstrom, A. and Fuxe, K. Evidence for the existence of monoamine-containing neurons in the central nervous system. I. Demonstration of monoamines in the cell bodies of brain stem neurons. *Acta Physiol. Scand. 62* (232); 1-36, (1965).

Dahlstrom, A., Fuxe, K, Kernell, D., and Sedvall, G. Reduction of the monoamine stores in the terminals of bulbospinal neurons following stimulation in the medulla oblongata. *Life Sci.* [*Oxford*] *4;* 1207-1212, (1964).

Delorme, F., Jeannerod, M., and Jouvet, M. Effects remarquables de la réserpine sur l'activité EEG phasique pontogeniculo occipitale. *C.R. Soc. Biol. 159;* 900-903, (1965).

Delorme, F., Froment, J.L., and Jouvet, M. Suppression du sommeil par la P. chloromethamphetamine et de la P. chloro-phenylalanine. *C.R. Soc. Biol. 160;* 2347-2351, (1966).

Dement, W.C. The biological role of REM sleep (circa 1968). *Sleep, Physiology and Pathology,* in, A. Kales, Ed., 1969, pp. 245-265.

Dement, W.C., Mitler, M.M. and Henriksen, S.J. Sleep changes during chronic administration of parachlorophenylalanine. *Rev. Cana. Biol., 31* (suppl.), 239-246, (1972).

Desiraju, T. Transformations of discharges of neurons of parietal association cortex during sleep and wakefulness in monkey. *J. Neurophysiol. 35*; 326-332, (1972).

Eccleston, D., Padjen, A. and Randic, M. Release of 5-hydroxytryptamine and 5-hydroxyindol-3-ylacetic acid in the forebrain by stimulation of midbrain raphé. *J. Physiol. [London] 201*; 22-23, (1969).

Evarts, E.V. Activity of neurons in visual cortex of the cat during sleep with low voltage fast EEG activity. *J. Neurophysiol. 25*; 812-816, (1962).

Evarts, E.V. Temporal patterns of discharge of pyramidal tract neurons during sleep and waking in the monkey. *J. Neurophysiol. 27*; 152-172, (1964).

Evarts, E.V. Methods for recording activity of individual neurons in moving animals. *Methods In Medical Research*, R.F. Rushmer, Ed., Medical Year Book Publishers Inc., Chicago, 1966, pp. 241-250.

Evarts, E.V. Activity of individual cerebral neurons during sleep and arousal. *Sleep and Altered States of Consciousness* (Res. Publ. Assoc. Nerv. Ment. Dis.), Vol. 45, in S.S. Kety, E.V. Evarts, and H.L. Williams, Eds., Williams and Wilkins, Baltimore, 1967a.

Evarts, E.V. Unit activity in sleep and wakefulness. *The Neurosciences—A Study Program*, in, G.C. Quarton, T. Melnechuk, and F.O. Schmitt, Eds., Rockefeller University Press, New York, 1967b, pp. 545-556.

Findlay, A.L.R., and Hayward, J.N. Spontaneous activity of single neurons in the hypothalamus of rabbits during sleep and waking. *J. Physiol. [London], 201*; 237-258, (1969).

Freedman, D.X. Effects of LSD-25 on brain serotonin. *J. Pharmacol. Exp. Therap. 134*; 160, (1961).

Graham, A.W. and Aghajanian, G.K. Effects of amphetamine on single cell activity in a catecholamine nucleus, the locus coeruleus. *Nature 234*; 100-102, (1971).

Gumulka, W., Samanin, R., Valzelli, L. and Consolo, S. Behavioral and biochemical effects following the stimulation of the nucleus raphis dorsalis in rats. *J. Neurochem. 18*; 533-534, (1971).

Harper, R.M. and McGinty, D.J. A technique for recording single neurons from unrestrained animals. *Brain Unit Activity During Behavior*, M.I. Phillips, Ed., C. Thomas, Springfield, Ill. 1973, pp. 80-104.

Harper, R.M. Relationship of neuronal activity to EEG waves during sleep and wakefulness. *Brain Unit Activity During Behavior*, in M.I. Phillips, Ed., C. Thomas, Springfield, Ill., 1973, pp. 130-154.

Hobson, J.A. Cellular neurophysiology and sleep research. *The Sleeping Brain*, in M.H. Chase, Ed., UCLA Brain Information Service, Los Angeles, 1973a, pp. 59-83.

Hobson, J.A. The cellular basis of sleep cycle control. Presented at meeting of the Assoc. for the Psychophysiological Study of Sleep, San Diego, Calif., May, 1973b.

Hobson, J.A. and McCarley, R.W. *Neuronal Activity in Sleep - An Annotated Bibliography*, UCLA Brain Information Service, Los Angeles, 1971a.

Hobson, J.A., and McCarley, R.W. Cortical unit activity in sleep and waking. *Electroenceph. Clin. Neurophysiol. 30*; 97-112, (1971b).

Hubel, D.H. Single unit activity in striate cortex of unrestrained cats, *J. Physiol. 147*; 226-238, (1959a).

Hubel, D.H. Single unit activity in lateral geniculate body and optic tract of unrestrained cats. *J. Physiol. 147*; 226-283, (1959b).

Hubel, D.H. and Wiesel, T. Integrative action in the cat's lateral geniculate body. *J. Physiol. 155*; 385-398, (1961).

Huttenlocher, P.R. Evoked and spontaneous activity in single units of medial brain stem during natural sleeping and waking. *J. Neurophysiol. 24*; 451-468, (1961).

Iskander, T.N. and Kaelbling, R. Catecholamines, a dream sleep model and depression. *Amer. J. Psychiat. 127*; 43-50, (1970).

Jacobs, B.L. A multidimensional approach to the study of unit activity in freely moving animals. *Brain Unit Activity During Behavior,* in M.I. Phillips, Ed., C. Thomas, Springfield, Ill. 1973, pp. 268-287.

Jacobs, B.L. and McGinty, D.J. Amygdala unit activity during sleep and wakefulness. *Exp. Neurol. 33*; 1-15, (1971).

Jacobs, B.L. and McGinty, D.J. Participation of the amygdala in complex stimulus recognition and behavioral inhibition: Evidence from unit studies. *Brain Res. 36,*; 431-436, (1972).

Jacobs, B.L., McGinty, D.J. and Harper., R.M. Brain single unit activity during sleep-wakefulness: A review. *Brain Unit Activity During Behavior,* in M.I. Phillips, Ed., C. Thomas, Springfield, Ill. 1973, pp. 165-178.

Jones, B., Bobillier, P. and Jouvet, M. Effects de la destruction des neurones contenant des catecholamines du mesencaphale sur le cycle veille-sommeil du chat. *C.R. Soc. Biol. [Paris] 163*; 176-180, (1969).

Jouvet, M. Recherches sur des structures nerveuses et les mécanismes responsables des différentes phases du sommeil physiologique. *Arch. Ital. Biol. 100*; 125-206, (1962).

Jouvet, M. Mechanisms of the states of sleep: A neuropharmacological approach. *Sleep and Altered States of Consciousness,* in S.S. Kety, E.V. Evarts and H.H. Williams, Eds., Williams and Wilkins, Baltimore, 1967, pp. 86-126.

Jouvet, M. Biogenic amines and the states of sleep. *Science* 32-41, (1969).

Jouvet, M. The role of monoamines and acetylcholine-containing neurons in the regulation of the sleep waking cycle. *Reviews of Physiology,* Springer-Verlag, New York, 1972.

Kasamatsu, T. Maintained and evoked unit activity in the mesencephalic reticular formation of the freely behaving cat. *Exp. Neurol. 28*; 450-470, (1970).

King, D. and Jewett, R.E. The effects of alpha methyl tyrosine on sleep and brain norepinephrine in cat. *J. Pharmacol. Exp. Therap., 177*; 188-194, (1971).

Kostowski, W., Giacalone, E. Garattini, S. and Valzelli, L., Electrical stimulation of midbrain raphé: Biochemical, behavioral, and bioelectric effects. *Eur. J. Pharmacol. 7*; 170-175, (1969).

Kuhar, M.J., Roth, R.H. and Aghajanian, G.K. Selective reduction of tryptophan hydroxylase activity in rat forebrain after midbrain raphé lesions. *Brain Res. 35*; 167-176, (1971).

McCarley, R.W. and Hobson, J.A. Single neuron activity in cat gigantocellualr tegmental field: Selectivity of discharge in desynchronized sleep. *Science 174*; 1250-1252, (1971).

McCarley, and Hobson, J.A. Simple spike firing patterns of cat cerebellar Purkinje cells in sleep and waking. *Electroenceph. Clin. Neurophysiol. 33*; 471-483, (1972).

McGinty, D.J. Encephalization and the neural control of sleep. *Brain Development and Behavior,* in M.B. Sterman, D.J. McGinty and A.M. Adinolfi, Eds., Academic Press, New York, 1971, pp. 335-357.

McGinty, D.J. Neurochemically-defined neurons: Behavioral correlates of unit activity of serotonin-containing neurons. *Brain Unit Activity During Behavior,* in M.I. Phillips, C. Thomas, Springfield, Ill. 1973, pp. 244-267.

McGinty, D.J. and Sterman, M.B. Sleep suppression after basal forebrain lesions in the cat. *Science 160*; 1253-1255 (1968).

McGinty, D.J., Harper, R.M. and Fairbanks, M. 5HT-Containing neurons: Unit activity in behaving cats. *Serotonin and Behavior,* in, J. Barchas and E. Usden, Eds., Academic Press, New York, 1973.

McGinty, D. and Sakai, K. Unit activity of the dorsal pontine reticular formation in the cat. *Sleep Research,* in M.H. Chase, Ed., Brain Information Service, UCLA, in press.

Mink, W.D., Best, P.J. and Olds, J. Neurons in paradoxical sleep and motivated behavior. *Science 158*; 1335-1337, (1967).

Moore, R.Y. Brain lesions and amine metabolism. *International Review of Neurobiology,* Vol. 13, in, C.C. Pfeiffer and J.R. Smythies, Eds., Academic Press, New York, 1970, pp. 67-91.

Morgane, P.J. and Stern, W.C. Monoaminergic systems in the brain and their roles in the sleep states. *Serotonin and Behavior,* in J. Barchas and E. Usden Eds., Academic Press, New York, 1973.

Moruzzi, G. Reticular influences on the EEG. *Electroenceph. Clin. Neurophysiol. 16;* 2-17. (1964).

Moruzzi, G. The sleep-waking cycle. *Reviews of Physiology,* Springer-Verlag, New York, 1972.

Mouret, J. and Delorme, F. Lésions du tegmentum pontique et sommeil chez le rat. *C.R. Soc. Biol.* 161, (1967).

Mukhametov, L.M. and Rizzolatti, G. The response of lateral geniculate neurons to flashes of light during the sleep-waking cycle. *Arch. Ital. Biol. 108;* 348-368, (1970).

Mukhametov, L.M., Rizzolatti, G. and Seitun, A. An analysis of the spontaneous activity of lateral geniculate neurons and optic tract fibers in free moving cats. *Arch. Ital. Biol. 108* (2); 325-347 (1970a).

Mukhametov, L.M., Rizzolatti, G. and Tradardi, V. Spontaneous activity of neurons of nucleus reticularis thalami in freely moving cats. *J. Physiol. 210;* 651-667, (1970b).

Noda, H., Manohar, S. and Adey, W.R. Spontaneous activity of cat hippocampal neurons in sleep and wakefulness. *Esp. Neurol. 24;* 217-231, (1969).

Noda, H. and Adey, W.R. Firing of neuron pairs in cat association cortex during sleep and wakefulness. *J. Neurophysiol. 33;* 672-684, (1970).

Nystrom, B., Olson, L. and Ungerstedt, U. Noradrenaline nerve terminals in human cerebral cortices: First histological evidence. *Science 176;* 924-926, (1972).

O'Keefe, J. and Bouma, H. Complex sensory properties of certain amygdala units in the freely moving cat. *Exp. Neurol. 23;* 384-398, (1969).

Olds, J. Operant conditioning of single unit responses. *Proc. XXIII Internat. Cong. Physiol. Union 4;* 372-380, (1965).

Oomura, Y., Ooyama, H. Naka, F. Yamamoto, T. Ono, T. and Kobayashi, N. Some stochastical patterns of single unit discharges in the cat hypothalamus under chronic conditions. *N.Y. Acad. Sci. An. 157;* 666-689, (1969).

Pin, C., Jones, B.E. and Jouvet, M. Les neurones contenant des monoamines dans le tronc cérébral du chat. I. Etude topographique par histofluorescence et histochimie. *J. Physiol. [Paris] 60;* 519-520, (1968).

Pompeiano, O. The neurophysiological mechanisms of the postural and motor events during desynchronized sleep. *Sleep and Altered States of Consciousness,* in S.S. Kety, E.V. Evarts and H.L. Williams, Eds., Williams and Wilkins, Baltimore, 1967, pp. 351-423.

Purpura, D.P. Operations and processes in thalamic and synaptically related neural subsystems. *The Neurosciences,* in G.C. Quarton, T. Melnechuk, and G. Adelman, Eds., Rockefeller University Press, New York, 1970, pp. 458-470.

Purpura, D.P., and Shofer, R.J. Intracellular recording from thalamic neurons during reticulocortical activation. *J. Neurophysiol. 26;* 494-505, (1963).

Rechtschaffen, A., Lovell, R.A., Freedman, D.W., Whitehead, K., and Aldrich, M. Effect of p-chlorophenylalanine on sleep in rats. *Psychophysiology 6;* 223, (1969).

Sakakura, H. Spontaneous and evoke unitary activities of cat lateral geniculate neurons in sleep and wakefulness. *Jap. J. Physiol. 18;* 23-42, (1968).

Sakakura, H. and Iwama, R. Effects of bilateral eye enucleation upon single unit activity of the lateral geniculate body in free behaving cats. *Brain Res. 6;* 667-678, (1967).

Sclabassi, R.J. and Harper, R.M. Laboratory computers in neurophysiology. *Proc. IEEE,* in press.

Sheu, Y., Chu, N.S. and Bloom, F.E. Unit activities of the brain stem raphé nuclei during wakefulness and sleep. Paper presented at the Internat. Meeting of the Assoc. Psychophysiological Study of Sleep, Bruges, Belgium, 1971.

Strumwasser, F. Long term recording from single neurons in the brain of mammals. *Science 127;* 469-470, (1958).

Towe, A.L., and Harding, G.W. Extracellular microelectrode sampling bias, *Exp. Neurol. 29;* 366-381, (1970).

Villablanca, J. The electrocorticogram in the chronic cerveau isole cat. *Electroenceph. Clin. Neurophysiol. 19;* 576-586, (1965).

Villablanca, J. Behavioral and polygraphic study of "sleep" and "wakefulness" in chronic decerebrate cats. *Electroenceph. Clin. Neurophysiol. 21*; 562-577 (1966).

Villablanca, J. and Marcus, R. Sleep-wakefullness, EEG and behavioral studies of chronic cats without neocortex and striatum, "the diencephalic cat." *Arch. Ital. Biol. 110*; 348-382, (1972).

Villablanca, J. and M.E. Salinas-Zeballos. Sleep-wakefulness, EEG and behavioral studies of chronic cats without the thalamus—the "athalamic cat." *Arch. Ital. Biol. 110*; 383-411, (1972).

Wyatt, R.J., Engelman, K, Kupfer, D.J., Sjoerdsma, A. and Synder, F. Effects of parachlorophenylalanine on sleep in man *Electoenceph. Clin. Neurophysiol. 27*; 529-532, (1969).

Advances in Sleep Research, Vol. 1
© 1974, Spectrum Publications, Inc.

CHAPTER 4

The Cellular Basis
of Sleep Cycle Control*

J. ALLAN HOBSON

I. INTRODUCTION AND GENERAL PROPOSITIONS

As is typical in a field which has grown up around a newly discovered phenomenon, neurophysiological studies of sleep have been pursued along largely descriptive or empirical lines and the results have been interpreted in loose mechanistic and functional frameworks. The first general proposition that I wish to make is that progress has reached an asymptote in the descriptive neurophysiology of sleep. The accumulation of more detailed data, (be it new spontaneous phenomena or new lesion and stimulation effects) is likely to be unproductive, most results being so readily predictable from those at hand as to be redundant or so confusing as to be uninterpretable. The corollary of this proposition is that progress in sleep research is now more likely to come from research dictated by explicit hypotheses, conducted according to systematic strategies, and interpreted in a tightly logical manner. In other words, I am asserting that it is intellectually high time to move from the descriptive to the analytic phase of investigative development. I think this assertion holds for most subdivisions of the sleep research field but is particularly true of neurophysiology.

In the area of neuroanatomical and electrophysiologic studies, the research conducted according to implicit (or nearly explicit) hypotheses that has been most productive has been the study of sleep control mechanisms. The second

*Position Paper on Neuroanatomy and Neurophysiology given at the 13th Annual Meeting of the Association for the Psychophysiological Study of Sleep May 3, 1973. San Diego, California.

Supported by USPHS grant Number MH 13,923.

general proposition that I wish to make is that more substantial progress has been made in localizing sleep control mechanisms than in understanding the functions of sleep. I believe that this imbalance is related to the power and limitations of existing methods and it will persist. For that reason, I do not plan to discuss functional questions further here.

Localization of sleep control mechanisms has been accomplished crudely, but in some cases fairly convincingly, by means of macroelectrode recording, stimulation, and lesion techniques. These techniques could be called macroscopic-multicellular to distinguish them from microscopic-unicellular and the submicroscopic-molecular levels of analysis. Thus, my third general proposition is that there are several reasonable candidates for central control structures in sleep. A corollary of this proposition (and proposition one) is that the macroscopic methods just enumerated may be expected to produce new candidates but are not likely to advance the candidacy of any one structure beyond the stage of the primaries. One might therefore move that nominations be closed and proceed to election, but unfortunately there are no procedural rules.

Rather than grapple with criteria of proof, many students of sleep control mechanisms have moved from the macroscopic-multicellular level to the submicroscopic-molecular plane. The descent from brain regions to chemical molecules is daring but dangerous and the same general logical problems that frustrated the physiologist await the intrepid chemist. Furthermore this shift skips the intervening cellular level of organization about which a great deal is known and one thereby fails to capitalize on an opportunity. My fourth proposition is that electrophysiological processes of unknown but almost certain relevance to events at the molecular level can be studied by cellular electrophysiology; furthermore, it is necessary to determine the interaction between these two levels if either is to be fully understood. The evidence from preliminary electrophysiological work conducted in a biochemical context justifies this concern as will be shown.

The fifth and final general proposition I wish to put forth is that the chronic microelectrode method is now a veritable *via regia* to unraveling the organization of sleep control mechanisms. Because it is capable of analyzing events at the level of single neurons, it can decode information almost certainly used by the nervous system in regulating its functional state. The single unit is the structural element that integrates the electrophysiological signal, intracellular metabolism, and intercellular transmission. In the balance of this paper, I hope to convincingly establish this final point by reviewing and developing a theory of sleep centers which can predict, evaluate, and integrate results of experiments conducted at the nuclear, cellular, and molecular levels. The theory will then be applied to data bearing on the central control of desynchronized sleep with the ultimate emergence of a general model for sleep cycle control.

II. CENTER THEORY OF SLEEP CYCLE CONTROL

A. The Center Concept is Heuristically Useful in Studying Sleep Mechanisms

The history of center theory was reviewed in detail in my 1971 report of the Bruges Symposium on Cellular Neurophysiology and Sleep Research (Hobson, 1972). To summarize, it was shown that the modern history of experimental sleep research, like all other branches of behavioral physiology, has been dominated by the notion of centers. When one considers the amount of work that has been motivated by the idea of centers and interpreted loosely in that framework, one is particularly impressed to notice the almost total neglect of the theory, a fact which probably explains the vagueness, fuzziness, or downright embarrassment that permeates writings on the subject. The word center is often placed in quotes to indicate that the user's tongue is in his cheek and words such as influence are sometimes used to avoid charges of naiveté and misplaced concreteness that open articulation of the center concept invites. However, the idea is so pervasive as to suggest that this hierarchical view of brain function is a category of the experimental mind if not of the observed brain. If this is so, it represents an important force in experimental work. Whether the idea is inspired or justified by the neurologic data is beside the point. The center idea may in fact be the product of an intellectual process more suited to the analysis of hierarchiarchal social organizations such as the church or the government than a tissue such as the brain. This could explain its relative popularity among the liberally educated scientists, the experimental psychologists, and the Europeans, and its relative disfavor among the technologically sophisticated, the bio-physicists, and the Americans. Whatever the reason, when faced with data from functioning brains man thinks in terms of centers—whether he knows it or not, whether he likes it or not. I believe that the notion therefore needs to be taken seriously.

This is neither sheer rationalization nor sheer rationalism. First and foremost, it permits recognition of observer bias. Secondly, it is an effort to characterize and measure that bias. Thirdly, it is a effort to control, reject, or capitalize on that bias. Only if the theory is made explicit can it be examined as logic and only when that is done can it be used creatively. It is validly argueable that the center concept, when specified and used with the same skepticism as any other scientific postulate, is a heuristically useful theory.

B. A Priori Criteria must be Established to Evaluate the Imputation of "Center" Function to Any Brain Region

Table I is an outline of a priori criteria for a behavioral control center revised slightly from my Bruges Symposium report where it was amplified by a full general explanation (Hobson, 1972). The discussion which follows here incorporates some of those points and also emphasizes efforts of the past two years to further clarify them, especially those criteria for which new data are available.

TABLE I

Criteria for a Behavioral Control Center

A. **Anatomical**

   1. Homogenous group of neurons
     a. transmitter specificity
   2. Strategically located
   3. Strategically connected

B. **Physiological—Spontaneous**

   1. Selectively active
     a. Mechanisms of selectivity
   2. Tonic latency
     a. negative before behavior
     b. negative after behavior
   3. Negative phasic latency
   4. Multiple cycle stability; periodicity
   5. Reciprocal interaction and/or
   6. Pacemaker activity

C. **Physiological—Responsive**

   1. Long-term stimulation produces
     a. increased incidence
     b. increased duration
     c. decreased latency
   2. Destructive lesions of "center" produce long-lasting
     a. decreased incidence
     b. decreased duration
     c. increased latency
   3. Interruption of pathways from "center" eliminates
     a. phasic events at peripheral sites distal to the lesion
     b. tonic events at peripheral sites distal to the lesion
     c. coordination of two or more peripheral events
   4. Isolation of "center"
     a. has no effect on spontaneous activity of component neurons (pacemaker hypothesis)
     b. progressively diminishes spontaneous activity of component neurons (self-reexcitation hypothesis)
     c. has same effects as 3.a.—c.
   5. Sensory stimulation
     a. is modality nonspecific
     b. demonstrates variable excitability (threshold)
     c. disrupts periodic activity if raised above threshold

1. Anatomical Considerations

a. *"Center" concept in anatomical terms.* What do we mean by a "center"? To distinguish the concept from that of reflexes or of systems, we mean a point of origin of electricity activity, a "trigger zone", which necessarily implies conversion from one information or energy system, say, the biochemical, to another, the electrical. By the term center we imply, at the anatomical level, a homogeneous group of neurons strategically located and connected so as to initiate and control the more widespread neuronal activity that forms the substrate of a behavior. Why homogeneous? Because it is assumed that a collection of cells that is functionally specialized will reflect that differentiation anatomically, it is further assumed that the cells will be close to one another and similar in size and shape to one another, as in a nucleus. Neural elements within a nucleus may be expected to use a single transmitter, that is, to be chemically coded. The phrase "strategically located" means spatially central to the several effector neurons that elaborate the behavior at the periphery (such as the relation of the pyramidal cells of the motor cortex to anterior horn cells of the spinal cord in the positive motor act). The phrase "strategically connected" means that there must be inputs to account for interruptions and delays in the behavior and direct, preferential, or one-way projections to the specific effector neurons at the periphery to account for the motor events that characterize the behavior.

The reticular formation of the brainstem has been imputed to be important in maintaining the sleep-waking cycle. Let us look at a few selected aspects of brainstem anatomy in the context of center theory. A translation of Cajal's observations on the pontine reticular substance (Cajal, 1952) is summarized here. Cajal distinguished three divisions: raphé, white, and grey.

i. The *raphé* contains medium and large sized cells which are concentrated near the commisures and tend to be more abundant rostrally and ventrally.

ii. The white contains *giant cells* with bifurcating axons extending rostrally and caudally.

iii. The grey contains *small cells.*

All three zones have extensive dendritic overlap and collateral axonal interaction with each other.

Thus there is a midline system (raphé) and two paramedian systems (white and grey). All appear to receive the same inputs. The midline system would seem to be situated so as monitor, integrate, and control activity in both paramedian systems. The giant cells of the white with their long axons would seem ideally suited to function as executive command or output elements influencing distant structures. The small cells of the grey with their laterally oriented dendrites would seem ideally situated to control access to, to monitor, and to control the ipsilateral paramedian system.

b. *The giant cells of the reticular white as possible executive elements of a sleep cycle control system.* The anatomy and physiology of the giant cells of the reticular formation (the gigantocellular tegmental fields or FTG of Berman) have been hitherto poorly understood. Brodal's book (1957) reviews the cyto-architecture and Golgi studies, as well as his own work with degeneration methods. Brodal found that neurons at the level of the pons have crossed and uncrossed ascending connections, but only ipsilateral descending connections. Medullary cells have both crossed and uncrossed efferents ascending and descending. Projections were found to the spinal cord from over half the neurons at all levels of the pontine and medullary reticular formation.

Pontine reticular cells in the FTG project to centromedian, intralaminar, and reticular nuclei of the thalamus, and to the hypothalamus. Afferents are described from spinal cord, principally the spino-reticular tract, the cerebellum, the superior colliculus, and the cerebral cortex. Brodal does not describe fibers from cranial nerve nuclei. The cerebral cortical fibers are mostly from the contralateral motor strip; no somatotopic organization was noted in their projections to reticular formation.

Further anatomical study of reticular formation has come principally from the Scheibels' Golgi studies (Scheibel and Scheibel, 1957). Their studies have characterized the medial reticular neuron as a large cell with unbranching dendrites oriented in a plane perpendicular to the neuraxis and subtending a large but circumscribed area. The axon is usually bifurcated with rostral and caudal projections of some length. In addition, there is a significant collateral innervation of areas adjacent to the soma. Thus, the neuron functions also as a Golgi-type II cell in this part of the reticular formation.

Structurally informative physiological studies by Magni and Willis (1963, 1964) have demonstrated antidromic stimulation from contralateral motor cortex and from spinal cord. The Scheibels, Mollica, and Moruzzi (1955) have noted convergence of many afferents on reticular neurons, i.e., cerebellar, somatosensory and auditory. No effect was seen from vagal stimulation and relatively little from optic stimulation. Lamarche et al. (1960) have demonstrated a strong input from trigeminal nerve, consisting mostly of bilaterally symmetrical, extensive receptive fields. Segundo's work achieved a similar result (Segundo et al., 1967, a, b). Lamarche failed to find any somatotopic representation of the periphery in the reticular formation (Lamarche et al., 1960).

The following are speculations which one might wish to make on the basis of the previously cited studies of the reticular formation. First, a regulatory or tonic role in many neural systems is suggested by its extensive projections. Second, a multi-faceted role is implied by its afferent connections; it would then be independent of particular sensory stimulation, but sensitive to many modalities simultaneously and, hence, indiscriminately. Lack of somatotopic distribution only confirms that this is not an area of sensory discrimination. Third, since one of its strongest inputs is its own axons, this region could be a substrate for pacemaker circuits, regenerative activity, etc. The peculiar "stacked chips" arrangement of its dendrites may also play a part in cyclical activity. Certainly the lack of rostral-caudal extensions of the dendritic field must be a significant finding.

The large neurons of the pontine reticular formation in the gigantocellular tegmental fields (FTG) are therefore possible candidates for a controlling role in sleep. Brodal has presented evidence that more than one half of the 3000-4000 giant cells in the cat FTG send descending axons beyond the midbrain, and more than one-half send descending axons into the spinal cord (Brodal, 1957). Included in these estimates are those cells that have both ascending and descending axon branches. These direct and widespread connections to regions outside the brainstem suggest that these cells could affect the ubiquitous and marked changes in brain and spinal neuronal activity that occur, especially during D (Rem) sleep. It is therefore significant that the FTG corresponds to the nucleus reticularis pontis caudalis, the very structure implicated by lesion and stimulation experiments to be important in the control of the desynchronized phase of sleep (Jouvet, 1962).

c. *Biogenic Amine containing neurons as possible excitability level setters for the brainstem.* By the application of the histo-fluorescent technique for biogenic amines, Dahlstrom and Fuxe have shown that the neurons in the brainstem fall into two chemically differentiated groups (Dahlstrom and Fuxe, 1965). One group, whose cell bodies concentrate 5-hydroxytryptamine (serotonin), is coextensive with the midline raphé nuclei of the pons rostrally. Another group of cells, rich in dopamine and norepinephrine, is situated more laterally. At the level of the brainstem, the locus coeruleus is composed exclusively of catecholamine-containing neurons. This dichotomy immediately suggested a functioning that was alluringly more simple than light-microscope observations on the brain could have predicted. It also provided a possible point of conversion from the biochemical to the electrical level so essential to the center concept.

Sleep was one of many complex functions waiting in the wings for this kind of cue, a structural-chemical dualism to match the peaks and troughs of the sleep cycle. Jouvet (1969) combined lesion techniques with biochemistry and showed that there was a three-way correlation between the extent of destruction of the serotonin neurons in the brainstem, the reduction of serotonin in the forebrain, and the reduction in sleep. Similarly, destruction of the locus coeruleus selectively eliminated D sleep, and depleted the forebrain of norepinephrine. Thus, it was boldly postulated that the raphé nuclei constituted a system with its own transmitter (serotonin), which when activated produced S (synchronized) sleep. A parallel system of which the locus coeruleus was a key part, was responsible for D sleep through the agency of a unique transmitter, (norepinephrine).

In the history of behavioral physiology other examples of anatomo-functional dualisms of this kind can be found. It is reminiscent of the sympathetic-parasympathetic dualism of Cannon (1929) and of the ergotrophic-trophotrophic subdivision of hypothalamic function by Hess (1954), notions that are still alive but not kicking very hard. Since it is possible that the biogenic amine hypothesis of sleep is another heuristically useful but short-lived oversimplification, it may be worth reviewing the inherent problems it faces and the tests it must withstand in establishing its veracity.

The first problem is logical: correlation is not causation. The second concerns the nonspecificity of lesion effects: animals with brainstem damage have more than insomnia, they are quadriplegic, cannot eat, and usually die within three weeks. Those with midline lesions also have more than their raphé nuclei destroyed: many decussating fibers of the brainstem are cut. (In the medulla midline, lesions abolish respiration even though the nerve cells of the respiratory "center" are in the paramedian reticular zones. Furthermore, all lesions of the posterior brainstem, whether or not in the midline, result in profound insomnia, and many of Jouvet's own control data reveal this to be true; this brings into question the specificity of the localization. Thirdly, stimulation of the raphé nuclei does not enhance S sleep, and stimulation of the locus coeruleus does not increase D sleep; these negative results are not fatal to the theory but they do not help it either. Fourthly, if the theory were correct, and assuming a positive correlation between cell firing and amine release, the cells of the raphé nuclei could be expected to discharge more rapidly in S sleep, and those of the locus coeruleus more rapidly in D sleep. Preliminary results to be discussed later failed to support the first of these predictions and are contradictory with respect to the second. Acceptance of the theory also awaits the demonstration that activation of the brainstem neurons directly results in changes of rate and pattern of other cells in the nervous system via the mediation of their transmitters.

The conservative basis of the Jouvet hypothesis, that amine specific neurons function as part of a complex level setting system for the brain is not, of course, damaged by the failure to support many specific predictions of the one-state, one-transmitter hypotheses. Rather, it would now seem indicated to take a step back to that conservative basis and then to go ahead with alternative models and more refined techniques for testing them. One such model, that of reciprocal interaction, is entirely consistent with the physiological data and is particularly appropriate to cellular studies as will be shown below. Anticipating that discussion, and integrating Cajal and Fuxe, it appears that the giant cells of the pontine tegmentum receive abundant synaptic input from both serotonergic and catecholaminergic systems to which they also project (Floyd Bloom, personal communication).

Advances in testing the general hypothesis that biogenic amine neurons are excitability level setters will go hand in hand with the more detailed anatomy needed to describe the brainstem to brainstem connections of these cells. In addition to further application of flourescent techniques and classical degeneration studies, radioactive labeling of intracellular protein and radioautographic histology appear to be promising techniques. Note that all of these anatomical methods are pursued at the miscroscopic level and are intended to differentiate between neurones! Clearly, the appropriate level at which to conduct correlative physiological experiments is also the microscopic. Only in this way can one hope to differentiate between neuronal groups functioning under physiologic conditions.

2. Physiological Considerations—Spontaneous Activity

When recording from cells in a putative center one would expect to find that firing highly correlated with the behavior in question; correlations could be negative, but to simplify discussion, will be assumed to be positive. Thus, firing rates of neurons should be differentially related to the behavior when compared with other behaviors. The degree of association between neuronal discharge and a behavior, or *selectivity*, can be quantified by the ratio of rates in several behaviors. To preserve the ratio scale for population means, the geometric mean is the statistic of choice in assessing selectivity. In some cases the association may be exclusive; that is, firing will occur if and only if the behavior is in progress.

The center concept includes functional specialization as indicated above. A corollary of centralization is diffusion of influence to the periphery. To influence many distant peripheral effectors, central neurons are likely to be large and will need to be unusually active to compensate for, or overcome, synaptic or conduction failures, thus insuring development of the behavior. Initiation of the process is likely to be time-consuming. Thus one can expect that a statistically significant change of activity in the center will lead (precede) in time such a change in peripheral neurons. This lead time can be called the *tonic latency*. It assumes that stable or background aspects of the behavior are the result of a net change in level of activity of a set of effector neurons brought about by a net change in level of activity or a set of central neurons. An example might be the postural tone that forms a necessary background for movement.

The tonic latency can be expected to be negative both before the onset of the behavior and before the termination of the behavior (where negative means earlier in time.) Obviously, it is necessary to have well-characterized determinants of a behavior so that time of onset and termination, t_0, can be precisely established. This is because the latencies of change in activity between two parts of the central nervous system may be on the order of milliseconds or at most a very few seconds.

If the behavior has phasic components, such as movements, these must be well-characterized and their occurences in time established so that *phasic latencies* can be measured. If the behavior originates in centers, latencies should of course again be negative and in this instance are almost certain to be shorter than one second and may be as brief as a very few milliseconds.

The onset of EMG activity is a particularly useful index of t_0 for phasic movements because individual action potentials can often be resolved even with macroelectrodes.

Cells in a putative center should show the properties of selectivity, and tonic and phasic latency consistently across *multiple cycles*. Long-term recording of single neurons allows the degree of *stability* of these measures to be checked quantitatively. Such recordings also allow tests of *periodicity* to be made; cells in a putative center controlling a cyclic recurrent phenomena such as sleep might be expected to show regularly periodic activation (whether or not the behavior was fully expressed.)

Criteria for pacemaker activity are well-developed from intracellular work with cardiac and invertebrate preparations, and some of these, being simply statistical, can be looked for in spike trains. In fact, Segundo detected evidence of pacemaker activity in his intracellular recording of reticular neurons, as evidenced by a positive slope in the resting potential (Segundo et al., 1967a). The Scheibels found cyclical changes in responsivity of reticular units to internal and external stimuli, related to the animal's waking and sleeping cycle (Scheibel and Scheibel, 1965).

More definitive tests of center theory at the cellular level will await the development of chronic intracellular recording techniques. Can there be initiation of action potentials without EPSPs as is true of cardiac cells or pacemaker neurons in lower animals? It is as yet unknown whether such mechanisms operate in behavioral control system of mammals, however it is difficult to account for the ebb and flow of excitation in the nervous system during the sleep cycle without considering intracellular mechanisms that could periodically alter membrane potentials and bring some cells to threshold. Here the basic issues of center theory and biological rhythm theory may converge. The cellular study of sleep may aid this integration and we believe that an extension of methods described below may soon make chronic intracellular recording of reticular neurons possible.

Another way in which a cyclic function might be controlled by nerve cells is by *reciprocal interaction* of two specialized cell groups. For example, cell group A might be self-excitatory and excitatory to cell group B while cell group B was self-inhibitory and inhibitory to cell group A. The time constant of the oscillation could be set by the variability in size (and hence threshold) within group A and/or group B or by a chemical mechanism regulating availability of transmitter A and/or B. This hypothesis will be developed in greater detail later.

3. *Physiological Considerations—Responsive Properties*

It will now be useful to reconsider lesion and stimulation methods. Despite their limitations, results generally support center theory and therefore direct attempts to test the theory at the cellular level to specific brain regions. If the results of cellular tests are positive, we will want to refine lesion and stimulation methods to examine more specific hypotheses and to combine cellular techniques with these methods.

Stimulation of a center should produce increased incidence, increased duration, and/or decreased latency to onset of a behavior thought to be under the control of that center. It should be possible to produce such results consistently and over long periods of time. To avoid current spread resulting in nonspecific (or antagonistic) effects, two intensities should be used. Pulses should be bipolar to avoid polarization of electrodes. High frequencies should be effective if tonic driving by the center is a supposed mechanism in its effects. Multiple electrodes and multiplexing may be necessary to avoid habituation in long-term applications of stimulation to regions such as the brainstem reticular formation. Stimulation through multiple microelectrodes is an obvious next step in refining this approach.

Destructive *lesions* of neurons in a center should produce effects opposite to those of stimulation, namely decreased incidence, decreased duration, and increased latency to onset of the behavior. The peripheral elements of the behavior should be retained but their coordination lost. Otherwise it would be possible to misinterpret the loss of specific components on which the definition of the behavior depends, e.g., through damage to pathways as opposed to damage to cell bodies of origin of activity. The effects of the behavior should outlast the dynamic changes (recovery) following intervention. Thus, as a general rule, observation periods should exceed one month before being considered to be of conclusive significance. Lesions destructive of central structures are particularly unsatisfactory because they are unselective and for that reason they are often followed by morbidity, which has its own unspecified or uninterpretable consequences. Here again multiple microlesions in cell-rich areas might be an improvement over large confluent macrolesions.

A promising approach for integration with unit recording experiments is the introduction of lesions between the center and the periphery. Interruption of pathways from the center should eliminate the tonic and phasic alterations of cellular activity at the peripheral site while leaving the central activity unchanged (assuming that the interruption is transsynaptic and there is no retrograde degeneration.) Coordination of tonic changes at two peripheral sites might also be temporarily disrupted if large, separate cell fields normally support each and depend on a third region, the center, for time-locking.

Complete isolation of the center from all inputs should have no effects on spontaneous activity if this activity is assumed to result from intracellularly regulated changes in membrane potential (the pacemaker hypothesis.) Naturally this criterion should be fulfilled even if all peripheral tissue is not only disconnected but also destroyed. Alternatively, if the activity is assumed to be input dependent, as in the self-reexcitation hypothesis, progressive isolation will result in progressive reduction of cell activity. It will be difficult to answer these questions in mammalian nervous systems, but by using some procedures developed in acute experiments it may not be impossible.

Sensory experiments are important because of the necessity of knowing how the activity of imputed pacemaker cells is sensitive to the outside world. One would like to repeat the Scheibels' work, measuring thresholds and sensitivity to sensory stimulation at various times during the cell's activity and relate this to the organism's state of arousal. One could then study the effect of sensory stimulation in changing the animal's sleep and waking cycle and the cell's rate of firing. One could use protocols similar to those used by investigators who have studied the rate of firing preceding EEG evidence of state change. One would also be interested in the effect of different frequencies of stimulation, which has been shown to be important in previous sensory studies and in studies of direct electrical stimulation of the reticular system.

Two particular sources of afferent input are worthy of further study. The cerebral cortex probably has a very significant role in the afferent supply of reticular neurons. The observation of several investigators that the trigeminal receptive fields are bilateral and symmetrical most probably indicates that this area is represented in reticular formation principally by cortical inputs rather than secondary sensory afferents. Furthermore, Jouvet (1960) has observed that the property of habituation to sensory stimuli noted in the reticular formation disappears in decerebrate animals. If a significant sensory role in the activity of the reticular formation is found, it would then be interesting to compare stimulation via peripheral nerves with stimulation via cortical cells, by stimulating cortical cells antidromically, say through the pyramidal tract or posteroventral lateral thalamic nucleus. The second particularly important afferent source is the reticular neurons themselves. They might best be studied by following up Brodal's observation that pontine reticular neurons do not have a crossed projection to the spinal cord (Brodal, 1957). One could then antidromically stimulate reticular neurons other than the one under study by stimulating the contralateral spino-reticular pathway.

C. Lesion and Stimulation Studies have Implicated Several Brain Regions as Centers in the Control of Sleep and Waking

Moruzzi (1972) has recently reviewed the lesion and stimulation experiments with reference to the central control of sleep. His interpretations and conclusions are summarized in Table II. The table is organized according to the behaviors, waking and synchronized sleep. For each behavior, the lesion and stimulation experiments most relevant to center theory are schematically illustrated. For each experiment, a concluding statement was selected to emphasize the implications for future work. Let us first examine data for synchronized sleep and waking, keeping in mind the criteria outlined above. The general thesis to be developed is that at the cellular level, virtually nothing is known about the adequacy of any of the center hypothesis advanced by Moruzzi for these two behaviors. Table III summarizes the available unitary data according to the criteria outlined in Table I. Desynchronized sleep will be considered in the following section where lesion and stimulation experiments will be integrated with cellular data.

1. *Sleep-Waking Rhythm* (Circadian Periodicity)

"The sleep-waking rhythm arises within the hypothalamus. Sleep-inducing neurons are localized in its anterior part while the waking center is localized in its posterior part."

This statement could be translated to read: The circadian clock is located in the hypothalamus; two cells groups, which are separate and distinct, make up an alternating system whose reciprocal activity forms the physiological basis of circadian rhythmicity. This hypothesis is testable using methods to be described below. If the hypothesis of anatomical discreteness is true, this is a site where multiunit recording, with chronic microwires might be particularly appropriate. Such an approach would allow neuronal activity to be monitored from one or both sites for days. Animals could then be isolated from time cues and the rhythm allowed to run free. Curves of unit activity could be used to characterize phase relationships between the two structures. The effects of stimulation could be examined under free-running conditions to assay the possibility or resetting the oscillator at various phases of endogenous cycle.

"Sleep-inducing neurons are localized in its anterior part": Findlay and Hayward (1969) reported that 10/21 anterior hypothalamus neurons increased rate with sleep onset while eleven decreased. The mean change was from 4.1 to 3.7 spikes per second. Anterior hypothalamus neurons thus show no constant rate change and as a group change rate in a direction opposite to that predicted by active control theory;

"The waking center is localized in its posterior part": Findlay and Hayward (1969) recorded 8 cells in the posterior hypothalamic area of rabbits of which 6 decreased rate in the W—S transition; the mean rate changed from about 4 spikes/sec to 3 spikes/sec. Vincent et al. (1967) reported no change in firing rate with sleep onset by slowing discharging units (<1 spikes/sec) in the premammallary hypothalamus of rabbits. These data are not dramatic but are consistent with the hypothesis of an active role in waking for the posterior hypothalamus.

III LESION EXPERIMENTS

WAKING

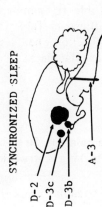

A-1a   A-2   B-1   A-1b

A-1a   Acute Cerveau Isolé
A-2   Chronic Cerveau Isolé
A-1b   Encephale Isolé
B-1   Midbrain Hemisection

A tonic influence arising, below the midbrain transection but above the spinal segments is necessary in order to maintain the sleep-waking cycle. (p. 13).

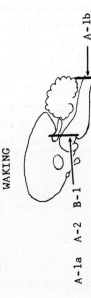

C-1 Mesencephalic Lesions resulted in a synchronized EEG. (p. 59)

SYNCHRONIZED SLEEP

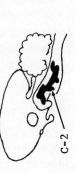

D-2
D-3c
D-3b

A-3

A-3 Pretrigeminal Preparation—in the lower brain stem there are structures oriented antagonistically to the activating reticular system (p. 31)
D-3c Basal Forebrain Area—striking insomnia produced by a lesion (p. 111)

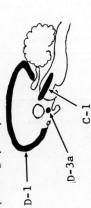

C-2

C-2 Raphe System—subtotal destruction followed by 3 to 4 days of complete sleeplessness (p. 63)

D-1 & D-2 The main conclusion of decortication (D-1) and of thalectomy (D-2) is the convincing demonstration that the sleep-waking cycle does not arise within the cortex and the thalamus (p. 83).
D-3 Sleep-waking rhythm...arises within the hypothalamus. Sleep-inducing neurons are localized in its anterior part (D-3b), while the waking center is localized in its posterior part (D-3a) (p. 83).

IV STIMULATION EXPERIMENTS

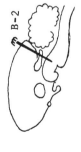

B-2 Electrical stimulation of the activating reticular system produces EEG and behavioral arousal (p. 98)

B-1 Electrical stimulation of the midline thalamus produced...sleep (p. 91)
B-2 Electrical stimulation of the solitary tract induced EEG synchronization (p. 100)
B-3 Basal Forebrain - EEG synchronization and behavioral sleep could be elicited with high rate stimulation (p. 102)

V DISCUSSION

The ascending reticular system and a group of neurons lying in the posterior hypothalamus are endowed with a tonic activating influence. They are probably concerned with...wakefulness. The lower brain stem and basal forebrain area contain structures with an opposing function which exert a tonic deactivating influence and lead ultimately to sleep. (p. 114)

TABLE II—Summary of Lesion and Stimulation Studies of Brain Structures Regulating Waking and Synchronized Sleep as Reviewed by Moruzzi [1972]. Section headings and page numbers are in reference to Moruzzi.

2. Waking

"A tonic influence arising in the pontomedullary brainstem is necessary in order to maintain the sleep waking cycle. The ascending reticular system and a group of neurons lying in the posterior hypothalamus are endowed with a tonic activating influence." The pooled data of Huttenlocher (1961), Kasamatsu (1970), and Manohar et al. (1972) support this hypothesis by showing relative selectivity of firing in waking when compared to synchronized sleep. Identification of cells has not been accomplished however, and localizations are not precisely documented in all studies. No other cellular criteria have been tested.

3. Synchronized Sleep

"The lower brainstem and basal forebrain area contain structures with an opposing function which exert a tonic deactivating influence and lead ultimately to sleep." In his concluding statement, Moruzzi does not make clear whether he includes both the raphé nuclei and the solitary tract in his lower brainstem theory. For our purposes, it will be convenient to separate them.

No data is available on spontaneous unit activity of the solitary tract. Location and identification of neurons in this small structure will be formidable.

Raphé Nuclei. McGinty's results (McGinty et al., 1972), using microwires to record neurons in the dorsal raphé nucleus, are contrary to the active control hypothesis for serotonergic neruons in synchronized sleep that Jouvet's evidence would predict (Jouvet, 1969). They fit very nicely, however, with a passive, permissive role and the raphé neurons could constitute one side of an oscillator for ultradian, within-sleep, periodicity. At last report only selectivity and phasic latency data were available for raphé neurons. Long-term recording should be a simple matter with McGinty's technique and more can be expected from this source. Physiological identification of those neurons has not yet been accomplished.

Basal Forebrain [Bfb]. Anecdotal evidence reported by McGinty and Harper (personal communication) indicates the possibility that selectivity and tonic latency criteria may be met by cells in the Bfb. Since the stimulation evidence is stronger for a positive Bfb role in sleep than for any other structure, this region must be regarded as a leading contender for a role in sleep induction. In addition, Bremer's studies have suggested that reticular inhibition may be the mediating mechanisms for Bfb's sleep-inducing effects (Bremer, 1970). Bremer's results suggest that antidromic activation from the reticular formation may be possible.

TABLE III
Results of Tests of Center Theory of Waking and
Synchronized Sleep at Cellular Level

Behavior and Structure	Criterion:			
	Selectivity	Tonic Latency	Phasic Latency	Perio dicity
Waking				
Post hypothalamus	W > S consistent with hypothesis	no data	no data	no data
Reticular activating system	W > S consistent with hypothesis	no data	no data	no data
Synchronized Sleep				
Anterior hypothalamus	W ≈ S contrary to hypothesis	no data	no data	no data
Dorsal raphe nucleus	W > S contrary to hypothesis	no data	no data	no data
Basal forebrain area	S > W consistent with hypothesis	yes	no data	no data
Lower brainstem	no data	no data	no data	no data

D. Satisfaction of Physiological Criteria Necessitates the Study of Sleep at the Cellular Level Under Natural Conditions

It should be clear from the foregoing survey that lesion and stimulation methods have in many cases reached the limit of their resolving power in studying the control of sleep and waking. Indeed, it could be argued that interpretations of the results of these experiments have actually gone beyond the power of the methods. Moruzzi (1972) has given a clear critique of the problems of the methods and I would agree with his inclusive but conservative reading of the evidence. In his paper, he has also reasonably likened the state of the art in experimental sleep research today to that in spinal cord physiology at the completion of Sherringtons' acute transection and chronic ablation work (circa 1930).

If the history of progress in that field can be taken as an indicator of where we should now move in sleep research, it will readily be appreciated that the detailed analysis of the reflex arc, of the gamma loop, and of the diverse supraspinal influences on the anterior horn cell and spinal interneurons, all depended upon the development of cellular neurophysiology in conjunction with microscopic anatomy. Progress from the application of microelectrode technology to spinal cord physiology is still forthcoming some 20 years after Renshaw's pioneering work and the end is not yet in sight.

Evarts' work in the analysis of single unit activity in sleep pointed up the feasibility of similar studies in the domain of behavior control (Evarts, 1967). It is interesting and ironic to note in passing that Evarts has now turned his attention to supraspinal motor control and that his own final comments on the unit approach to sleep physiology were pessimistic. However, it should also be appreciated that Evarts' work on sleep was pursued from a functional theoretical position and that he did not broach questions regarding central control mechanisms.

Application of Evarts' methods could provide data necessary to complete Table III and thereby strengthen or weaken the case for a central control function for each of the structures named. In the following section, I will show that such an approach—which we have taken in the study of desynchronized sleep—not only supports the center hypothesis for the pontine brainstem but also give clues as to the nature of the control mechanisms obtainable in no other way. I suspect that the same would be true of brain regions implicated in the control of waking and synchronized sleep.

III PONTINE RETICULAR FORMATION AS A DESYNCHRONIZED SLEEP CENTER

Table IV summarizes the lesion and stimulation evidence implicating the pontine brainstem in D sleep control as reviewed by Moruzzi (1972). Perhaps the most cogent evidence is the fact that the pontine cat shows periodic atonia with rudimentary eye movements. The atonia was first described by Bard and Rioch (1937) and replicated, extensively documented, and interpreted in the context of D sleep center theory by Jouvet (1962). Subsequent work by others has confirmed the persistence of atonia but the regular periodicity and quantitatively normal amounts of D sleep reported by Jouvet have not been replicated as yet in similar preparations (Hobson, 1965). In fact, as will be shown below, one would not expect the system to be unaffected by anterior brainstem transections so that the drastic reductions in amount of D sleep as lesions approach the mid-pons do not seriously weaken the theory.

That small rostral pontine lesions disrupt atonia seems well established (Jouvet, 1972) though there is still considerable disagreement about whether small lesions effectively abolish atonia (Carli and Zanchetti, 1965). As in other studies of sleep, it may be that the limits of the methods are being exceeded by attempts to implicate increasingly small subdivisions of various nuclei in controlling various aspects of D sleep. In any case, it appears that a point of diminishing returns has been reached and one can only safely conclude that the lesion criterion for D sleep control is generally satisfied by the pontine reticular formation (PRF).

The reservations stated above apply as well to attempts to delineate phasic activity generation. In particular, the conclusion reached by Pompeiano (1967) regarding the participation of vestibular nuclei (often misquoted by others as indicating phasic activity generation) seems doubtful in view of new contrary evidence by Perenin et al. (1972). At present, there seems to be no compelling reason to reject the parsimonious hypothesis that phasic and tonic events are both under the control of the PRF.

III LESION EXPERIMENTS

DESYNCHRONIZED SLEEP

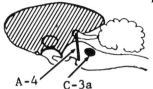

A-4   C-3a

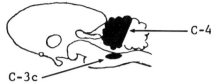

C-3c   C-4

A-4 Chronic Decerebration (Pontine Cat).
Same triggering neurons responsible for
cataplexic episodes after decerebration and
for paradoxical sleep of intact cat (p.38)
C-3a Pontine Lesions—Structures in rostral
half of pons contribute of origin of
paradoxical episodes (p. 65)

C-3c Vestibular Lesions—Phasic events
abolished when medical descending vestibular
nuclei are destroyed (p.66)
C-4 Cerebellar Anterior Lobe Ablation (with
A-4)—Mechanisms for sleep atonia overcome
alpha and gamma rigidity (p. 68)

IV STIMULATION EXPERIMENTS

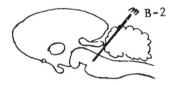

B-2

B-2 Prolonged stimulation of the pontine tegmentum was followed by a reduced latency to
paradoxical sleep and an increase in the total amount of paradoxical sleep (p. 99)

V DISCUSSION

An accumulation followed by dissipation of chemical substances within a pontine "center" is
likely to be the cause of the onset and of the end of each paradoxical episode (p. 119)

TABLE IV—Summary of Lesion and Stimulation Studies of Brain Structures Regulating
Desynchronized Sleep as Reviewed by Moruzzi (1972). Section headings and page numbers are
in reference to Moruzzi.

Chronic high frequency stimulation of the PRF is one of the very few
experimental treatments known to increase D sleep (Frederickson and
Hobson, 1970). This phenomenon should be replicated and studied in greater
detail since it would be enormously helpful in analytic neurophysiologic work
to be able to turn on the D sleep system instead of waiting for it to occur or
resorting to deprivation to increase its probability of occurrence. Thus the
PRF is one of only two structures in the brain (the other is the basal forebrain
area) which satisfies a high frequency stimulation criterion of sleep control.

Taken together, the foregoing results constitute one of the most consistent
stories of localization of behavioral control in the lesion-stimulation

literature. In addition the anatomy of the region, especially the size, location and axonal projections of the giant cells, makes this region especially attractive as a target for single cell studies. In the subsequent section findings suggesting that the neurons of the PRF are indeed involved in D sleep generation will be reviewed. These and other unit data will be used to begin to construct a model for a D sleep control system.

A. **Control of Desynchronized Sleep Appears to be Localized in the Pontine Brainstem. Cellular Studies Suggest that the Tegmental Giant Neurons may be an Output Element of the Center**

The sections following list the various criteria satisfied.

1. *Selectivity Criterion*

Data on the selectivity criterion have been published (McCarley and Hobson, 1971). In summary, of 69 brainstem neurons recorded, the 34 neurons in the gigantocellular tegmental field showed a high degree of selectivity of firing in D. Ten FTG neurons did not discharge at all in W and 6 of these and one other were silent in S. To quantify this property, we calculated geometric means and the ratios of the means in D over those in W or S. FTG neurons had a D/S ratio of 50:1, and a D/W ratio of 100:1. These ratios are more than 5 times higher than those in other tegmental fields (13 neurons) and more than 10 times higher than those of the pontine grey (8 neurons) and the pontine reticular nucleus (14 neurons). The ratios are 25 to 30 times higher than corresponding values computed from our own previously collected data on cerebral cortex and cerebellar neurons. The marked selectivity of firing of FTG neurons in D and the large differential values attained by them in D are compatible with their playing an active and central role in the production of rate changes elsewhere in the nervous system during D sleep. We have recently done several other studies in an effort to validate and explain FTG selectivity.

a. *Selectivity is stable across cycles* (McCarley et al., 1972). If FTG units were responsible for generating desynchronized sleep episodes, the marked rate increases during D and the concentration of firing in D should be consistent for a given cell from cycle to cycle. Multiple cycle data also permit detection of rate modulation at phases of the cycle other than the S-D transition to which we had previously restricted our attention (see tonic latency, periodicity, and model).

Our technique now allows us to record from single cells, without loss of resolution, for an indefinite length of time. In four units of which data analysis is complete, the firing rate increases in D were found to be consistent throughout each of the 10 to 16 successive cycles recorded. The overall tendency of the units firing selectively in D is reported in Table V.

TABLE V

Unit #	Hours Obs.	# D Cycles	Total Firings	Firing in D #	%	% Time in D	Rate [s/s] D	Non-D	Rate Ratio D/Non-D
531*	5.0	10	11,831	10,685	90.3	17.5	3,387	.07730	43.8
568	4.2	13	59,212	48,652	82.2	24.9	12.87	.9255	13.9
585	5.3	11	4,365	4,255	97.5	16.7	1.326	.006877	193.0
610	10.5	16	77,078	58,721	76.2	13.7	11.47	.5644	20.3

* Histological study reveals this to be an FTC neuron. The others are FTG neurons.

Three of the four units showed rate increases beginning about 4 minutes prior to the onset of D. Rates accelerated rapidly in the minute before D, reach a peak within the first portion, then declined slowly with an abrupt decrease as D ended. Still further decreases continued until about 3 to 5 minutes after D, with rates at this time reaching their lowest levels. This was followed by a gradual return to the average non-D firing rates.

The time course of firing was plotted as an activity curve for each of the four cells. For each D period, the rates were computed for 1 minute epochs during the 10 minutes before and after D and these rates were averaged over all D cycles. We normalized the time duration of each D sleep period to 5 minutes. That is, longer D sleep periods were compressed to 5 minutes and D sleep periods shorter than 2 minutes were exluded. Thus each D bin represented the average firing rate during each fifth of the recorded episodes.

Each of the four curves represented recording of one cell from 4 to 10 hours, the total number of D periods was 50 (with a minimum of 10 for each cell), and the total number of firings was over 100,000. This data, composed of averages from many D cycles from a few cells, showed consistent selectivity of firing during D. In addition, the method revealed a previously unsuspected suppression of firing *after* D for some of the cells. The curves are strikingly similar to those describing the activity of a relaxation oscillator as will be discussed below.

b. Is FTG selectivity a function of phasic bursting? Cells in the FTG show intense bursts associated with the eye movements of D but some of those that do are *also* tonically active. We wished to know the relative contributions of tonic and phasic rate increases to the selectivity criterion. To answer the question for the whole pool of FTG neurons, we determined the degree to which the FTG rate increase in D was a function of rich eye-movement and poor eye-movement segments. We then calculated and pooled the rate for each subset and compared them with the figures for W, S, and D. The rich eye-movement portion of D has about four times as much firing as the poor eye-movement portion; the latter in turn, had rates about equal to those in waking, i.e., about half again as high as those found in S. From these figures it could be concluded that the tonic contribution to the rate increase of D was small for FTG neurons and that the high rates D (and hence selectivity) were almost exclusively a function of bursts of unit firing.

c. *Is selectivity a function of cell position and/or size?*   Our histological localization technique allowed us to establish 3 stereotaxic coordinates (to the nearest 0.1 mm) for all 74 FTG cells used in quantitative rate determination. Selectivity was plotted against each of the three dimensions of space to determine the distribution of the physiological property in tissue space. Only the horizontal position (i.e., distance from the midline) significantly differentiated selectivity within the FTG. When a plot was made, it was apparent that selectivity peaked at between 1 and 2 mm from the midline, corresponding to the part of the field where the largest neurons are found. It thus seems possible that cell position and/or size, which is known to determine the excitability and inhibitability of spinal montoneurons, determines selectivity. Consequences of this possibility will be discussed below.

d. *Selectivity is a function of endogenous excitability change* (Freedman et al., in press).   Sensory studies of cat pontine brainstem neurons were undertaken to obtain a more complete characterization of cells thought to be active in the genesis of desynchronized sleep. Twenty-eight cells were studied in three cats. The animals were stimulated while in waking or drowsiness with visual, auditory, and tactile stimuli. Twenty-three of 28 neurons responded in some degree to all three modalities. The tactile stimulus, which was designed to be annoying, but not painful, was generally the most effective and light was generally the least effective. Responses varied in magnitude from one firing to bursts of up to 100/sec. Inhibition, i.e., a complete cessation of firing for 0.5 to 1.0 sec, was seen only in cells with high tonic rates of activity. Most cells with a high degree of selectivity for firing in D responded with fewer than 20 spikes even to the tactile stimulus.

Seven cells, from one cat, were studied in more detail to investigate the latency of response. The latency of response, i.e., the interval between the stimulus and first firing, was generally between 5 and 30 msec. The variability between repeated trials was quite marked. Three units showed a consistent 10 msec increase in latency when responses from the contralateral tactile stimuli were compared with ipsilateral stimuli. One of them showed the same difference for auditory stimuli as well.

Twelve of the 28 tested neurons were histologically localized to the FTG, a cell group with unparalleled selectivity for firing in D sleep compared to waking or synchronized sleep. As a more stringent test of the selectivity criterion, mean firing rates during stimulation were determined for each cell by pooling the firings in the first three successive 0.5 sec/poststimulus intervals for each modality. A mean rate of 7.031 spikes/sec was obtained for waking with stimulation, a 40% increases over the rate in unstimulated waking but still less than one-third of that found for the same neurons in D (25.0285).

These findings show that FTG neurons have a multisensory, variable latency input, which is capable of driving them in a minimal way. The very selective cells respond with a maximum of 3-4 spikes per stimulus and often did not follow repeated stimuli. None of the conditions of stimulation that we tried evoked activity comparable to the phasic activity of D sleep, even though the tactile stimuli were annoying enough to elicit movement responses, such as head turning and limb retraction. The cells' inactivity in quiet wakefulness bespeaks their inattention to sensory phenomena in all but the most unusual circumstances and suggests that the selectivity of firing in D previously reported for these neurons is a genuine and significant variable denoting massive shifts in FTG excitability during the sleep cycle.

e.   *Selectivity is a property of cells with axonal projections to spinal cord* (Wyzinski and Hobson, in press). One would expect the hypothesized driving role of FTG neurons to be reflected in their morphology. Studies of retrograde changes in reticular formation neurons following various lesions of the CNS have revealed that the majority of their axons ascend beyond the mesencephalon and/or descend to at least the thoracic segments of the spinal cord (Brodal, 1957). It has not yet been demonstrated that the FTG neurons exhibiting selective firing during D are the same RF neurons which project their axons long distances rostrally and caudally and are thereby able to control extensive regions of the CNS. We wished to explore this possibility.

Under acute conditions, Magni and Willis (1963) showed that over one-third of the neurons recorded intracellularly in the medial part of the pontine and medullary RF could be antidromically invaded from the first lumbar segment of the spinal cord. In order to study the spontaneous activity of these neurons during the sleep-wakefulness cycle, it was necessary to develop a technique for chronic implantation of electrodes in the spinal cord (see Fig. 1). The fourth cervical vertebra was chosen because the lamina has a large surface area and is relatively flat; this permits four wire electrodes in the cord to be fixed in place with dental cement. The vertebra is held rigidly by two metal supports extending from a special fixture attached to the stereotaxic apparatus and the spinous process is ground down before the electrodes are inserted through the dura to the desired points. Various landmarks are used to position the electrode tips with respect to the three Cartesian coordinates and the usual histological methods are used to verify the placement. Cats which recovered from surgery showed no neurological impairment during survival periods of up to three weeks.

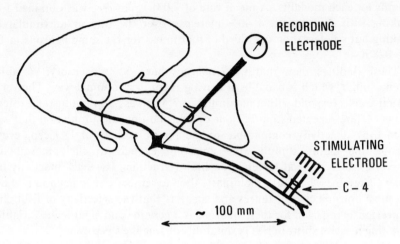

Figure 1—Technique for Physiological Identification of Reticulospinal Neurons by Antidromic Activation. Stimulating electrodes are chronically and stereotaxically located in the anterior horn of the spinal cord and fixed to the arch of the fourth cervical vertebra. When a brain stem neuron has been isolated by the moveable recording microelectrode, the possibility of antidromic invasion is tested by stimulating the cord. Such neurons can thus be identified as reticulospinal and computation of conduction velocities allows further analysis of the cells' discharge properties according to size.

FTG neurons were found to respond antidromically and synaptically at short and long latencies to stimulation of the spinal cord. Antidromic responses are the most revealing because they can be recognized with certainty and they give positive evidence regarding the axonal projections of the recording neuron. This technique thus allows physiological identification of brainstem neurons under the chronic conditions essential to the study of natural sleep. Preliminary results show that those neurons which are antidromically activated are also highly selective, strengthening the hypothesis that the influence of selective firing by FTG cells in D is direct and widespread.

2. *Tonic Latency* (Freedman et al., in press)

a. *FTG neurons increase rate before cortical neurons in pre-D transition.* Averaged data from long-term recording of neurons in the cat gigantocellular tegmental field (FTG) have revealed tonic increases in firing rate as long as 4 minutes before the onset of a desynchronized sleep period (D). This phenomenon has been called the tonic latency (Hobson, 1972). The pooled curves of FTG neurons revealed significant rate increases some 10 seconds earlier than data from a population of cerebral cortical neurons. The earlier increases in firing rate by FTG neurons fulfills the tonic latency criterion for the FTG in the active central control theory of D sleep.

b. *Individual rate curves are distinctive for each FTG neuron.* Using the data from cells which have been recorded for multiple cycles, we have looked more closely at tonic latency by seeing 1) how the tonic latency of an individual cell varies between transition periods, 2) how the range of tonic latencies differs from cell to cell, and 3) how tonic latencies are distributed across the entire cell population. The tonic latency was established for a given transition period by noting the time of a statistically significant increase in firing over a baseline period. In general, once the firing rate had increased beyond the level of significance, it did not decrease below that level, but the increase in firing rate was not strictly monotonic, and was occasionally seen to return to the baseline level.

The time of onset of sustained firing varied widely over different transition periods as demonstrated by cumulative histograms for individual neurons. The widest range for one cell was from t_{-225} sec to t_{+25} sec where t_0 is defined as the time of the first eye movement of D. All cells increased their firing rate before D onset during at least some transition periods, and most cells showed both positive and negative latencies. Thus, rather than firing at a fixed and constant time before D onset, each neuron had a distribution of latencies which was unique to itself. For example, two units exhibited different curves from one another, although both had a similarly wide range of latencies. The mean tonic latency for a given cell was not related to anatomical localization or to baseline firing rate.

c. *Pooled rate curve of FTG neurons is exponential suggesting self-excitation.* A cumulative histogram for the population of cells studied was constructed, weighting each cell equally. Sixty transition periods were included. The experimental curve was fit well by the equation for the exponential growth, $y = e^{kt}$. It could not be fitted by the equation for the normal distribution. Thus, the shape of the histogram does not reflect a random distribution of tonic latency times, but rather suggests that the tonic latencies of these cells are dependent upon each other. In its differential form, the exponential growth equation states that the number of cells increasing their firing rate at any time is proportional to the number which have already so increased, i.e., $dy/dt = ky$. This observation is in accord with the anatomical evidence that a large source of input to FTG neurons are the ramifications of axons of other FTG neurons and is therefore compatible with a self-reexcitation process within the FTG during pre-D transition periods.

3. *Phasic Latency and Rhythmicity*

a. *FTG bursting begins before eye movements.* Previous investigations of cellular activity in the pontine reticular gigantocellular tegmental field (FTG) have established that these cells show a phasic rate increases prior to isolated eye movements (EMs) during D (Hobson et al., in press). Furthermore, these rate changes have been shown to precede rate changes in cortical neurons recorded under similar conditions. Phasic rate changes in FTG neurons have now been compared with those of adjacent reticular areas to test the phasic latency criterion more rigorously.

b. FTG bursting begins before that of other brainstem units (Pivik et al., in press). Isolated EMs were defined as EOG deflections of 35 μ V separated from similar deflections by at least 1 sec. The data were analyzed on a PDP-12 computer utilizing a program which determined EM onset (t_o), summed the number of unit discharges in consecutive 10 msec bins 500 msec before and after t_o, and rectified, scaled, and summed the EOG voltages. Subsequently the data was collapsed into 20 consecutive 50 msec bins for further analyses.

Sequential interval histograms were constructed from pooled data and revealed prominent rate increases (greater than 30% increment over the mean of the preceding 450 msecs) in FTG, tegmental reticular nucleus (TRN), and other tegmental field (FT) neurons in the 50 msec prior to t_o which were sustained through t_{+100} for these three reticular areas. Activity of pontine grey (PG) neurons remained unchanged during isolated EMs. Peak periods of activity for the three areas showing EM-related firing occurred at t_{-50} and t_{+50} (FTG), t_{+100} (other FT areas), and t_{+50} (TRN). Although all three reticular areas showed increases 50 msec prior to t_o, increments in FTG neurons were evident at t_{-150}. With the exception of PG neurons, all nuclear groups had more firings after than before t_o, with the intergroup proportions being nearly exactly the same.

The data indicate that neurons of both the pontine tegmental fields and nuclei show EM related firing, whereas those of the pontine gray do not. FTG neurons are distinguished however, by increments and peak activity in advance of the other groups. The data are thus consistent with the theory that FTG neurons are at or near the source of the phasic excitation characteristic of D sleep.

c. FTG bursting is rhythmic prior to PGO spikes (McCarley et al., in press). It was of interest to examine the nature of phasic FTG neuronal firing in greater detail and with greater precision with a view to understanding the physiology of phasic bursting at the cellular level. The temporal relationship between FTG neuronal firing and a phasic event of D, the PGO (pontogeniculate-occipital) wave in the transcortical EEG, was studied by the method of cross-correlation.

Three histologically localized FTG neurons, recorded by extracellular microelectrode techniques in chronic cats, were studied. All were characterized by selective, clustered firing in D. PGO spikes were detected by a PDP-12 computer from a record digitized at 100 samples/sec. Two successive D periods were used for each analysis.

The average waveform of 144 PGO spikes was plotted. A broad peak lasting about 200 msec, which constitutes the waveform of the "classic" PGO spike, was observed. Noted also in the average waveform wave were smaller peaks of about 70-80 msec duration that may represent the fundamental period of the PGO spikes.

d. FTG neuronal burst rhythm has same period as PGO spikes (McCarley et al., in press). Cross-correlation functions (CCF) between PGO spikes and unit activity were then made. Time zero marked the occurrence of a peak of the PGO spike. The unit firings were summed in 10 msec bins in relation to this event. The most striking feature of the CCFs was the rhythmic peaking of unit activity preceding the occurrence of a PGO spike. The tightest phase locking of unit firing with PGO spikes was shown by the peak closest to the PGO spike, where unit firing showed more than 8-fold increases at the peak over the rate at the nadir. The period of the peaks of unit firing preceding the PGO spike was 70-80 msec, the same as the fundamental period of PGO spikes.

The temporal precedence, tight phase-locking, and rhythmic firing at the fundamental period of PGO spikes suggest that FTG units may generate PGO spike activity. The 70-80 msec range of periods for the bursts of unit activity is within the time range for EPSP-IPSP sequences which may underlie this rhythmic neuronal firing.

B. Reciprocal Interaction as a Possible Basis for Sleep Cycle Control

1. *Periodicity* (McCarley et al., 1972)

As evidence has accumulated suggesting that activity of cells in the gigantocellular tegmental field (FTG) of the pontine reticular formation may underlie the generation of desynchronized sleep (D), we have begun to consider estimation of the parameters in the time course of firing throughout the sleep cycle and from one cycle to the next.

We have analyzed the time course of activity of four histologically localized FTG neurons, each with continuous extracellular recordings of 10 or more successive D cycles. Two kinds of detailed analysis of the time course of the activity have been done.

a. FTG activity curves are nonsinusoidal First we have estimated the "average" time course of firing over a complete D cycle. The start of a cycle is the electrographically defined end of a D period, and the cycle continues until the end of the next D period. Because of variation in cycle duration we have normalized each cycle to a constant duration, then computed for each cycle the unit activity at 100 points during the cycle, and averaged all the cycles to obtain the average time course of firing. The average time course of activity is strongly nonsinusoidal and consists of a nadir occurring shortly after the end of D, a gradual increase, then an explosive acceleration of activity with a peak during the D period, and then a rapid deceleration during the last fraction of the D period.

We believe that the average time course curve of pooled FTG neurons will yield a reasonable estimate of the average membrane potential of the pool. Since exogenous input can be assumed to be constant, the regular changes in membrane potential must be endogenous. As such they could reflect rhythmic intracellular processes currently inaccessible to analysis, or they could represent rhythmic intercellular process that might be detectable by comparing activity of FTG cells with one another or with other groups of cells.

b. FTG Activity Curves are Periodic. The second kind of temporal analysis was directed toward quantitative documentation of the nonsinusoidal periodicity observable in the activity curves of the units through serial correlation coefficients and spectral analysis. Periodicity was indicated in the serial correlation coefficients by regular peaks and in the power spectral density by a dominant peak. The nonsinusoidal nature of the periodicity was indicated by smaller peaks in the power spectral density at multiples or harmonics of the frequency represented by the dominant peak. Thus the average membrane potential of the FTG pool must be under the control of a periodic oscillator. This result could be confidently predicted from the ultradian rhythmicity of D sleep but we feel that establishing periodicity at the neuronal level represents an important step toward understanding the mechanism of its control.

2. Reciprocal Rate Changes in FTG and Loeus Coelruleus (LC) Neurons (Hobson et al., in press)
Massive shifts in excitability of FTG neurons during the sleep cycle are suggested by several of the findings previously discussed. Moreover, self-reexcitation is a possible mechanism for producing the bursts of discharge seen once the FTG neurons are tonically brought to threshold. This tonic change could occur either by an increase in excitatory input from another source (the true active half-center) or by withdrawal of tonic inhibition from another source (the passive half-center). If the latter mechanisms exists, one would expect to see a reciprocal relation of tonic firing by FTG and other neurons.

In our first 75 microelectrode explorations of the brainstem of 10 cats we found only 10 of 100 neurons to have rates of discharge that were lower in D sleep than in waking or synchronized sleep (S). We were thus interested to note that 8 of those 10 cells came from 3 descents that passed through the anterior pontine tegmentum and could be further localized to the posterior pole of the nucleus locus coeruleus (LC) and the nucleus subcoeruleus. The mean rate of these 8 LC neurons yielded selectivity ratios of D/S=0.3, values which are 500 times less than those of the FTG (D/W 100, D/S 50.) In addition, the time course of the rate deceleration for LC neurons in transition from S to D was found to be the mirror image of the acceleration characteristic of FTG neurons.

We have now made an additional eleven descents in two cats aiming to hit the LC by intention. Of 47 neurons recorded, 14 showed a rate decrease in transition from S to D. This yield is more meager than initial experience has led us to expect but it is still some 17 times greater than the incidence of such neurons in other parts of the brainstem explored by us (see Table VI).

TABLE VI

	No. of descents	No. of cells D < W, S. over total	% showing decrease	Ratio LC/ Non-LC
LC Descents	14	22/58	37.80	16.8
Non-LC Descents	72	2/89	2.25	1

Quantitative rate determinations and detailed histological examination now in progress may force some revision of these figures but it does appear likely that some neurons which have reciprocal rate relations with the FTG may be localized in or near the LC. This finding suggests the possibility of a functional interaction between the two cell groups. If verified, this interaction could provide a basis for sleep stage oscillation.

3. A Preliminary Model for Sleep Cycle Oscillation (McCarley, in press)

In the light of reciprocal rate changes by LC and FTG neurons, we have begun work on a model that assumes interaction of two populations of cells and yields results that mimic the time course of firing of FTG units. The model is intended to show a way that nonsinusoidal periodicities could arise from two populations of units. It is to be noted that many of the assumptions of the model are unproven physiologically, and the model is offered as a working hypothesis rather than as a description. It is likely that substantial alterations in the model will prove to be necessary as more data is collected.

Table VII summarizes the fragmentary physiological characteristics of brainstem neuronal groups which may interact reciprocally. In this chapter we have summarized evidence that the FTG is selectively active in D and have advanced our reasons for thinking that FTG neurons are self-excitatory. It has been shown that cholinomimetic substances can potentiate D sleep and we are currently investigating the possibility that FTG neurons are cholinergic and cholinoceptive. To account for the silence of FTG neurons in W we now propose tonic inhibition by other cell groups for which the leading candidates are the DRN and the LC. The rate data reported by us (Hobson et al In Press) and by McGinty and Harper (McGinty and Harper 1972) are consistent with this hypothesis. It is interesting to note that ACh has been hypothesized to be excitatory centrally as well as peripherally and that both NE and 5HT have been presumed to be inhibitory transmitters. The question marks in Table VII indicate assumptions for which there is no evidence. We believe, however, that simple extension of the methods outlined here will allow them to be tested.

TABLE VII

Physiological Characteristics of a Model for Reciprocal
Interaction Underlying Sleep Cycle Oscillation

	Cell Group A	Cell Group B
Anatomical substrate	FTG	LC, DRN
Transmitter	ACh (?)	NE, 5HT
Excitatory to self	+	— (?)
Excitatory to other	+ (?)	— (?)
Inhibitory to self	— (?)	+ (?)
Inhibitory to other	— (?)	+ (?)

The model assumes that FTG units are self-excitatory and excitatory to the LC units. The LC population is assumed inhibitory to FTG units and to itself. Interactions between the two populations are assumed to be nonlinear in that the effect of inputs is proportional to the current level of activity (see Fig. 2). Let x=activity level in FTG units, let y=activity level in the LC units, and let a, b, c, and d be positive constants representing potency of interactions. The resulting system of equations is

$$dx/dt = ax - bxy$$
$$dy/dt = cy + dxy$$

These equations were solved for x by the method of continuous analytic continuation. The time course of activity for x as produced by one set of constants was graphed. A gradual increase of activity, an abrupt rise to a

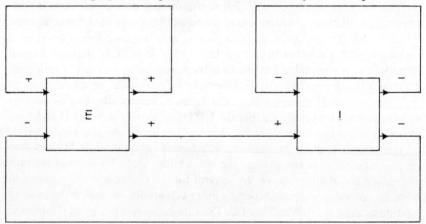

FIGURE 2—Simple Model Yielding Non-Linear Differential Equations of the Volterra-Lotka type. In the diagram, E cells are assumed self-excitatory and excitatory to I cells, while I cells are assumed self-inhibitory and inhibitory to E cells. In the text, it is emphasized that the model does not make specific assumptions about the mechanism of interaction: these could be either biochemical or synaptic or both. It is our working hypothesis that FTG neurons may be E cells, reciprocally interacting with LC neurons which may be I cells.

peak, and subsequent sudden fall reproduced rather well the actual time course of FTG unit activity.

The system of equations is well known as the Volterra-Lotka equations; in population biology they are used to describe the oscillations of the number of members of populations of predator and prey. Again, it is to be emphasized strongly that many features of the model are only assumptions. However, these features are open to experimental verification, rebuttal, or modification and indeed, the model suggests experiments. A final comment is that the model does not make specific assumptions about the mechanisms of interaction; these could be biochemical as well as electro-physiological.

SUMMARY AND CONCLUSIONS

The field of sleep research is characterized by an explosive increase in descriptive information regarding psychological and physiological phenomena. Macroscopic methods of neuroanatomy and neurophysiology have provided data of relevance to the question of mechanism, especially the localization of brain structures involved in sleep control. This exploratory work has been conducted and interpreted in loose or unspecified logical frameworks with the result that there are many sleep "centers" but no means to determine how they may act or interact in the generation of sleep. The recent emphasis on biogenic amine systems has carried this problem to the level of putative transmitters without answering the fundamental question of how sleep is produced.

Further progress in this line of research may be aided by the development of a theory of central control which includes elaboration of specific anatomical and physiological criteria against which experimental data could be quantitatively compared. A theory is offered which emphasizes the microscopic level of analysis. The methods of cellular neurophysiology are seen as offering theoretical and practical solutions to the question of mechanism because they take account of a cardinal organizational feature of the nervous system, the individual neuron.

The stimulation and lesion literature was surveyed and the structures implicated in sleep control were outlined. Evidence regarding the activity of nerve cells in each structure was ordered according to the set of quantitative physiological criteria that are the heart of the theory. The cellular control of waking and synchronized sleep was represented as a terra incognita with only scanty evidence at the cellular level bearing on how these behaviors might be regulated.

The cellular control of desynchronized sleep was seen to be somewhat better understood. The evidence implicating the giant cells of the pontine reticular formation as part of a control system for this behavior was reviewed in detail: 1) the firing of the giant neurons is highly selective for desynchronized sleep; 2) tonic rate increases anticipate each episode by many minutes; 3) phasic rate increases lead the eye movements and EEG events by many milliseconds; 4) the changes are consistent from cycle to cycle and are strongly periodic.

The mechanism of the periodic activation of the giant cells remains to be determined. Reciprocal rate changes by amine specific neurons of the brainstem suggest that reciprocal interaction between two cell groups may occur. A model for such interaction has been developed which accurately describes giant cell activity curves. The model serves both to test and to generate other hypotheses about the control of sleep cycle oscillation.

It is hoped that the approach outlined here may prove useful in exploring other aspects of sleep control, especially circadian alternations of sleep and waking. It might also be applied to other oscillatory behaviors.

REFERENCES

Bard, P. and Rioch, D. Mck. Study of four cats deprived of neocortex and additional portions of the forebrain. *Bull. Johns Hopkins Hospital 60,* 73-147 (1937).

Bremer, F. Preoptic hypnogenic focus and mesencephalic reticular formation. *Brain Res.* 21, 132-134 (1970).

Brodal, A. *Reticular Formation of the Brain Stem. Anatomical Aspects and Functional Correlations.* Oliver & Boyd, Edinburgh, 1957.

Cajal, R. Intrinsic nuclei and pathways of the bulb. in, *Histologie Du Systeme Nerveux.* Vol. 1, CSIC, Madrid, 1952, pp. 948-954.

Cannon, W.B. Organization for physiological homeostasis. *Physiol. Rev. 9,* 399-431 (1929).

Carlie, G. and Zanchetti, A. Study of pontine lesions suppressing deep sleep in the cat. *Arch. Ital. Biol. 103,* 751-788 (1965).

Dahlstrom, A. and Fuxe, K. Evidence for the existence of mono-amine-containing neurons in the central nervous system I. Demonstration of monoamines in the cell bodies of brain stem neurons. *Acta Physiol. Scand. 62* (Suppl. 232), 1-25 (1964).

Evarts, E.V. Unit activity in sleep and wakefulness. in, *The Neurosciences—A Study Program,* G.C. Quarton, T. Melnechuk, and F.O. Schmitt, eds., Rockefeller Press, New York, 1967, pp. 545-556.

Findlay, A.L.R. and Hayward, J.N. Spontaneous activity of single neurones in the hypothalamus of rabbits during sleep and waking. *J. Physiol [London] 201,* 237-258 (1969).

Fredrickson, C.J. and Hobson, J.A. Electrical stimulation of the brain stem and subsequent sleep. *Arch. Ital. Biol. 108,* 564-576 (1970).

Freedman, R., Hobson, J.A., McCarley, R.W. and Pivik, R.T. Characterization of the rate increase of cat pontine brain stem neurons in the transition period prior to desynchronized sleep. *Sleep Res. 2,* in press.

Freedman, R., Hobson, J.A., McCarley, R.W. and Pivik, R.T. Sensory responsiveness of cat pontine brain stem neurons as a function of selectivity for firing in desynchronized sleep. *Sleep Res. 2,* in press.

Fuxe, K. Evidence for the existence of monoamine neurons in the central nervous system. IV. Distribution of monoamine nerve terminals in the central nervous system. *Acta. Physiol. Scand.* (Suppl. 247), 37-84 (1965).

Hess, W.R. *Diencephalon. Autonomic and Extrapyramidal Functions.* Grune & Stratton, New York 1954.

Hobson, J.A. The effect of chronic brain stem lesions on cortical and muscular activity during sleep and waking in the cat. *EEG Clin. Neurophysiol. 19,* 41-62 (1965).

Hobson, J.A., McCarley, R.W. and Pivik, R.T. A comparison of phasic rate changes in brainstem and cortical neurons associated with eye movements of desynchronized sleep. *Sleep Res. 1,* 21, (1972).

Hobson, J.A., McCarley, R.W., Wyzinski, P.W. and Pivik, R.T. Reciprocal tonic firing by FTG and LC neurons during the sleep-waking cycle. *Sleep Res. 2,* in press.

Hobson, J.A. Cellular neurophysiology and sleep research, in *The Sleeping Brain,* M. Chase, ed., UCLA Brain Information Service, Los Angeles, op. 59-83, 1972.

Huttenlocher, P.R. Evoked and spontaneous activity in single units of medial brain stem during natural sleep and waking. *J. Neurophysiol. 24,* 451-468 (1961).

Jouvet, M. Approches neurophysiologiques des processus d'apprentissage. *Biol. Med. 49,* 282-360 (1960).

Jouvet, M. Recherches sur les structures nerveuses et les mecanismes responsables des differentes phases du sommeil physiologique. *Arch. Ital. Biol. 100,* 125-206 (1962).

Jouvet, M. Biogenic amines and the states of sleep. *Science 163,* 32-41 (1969).

Jouvet, M. The role of momoamines and acetycholine-containing neurons in the regulation of the sleep-waking cycle. *Ergebnisse Physiol., 64,* 166-307 (1972).

Kasamatsu, T. Maintained and evoked unit activity in the mesencephalic reticular formation of the freely behaving cat. *Exper. Neurol. 28,* 450-470 (1970).

Lamarche, J., Langlois, J.M. and Heon, M. Unit study of the trigeminal projections in the reticular formation. *Can. J. Biochem. Physiol. 38,* 1163-1166 (1960).

Magni, F. and Willis, W.D. Identification of reticular formation neurons by intracellular recording. *Arch. Ital. Biol. 101,* 681-702 (1963).

Magni, F. and Willis, W.D. Cortical control of brain stem reticular neurons. *Arch. Ital. Biol. 102,* 418-433 (1964).

Manohar, S., Noda, H. and Adey, W.R. Behavior of mesencephalic reticular neurons in sleep and wakefulness. *Exper. Neurol. 34,* 140-157 (1972).

McCarley, R.W. and Hobson, J.A. Single neuron activity in cat gigantocellular tegmental field: Selectivity of discharge in desynchronized sleep. *Science 174,* 1250-1252 (1971).

McCarley, R.W. A model for the periodicity of brain stem neuronal discharges during the sleep cycle. *Sleep Res. 2,* in press.

McCarley, R.W., Hobson, J.A. and Pivik, R.T. Time course of firing of brain stem neurons over the sleep cycle. *Sleep Res. 2;* in press.

McCarley, R.W., Hobson, J.A. and Pivik, R.T. Activity of individual brain stem neurons during repeated sleep-waking cycles. *Sleep Res. 1;* 26 (1972).

McCarley, R.W., Hobson, J.A. and Pivik, R.T. Relationships between discharges of neurons in the pontine reticular formation and PGO waves recorded at occipital cortex. *Sleep Res. 2,* in press.

McGinty, D.J. and Harper, R.M. 5HT-containing neruons: Unit activity during sleep. *Sleep Res. 1,* 27 (1972).

Moruzzi, G. The sleep-waking cycle. *Ergebnisse Physiol. 64,* 1-165 (1972).

Perenin, M.T., Maeda, T., and Jeannerod, M. Are vestibular nuclei responsible for rapid eye movements of paradoxical sleep? *Brain Res. 43,* 617-621 (1962).

Pivik, R.T., Hobson, J.A. and McCarley, R.W. Eye movement associated rate changes in neuronal activity during desynchronized sleep: A comparison of brain stem regions. *Sleep Res. 2,* in press.

Pompeiano, O. Sensory inhibition during motor activity in sleep. In, *Neurophysiological Basis of Normal and Abnormal Motor Activities,* M.D. Yahr and D.P. Purpura, eds., Raven Press, New York: 1967, pp. 323-375.

Scheibel, A.B., Scheibel, M.E., Mollica, A., and Moruzzi, G. Convergence and interaction of afferent impulses on single units of reticular formation. *J. Neurophysiol. 18;* 309-331, (1955).

Scheibel, M.E., Scheibel, A.B., Structural substrates for integrative patterns in the brain stem reticular core. in, *Reticular Formation of the Brain,* H. Jasper et al. eds., J.A. Churchill, London, 1957, pp. 31-56.

Scheibel, M.E. and Scheibel, A.B. Response of reticular units to repetetive stimuli. *Arch. Ital. Biol. 103,* 279-299 (1965).

Segundo, J.P., Takenaka, T. and Encabo, U. Electrophysiology of bulbar reticular neurons. *J. Neurophysiol. 30,* 1194-1220 (1967).

Segundo, J.P., Takenaka, T. and Encabo, H. Somatic sensory properties of bulbar reticular neurons. *J. Neurophysiol. 30,* 1221-1238 (1967).

Vincent, J.D., Benoit, O., Scherrer, J., and Faure, J.M. Activites elementaires recueillies dans l'hypothalamus au cours de la veille et du sommeil chez le lapin chronique. *J. Physiol. [Fr.]* (suppl. 4) 59, 527 (1967).

Wyzinski, P.W. and Hobson, J.A. Technique for chronic implanation of spinal electrodes. *Sleep Res. 2,* in press.

Advances in Sleep Research, Vol. 1
© 1974, Spectrum Publications, Inc.

CHAPTER 5

Central Neural Control of Brainstem Somatic Reflexes During Sleeping and Waking

MICHAEL H. CHASE

INTRODUCTION

The somatic reflex is a basic component of behavior. Since sleep and wakefulness are behavioral states, we have examined state-dependent changes in somatic reflex activity in an effort to understand the central neural mechanisms which operate to assure the appropriate array of physiological processes which comprise sleep and wakefulness. In turn, such information we hoped would lead to an increased understanding of the factors responsible for the initiation and maintenance of the states themselves.

There are a number of specific reasons for choosing to study somatic reflex activity, and in particular brainstem reflexes, rather than other physiological processes which comprise sleep and wakefulness. Some of these reasons are practical, relating to our goal-oriented research strategy, while others are based on historical precedent, relating to our prior experiences, surgical skills, and a general fondness for the brainstem masseteric and digastric reflexes.

An important reason for choosing to study somatic reflex activity is that the response, i.e., contraction of a somatic muscle, is easily recorded in freely moving animals as a discrete time-locked event following afferent stimulation. The fluctuations in its amplitude are consistent across states, between animals, and over time. Reflex activity is therefore stable and to a great extent does not appear to reflect variations in the exteroceptive (e.g., visual) or interoceptive (e.g., heart rate) environments. Moreover, the factors which modulate the somatic reflex can be analyzed in a relatively straightforward fashion, because the response is solely dependent upon the excitability of presynaptic afferent terminals and the postsynaptic motor neurons.

When describing somatic reflex activity, a number of points must be kept in mind, perhaps the most important of which is the reciprocal nature of the innervation of somatic musculature. Were one to lose sight of this fact, one might, for example, examine a test somatic reflex, find its amplitude reduced by the experimental manipulation, and generate an hypothesis that the effect of the experimental manipulation was to produce reflex inhibition; or, one might as reasonably assume that the experimental manipulation facilitated the antagonistic reflex producing, in turn, reciprocal inhibition of the test reflex, in which case the experimental manipulation would be directly related to reflex facilitation, rather than to inhibition. Therefore, in order properly to examine the response of somatic reflexes, an analysis of the amplitude of the agonist as well as the antagonist reflex must be included in the experimental design.

Another important point to bear in mind when investigating spinal somatic reflex activity is that amplitude is critically dependent upon posture. Since each posture loads certain muscles and unloads others, reflex excitability *may* reflect postural-dependent patterns rather than state-dependent processes. In order to eliminate the difficulties inherent in examining spinal cord somatic reflexes, we decided to study the brainstem masseteric and digastric reflexes. The masseteric reflex is monosynaptic, and is involved in jaw closure, while the digastric reflex is polysynaptic, and its action is to open the jaw. These, then, are antagonistic brainstem reflexes which are not directly influenced by postural variations and, in addition, provide information regarding the excitability of both mono- and polysynaptic circuitry.

The monosynaptic masseteric reflex is comprised of: 1) muscle spindles and their sensory innervation; 2) gamma motoneurons which innervate the intrafusal muscle fibers within the spindles; and 3) alpha motor neurons whose fibers leave the brainstem to innervate the extrafusal fibers of the masseter musculature (Fig. 1). The monosynaptic connection is located entirely within the brainstem. Thus, fibers whose cell bodies lie within the mesencephalic nucleus of the 5th nerve connect the proprioceptive receptors within the masseter muscle with the trigeminal (alpha) motor neurons. Excitation of these motor neurons leads to contraction of the masseter muscle. The degree of contraction is dependent upon the discharge of the alpha motor neurons which in turn is regulated by muscle spindle afferent and presynaptic terminal discharge. In our studies, the masseteric reflex was induced electrically by excitation of the sensory cells of the mesencephalic nucleus of the 5th nerve, by-passing the proprioceptive endings which normally induce activity in these cells and their fibers. The monosynaptic reflex response was recorded either from the motor (masseter) nerve innervating the masseter musculature or directly from the musculature itself.

The polysynaptic digastric reflex is also organized entirely within the brainstem (Fig. 1). However, unlike the masseteric reflex, it lacks muscle spindles and gamma motor neurons. Thus, stimuli adequate to initiate the reflex response arise not from receptors within musculature but from receptors located in the periodontal area. These sensory receptors in the buccal cavity project to the brainstem via fibers of the 5th cranial nerve, thus forming the afferent limb of the reflex arc. The efferent limb consists of the mandibular portion of the 5th nerve which in turn becomes the digastric (mylohyoid) nerve, innervating the anterior belly of the digastric muscle. In our studies we induced the digastric reflex electrically by stimulating fibers issuing from the periodonal receptors. The reflex response was recorded either from the digastric nerve or the digastric muscle.

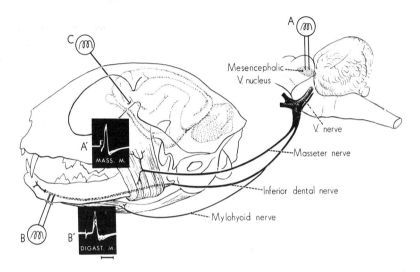

Fig. 1. Reflex activity within the masseter (A′) or digastric (B′) musculature was obtained by electrical stimulation of the ipsilateral mesencephalic nucleus of the Vth nerve (A) or the inferior dental nerve (B), respectively. The effect of orbital cortical stimulation (C) upon the spontaneous and reflex-induced activity of these muscles was examined. The bipolar recording electrodes within the digastric and masseter musculature are not shown. Calibration line: 10 msec and 200 μ V. (From Chase and McGinty (1970b).)

By including in our experimental paradigm studies of the adult as well as the neonatal animal, it was possible to determine when patterns of reflex activity mature. Through a combination of development-dependent and state-dependent analyses, we sought to obtain a comprehensive understanding of somatic reflex activity, including its emergent control in the newborn and the adult pattern of modulation. We also hoped that this type of analysis of central neural activity would provide information as to the dynamic processes responsible for the initiation and maintenance of the states of sleep and wakefulness themselves. In an endeavor to implement the preceding approach to the study of the central nervous system's functional organization during sleep and wakefulness, we carried out the following group of experiments (see Table I for an overview).

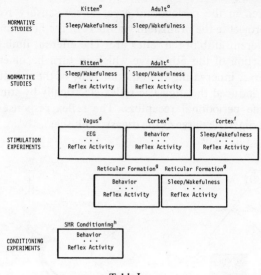

Table I

a Chase and Sterman (1967), b Chase (1970, 1971, 1972b).
c Chase et al. (1968); Chase (1970, in press).
d Chase et al. (1966, 1967); Chase and Nakamura (1968a,b); Chase et al. (1970a,b).
e Clemente et al. (1966); Chase and McGinty (1970a); Chase et al. (in press).
f Chase and McGinty (1970a); Chase (in press).
g Chase and Babb (in press); Watanabe and Chase (in press).
h Chase (1972; in press).

DEVELOPMENT OF SLEEP AND WAKEFULNESS IN KITTENS

Introduction

The developing animal sleeps and is awake. When the developmental period is over, the animal continues to demonstrate these states, but their accompanying physiological activity is very different. The interaction between the factors which govern the development of sleep and wakefulness and the forces which govern the development of physiological processes results in constantly changing complex patterns of activity in immature animals which are quite different and more variable than those found in adults.

In 1967 we published a study of the development of sleep and wakefulness in kittens which utilized prolonged recordings and strict environmental controls (Chase and Sterman, 1967). We hoped that a careful analysis of this data would further our understanding of the developmental process, provide a foundation for manipulative ontogenetic research and, most important, enable us to understand the adult state by determining its origins, i.e., "how it got that way." Previous studies of the development of sleep and wakefulness had utilized short and variable recording sessions, which placed obvious limitations on the data analysis (Jouvet, 1963; Valatx et al. 1964). In the present study, by recording for periods of 24 hours, we attempted to attain statistically significant descriptions of the development of the alert, drowsy, quiet sleep, and active sleep states in the maturing kitten (Fig. 2).

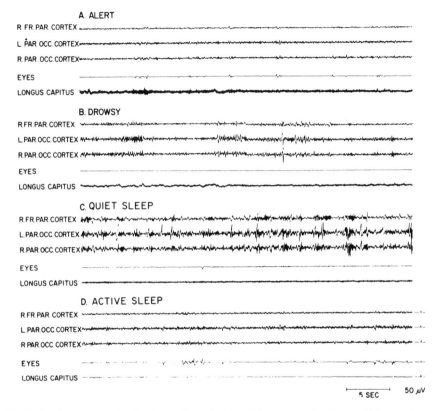

Fig. 2. This figure illustrates the four patterned states of sleep and wakefulness which served as the basis for our analyses. These tracings were obtained from a 4-month-old kitten. We observed no difference in the waveform or frequency characteristics of the EEG in any of the animals in our population. Additionally, these patterned states were clearly distinguishable in both the young and older animals. (From Chase and Sterman (1967).)

Methods

A group of 14 kittens was utilized, ranging in age from 36 to 208 days. All animals were weaned prior to experimentation. In order to record from freely moving and unanesthetized kittens, we implanted permanently placed chronic recording electrodes while the animals were anesthetized with sodium pentobarbital (Nembutal—35 mg/kg given as a dilute 10 mg/ml solution).

After anesthetization, the skin overlying the dorsal calvarium was reflected and 1/8 in. stainless steel screws were inserted in the calvarium overlying the frontal, parietal, and occipital areas of the cortex to record electroencephalographic (EEG) activity. Electroocular (EOG) activity was monitored with stainless steel balls (1/8 in diameter) sutured bilaterally into the faciae bulbi of the eyes. The electromyographic activity (EMG) of the longus capitus neck musculature was monitored with stainless steel balls sutured into the muscle parenchyma. Insulated leads from all recording electrodes were soldered to a Winchester plug which was subsequently affixed to the calvarium with acrylic cement. After recovery from the operative procedures, the kittens were habituated to a chamber which maintained a constant visual, auditory, and olfactory environment so as to minimize variations in external cues. Food and water were provided *ad libitum*. During recording sessions the animal was connected to a counter-weighted cable and slip-ring assembly which allowed free movement within the chamber. Twenty-four hour recordings were obtained on a polygraph equipped with a laboratory-manufactured "glamour hammer" (a paper collection device which collects and folds a continuous 24-hour flow of EEG paper at the rate of 15 mm per sec.).

We discussed at length the advantages and disadvantages of recording from kittens that were weaned, removed from their mothers and placed in an isolated environment. Although we realized that this was not the normal environment for the animal, we felt that the variables which would otherwise have had to be taken into account were too difficult to control. For example, when recording from kittens while they are with their mothers and litter mates, variations in maternal and litter mate sleep and waking cycles would undoubtedly have influenced cycles in the developing kitten. Such factors as the number of litter mates and their behavior would be not only beyond our control, but would have varied from litter to litter and laboratory to laboratory, as would maternal behavior. We therefore felt that the optimal method for obtaining reliable data would be to generate a standard environment which could be controlled by ourselves and duplicated by others. In addition, the environment was similar to that utilized for data obtained in complementary studies of sleep and wakefulness in adult animals (Sterman et al., 1965).

In order to perform statistical tests, we divided the animals into three groups: a) a youngest group of 7 animals ranging in age from 36 to 78 days (mean = 1.7 months); b) an intermediate group of 4 animals ranging in age from 119 to 150 days (mean = 4.6 months); and c) an oldest group of 3 animals ranging in age from 189 to 208 days (mean = 6.5 months).

The key feature in this study was the 24-continuous recording of sleep and waking patterns (actually 23 hr, since we omitted the first hour of our analyses to compare our data with that reported for the adult cats). We assigned each minute of the 23 hours to one of four states: a) alert, b) drowsy, c) quiet sleep, or d) active sleep (see Chase and Sterman [1967] and Chase

[1972a]) for a description of the states and clarification of their nomen-clature). Both analysis of variance and the student t-test for small groups with unequal Ns were applied to determine the changes in the following variables as a function of age: a) percentage occurrence of the basic patterns of sleep and wakefulness; b) frequency and duration of individual episodes of the four states; and c) their circadian distribution.

Results

By 110 days of age the percentage of the alert, drowsy, quiet sleep, and active sleep states was similar to adult values (Fig. 3). The youngest group of animals exhibited a significantly higher percentage of active sleep (decreasing with age) and a lower percentage of alert and drowsy patterns (increasing with age) (Fig. 3). The amount of quiet sleep did not change within the age limits of the animals employed in this study (Fig. 3).

The increase in the alert state followed an asymptotic function ($r = 0.66$), as did the increase in the drowsy state ($r = 0.89$). However, the curve of best fit for the drowsy state was an increasing linear function ($r = 0.92$). Active sleep exhibited a symptotic decrease in percentage occurrence ($r = 0.90$). The pattern percentage of quiet sleep for the age groups studied was not significantly different, and its low correlation with the curve of best fit ($r = 0.36$) indicated that the distribution of the data points was random.

Since this chapter is devoted to an overview of the development of sleep and wakefulness with respect to somatic reflex activity, our detailed analysis of the changes in sleep and waking patterns which occur during maturation will not be recapitulated (Chase and Sterman, 1967). Instead, a brief sum-mary of the major findings will be presented.

In order to determine the bases for the developmental changes in the pattern percentages described above, we performed an analysis of the variations in episode length of sleep and wakefulness as a function of age. It was discovered that episodes of long duration, that is, 7 minutes or more in length, did not change as a function of age. All of the developmental changes in pattern percentage were due to variations in the amount of time spent in episodes of short duration, that is, less than 7 minutes in length. The in-creased time spent in the alert and drowsy states, as well as the decreased time spent in active sleep, were accounted for solely on the basis of changes in the frequency of the short duration episodes. There were no changes in the frequency of either long or short episodes of quiet sleep, nor was there a corresponding change in the total percentage occurrence of this state as a function of age.

The recurrent circadian and ultradian patterns of sleep and wakefulness, described in the adult (Sterman et al., 1965), were also observed in the oldest group of kittens (Fig. 4), and we were able to plot their development beginning with the youngest group. The recurrent patterns of sleep and wakefulness which developed were due to the grouping or reshuffling of the

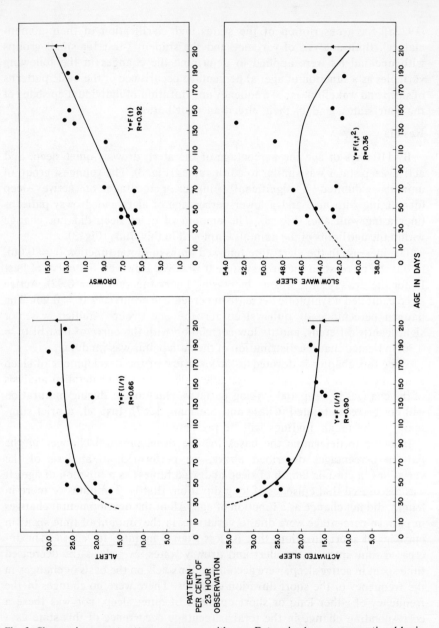

Fig. 3. Changes in percent pattern occurrence with age. Determined on a cross-sectional basis, curves of best fit were generated for the total percentage values of each state for the animals within our population. The mathematical functions for the alert and active sleep states were the same; however, the alert pattern was a positively accelerating function while active sleep was negatively accelerating. Asymptotes for both were reached at approximately the same age. The analysis of the quiet sleep pattern showed no systematic trend with age since the curve of best fit indicated no significant correlation with data. (From Chase and Sterman (1967).)

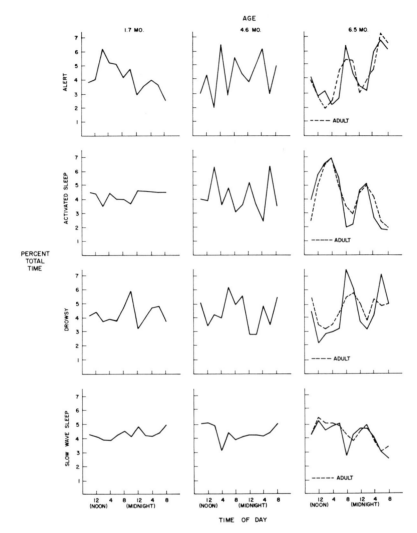

Fig. 4. The ontogenetic development of adult circadian cycles in the various patterns of sleep and wakefulness is demonstrated by curves showing the distribution of each pattern over a 23 hr. period for three age groups. A periodicity was noted for the alert, drowsy, and active sleep patterns by the 4th month of life. By 6 months, the bimodal pattern previously described for adult cats in our laboratory was achieved. (From Chase and Sterman (1967.)

episodes of long duration. Short duration episodes (which were responsible for the development of total pattern percentages) played no part in the development of circadian or ultradian rhythms.

An analysis of sleep cycle time was also carried out. The mean cycle time for the youngest group of animals was 19 minutes, while that for the oldest group was 24 minutes (similar to that of adult cats). Kittens in the intermediate age group exhibited a sleep cycle time of 31 minutes. This increase in sleep cycle time in the intermediate age group might be accounted for by the slight decrease observed in active sleep time for this group. It is interesting to note that a similar decrease in active sleep time has been observed in humans during early adolescence (Roffwarg et al., 1966).

To recapitulate, during the period of maturation dynamic changes occurred in almost all aspects of our analyses. The total percentage of active sleep decreased, while the percentages of the alert and drowsy states increased. These changes in total pattern percentages were due to decreases and increases of episodes 6 minutes or less in duration. The circadian and ultradian rhythms which developed were due to the systematic grouping of episodes of long duration (greater than 6 min. in length), the frequency of which did not change as a function of age. There were no significant changes either in the percentage occurrence of quiet sleep or in the frequency or duration of its episodes.

In every parameter of our analysis a negative correlation was observed between the active sleep and alert states. As the percentage occurrence of the alert pattern increased, a parallel and statistically significant decrease in the percentage occurrence of the active sleep pattern took place. As the frequency of short duration episodes of the alert state increased, there was a significant decrease in the percentage occurrence of active sleep episodes of less than 7 minutes duration. Similar negative correlations were obtained for data relating to the development of the circadian and ultradian distribution of these two states.

Discussion

The changes in percentage, duration, frequency, and distribution of sleep and wakefulness appear to reflect the development of the mechanisms responsible for the states themselves rather than the maturation of specific physiological processes. This view is supported by the facts that the wave form and frequency characteristics of the EEG are well developed by the first month of life (Scheibel, 1961; Jouvet, 1963; Scheibel and Scheibel, 1964) and that the epiphenomena of sleep and wakefulness, for example, muscular twitches and rapid eye movements, are present in even the youngest group of animals studied. In addition, the modulation of reflex activity has matured before kittens are 36 days old, the beginning of the period of this analysis (see the following section). Thus, it is reasonable to assume that the mechanisms responsible for the development of the physiological processes which comprise sleep and wakefulness are essentially mature by the second month of life. In kittens from 36 to 208 days old, changes in the duration of the episodes of the states and the grouping of episodes of each state into an adult pattern of sleep and wakefulness are the striking developmental characteristics.

As was mentioned earlier, in every aspect of our analysis, the alert state correlated negatively with active sleep. The curve of best fit for the development of these two patterns was generated by the same mathematical function, but with an opposite direction of change. A negative correlation was also observed between the alert and active sleep states for the changes in duration and frequency of the episodes, as well as for their circadian distribution. This may reflect a functional antagonism between the systems responsible for these states, or it may indicate the development of a single system underlying both states but able to generate only one state at a time. It seems, at any rate, that the functions, processes, mechanisms, and drives underlying wakefulness and active sleep are mutually exclusive.

In the next section, which is concerned with the development of somatic reflexes, we will note once again the functional antagonism between wakefulness and active sleep, as reflected in the development of adult patterns of state-dependent reflex modulation.

Having determined that a stable distribution of sleep and waking patterns is reached in the developing kitten by approximately 110 days of age, we became interested in correlating this development with that of somatic reflex activity. We believed that somatic reflex activity would also change during development, reaching an adult pattern sometime during the period when the adult configuration of sleep states was achieved. We chose to study the development of two brainstem reflexes, the masseteric (jaw closing) and the digastric (jaw opening), for the reasons discussed in the Introduction. We wished to determine the fashion in which the adult pattern was achieved. We found, contrary to our expectations, that all state-dependent changes in these somatic reflexes reached their adult level *before* the kittens were two months of age. A description of their development is presented in the next section.

THE DEVELOPMENT OF REFLEX ACTIVITY IN KITTENS

Introduction

While investigation of somatic activity goes back to at least 1651, when Harvey described motor activity in the hen embryo (Harvey, 1651), it was not until early in this century that the phenomenon of reflex activity during sleep began to be seriously studied (Pieron, 1913). At that time, since sleep was believed to be a homogeneous state rather than one consisting of two distinct phases, not surprisingly, widely conflicting results were reported. Only in the 1950's, when the two states of sleep were recognized and described, could a rigorous basis be laid for the analysis of somatic reflex activity during sleep in the adult, and, subsequently, in the developing animal.

In analyzing the development of somatic reflex activity, two key issues must be kept in mind. First, there is progressive maturation of the component parts of the reflex arc. Second, regardless of the extent to which the component parts of the reflex arc are developed, there is progressive maturation of the suprasegmental systems which control its excitability. The resultant complex interaction between maturation of the component parts of the reflex arc and maturation of the suprasegmental control of reflex activity must be considered in any investigation of the development of state-dependent somatic reflex processes.

Patterns of reflex activity in young animals which probably underly immature *segmental* structure and physiology are illustrated by the following observations: 1) The structure of primary sensory terminals is different in the young animal from that in the adult (Skoglund, 1960). 2) There is no post-tetanic potentiation of spinal monosynaptic reflexes in kittens (Skoglund, 1960c; Eccles and Willis, 1965). 3) The pattern of response to exteroceptive stimuli is different in the young animal than in the adult (Langworthy, 1924; Pollock and Davis, 1931; Skoglund, 1960b). (In neonates there are mass reflexes, bilateral flexion with extensor thrusts, etc.) 4) Flexor tone predominates in the newborn animal whereas extensor tone is dominant in the adult (Schulte and Schwenzel, 1965; Skoglund, 1966). There are many other examples of differences in somatic reflex activity between newborn animals and adults which appear primarily dependent upon immaturity of the reflex arc (Vlach, 1968; Chase, 1972b).

However, in the newborn it is also probable that the pattern of reflex response differs from that of adult cats not only because the component parts of reflexes are immature, but because they exist in an "immature" organism, (in the present context an animal in which the descending *suprasegmental* influences on somatic reflex activity are immature, i.e., different than that in the adult). Patterns of reflex response may therefore be immature even though the component parts of the reflex arc are no different than those of the adult. The Babinski response is an example of an activity pattern occurring in the neonate which disappears during the process of development. It reappears in the adult when the central nervous system is damaged and the normal pattern of descending suprasegmental influences is disrupted. Similarly, grasp and sucking reflexes reappear in the adult after forebrain damage, indicating that suprasegmental rather than segmental processes are critical to developmental changes in these reflex patterns (Bieber, 1940; Ausubel, 1966).

When we add to the complex developmental interaction of segmental and suprasegmental influences the development of the systems which promote and maintain sleep and wakefulness, we arrive at a proliferation of possible explanations for state- and development-dependent variations in muscle contraction following afferent stimulation, i.e., reflex responsiveness. Perhaps the most predictable finding in our developmental study was that state-dependent reflex modulation in the maturing kitten was dynamically changing and complex, with no evidence that somatic reflexes reach their adult configuration via a smooth transition along a straight line extending from an immature to a mature pattern. In fact, during the postnatal period, patterns of reflex response were diametrically opposed to those observed in the adult. In order to reach the adult pattern, the state-dependent configurations in the neonate had to reverse their field and, in doing so, complex interactions emerged.

Methods

A total of 18 kittens, studied at ages ranging from 1 to 8 weeks, were utilized to examine the development of state-dependent variations in the amplitude of the masseteric and digastric reflexes. Each kitten was initially anesthetized and prepared for recording in the freely moving condition according to procedures described in the previous section. In addition to the standard array of electrodes used to record EEG, EOG, and EMG activity, electrodes were implanted to induce and record the masseteric and digastric reflexes (Fig. 1). In order to place a bipolar stimulating electrode in the mesencephalic nucleus of the 5th nerve, the kittens were first placed in a modified stereotaxic instrument. The location of the mesencephalic nucleus was determined by approximating adult coordinates and inducing the reflex during the period of implantation. The reflex was recorded by bipolar wire loop electrodes sutured into the parenchyma of the masseter musculature. The digastric reflex was induced by stimulation of the inferior dental nerve with a pair of stainless steel screws placed in the mandibular canal. The reflex was recorded by bipolar wire loop electrodes sutured into the parenchyma of the anterior belly of the digastric muscle.

After recovery from these procedures, the animals were placed, as in the previous experiment, in an environmental recording chamber. For each animal the amplitude of the masseteric and digastric reflexes was analyzed during consecutive sleep cycles on at least four separate days. While the animals were within the recording chamber either the masseteric or digastric reflex was evoked repeatedly at rates ranging from 0.5 to 1.0 per second. For each reflex, a level of excitation was employed which was adequate to maintain a response during all states of sleep and wakefulness, but was not sufficient to yield a supramaximal response during any state. The response was monitored oscilloscopically and recorded on an ink-writing polygraph along with the EEG, EOG, and EMG. It was possible to record the reflex polygraphically by employing a window circuit to isolate the response from the artifact and other movement phenomena and a peak-reading, time-expanding circuit to prolong the response (allowing the polygraphic pen to be deflected to an extent comparable to the reflex amplitude). For this and the following experiments, a histologic verification of the site of the stimulating and recording electrodes within the brain parenchyma was carried out.

Although state-dependent physiological processes in kittens 1 to 4 weeks of age are different than those observed in the adult, it was possible to differentiate states of wakefulness, quiet sleep, and active sleep (Figs. 5, 6, 7). Wakefulness was typified by periods when the animals were moving about or attending to the environment, while active sleep was evidenced by the absence of muscle tone, rapid eye movements, and muscular twitches. The most

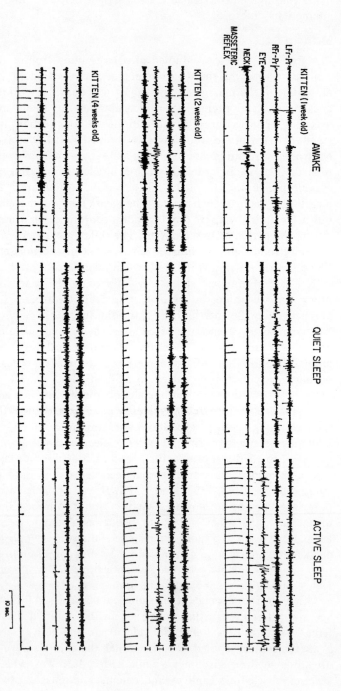

Fig. 5. Masseteric reflex modulation in the one, two and four-week old kitten. This reflex was of greatest amplitude during active sleep in the one and two-week old kittens. By four weeks of age the mean amplitude of the reflex was largest during the awake state and smallest during active sleep. Note the lack of clearly differentiable state-dependent EEG pattern in the one-week old kitten. Stimulation parameters: Masseteric reflex—3 V, 0.5/sec. Calibration: EEG,EOG, EMG, 50 μV; Reflex, 500 μV.For this and subsequent figures the following abbreviations for the cortical recording sites were employed: LFr-Pr, left frontal to left parietal; RFr-Pr, right frontal to right parietal; Trans-Fr, transfrontal. (From Chase (1971).)

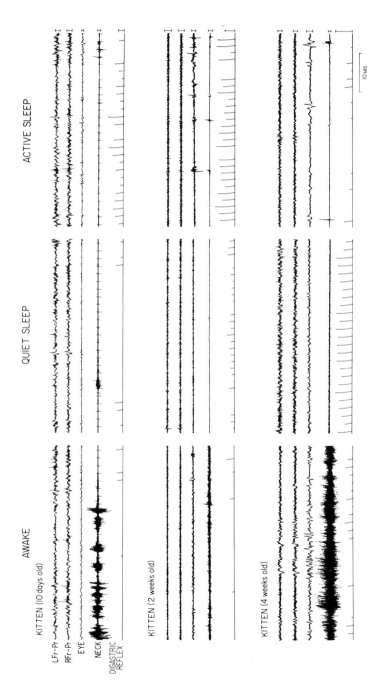

Fig. 6. Digastric reflex modulation in the ten-day, two-and four-week old kitten. The mean amplitude of both waves of the digastric reflex fluctuated in parallel during sleep and wakefulness. The records shown in this figure represent the amplitude of the initial component of the reflex response which was reduced in all age groups during the awake state compared with quiet sleep. In the ten-day and two-week old kittens it was largest during active sleep, whereas it was greatest during quiet sleep in the four-week old animal. By three to four weeks of age the adult pattern of modulation was present. Stimulation parameters: Digastric reflex—6 V, 0.75 msec (10 days); 5 V, 1 msec (2 weeks); 2 V, 0.5 msec (4 weeks); 0.5/sec. Calibration: EEG, EOG, EMG, 50μV; Reflex, 500μV. (From Chase (1971).)

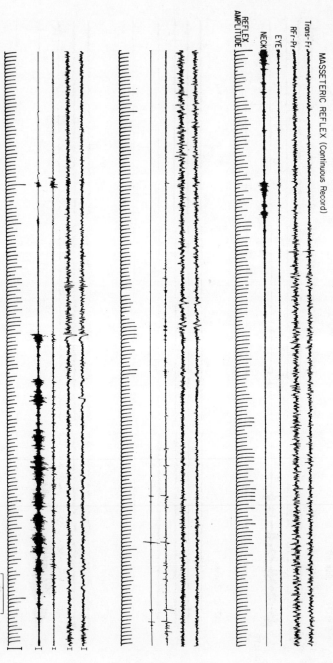

Fig. 7. At approximately three weeks of age the masseteric reflex exhibited only minor variations in amplitude as the animal changed state. Apparently at this point in development those factors which lead to progressively greater responses during the awake state are equal to those processes which tend to suppress activity during active sleep. This pattern is observed for only a very short time, usually less than a few days. Stimulation parameters: Masseteric reflex—4 V, 0.5 msec, Calibration: EEG, EOG, EMG, 50 μV; Reflex, 1 mV. (From Chase (1971).)

difficult state determination to make was quiet sleep. As reported previously, the EEG is not a good indicator (Jouvet-Mounier et al., 1970). Moreover, muscle tone during quiet sleep is diminished to almost the same extent as that of active sleep. Because of the lack of positive indicators we were forced to designate as quiet sleep those periods when the animal was neither awake nor in active sleep; of course, we utilized EOG, EMG and postural criteria as well in making all state determinations. Generally, there was little difficulty in differentiating between these basic states. (We did not include an analysis of the drowsy state since it was not possible to differentiate it from the alert or quiet sleep states.)

Results

Kittens Less Than Three Weeks of Age

In kittens less than 3 weeks of age, the masseteric and digastric reflexes followed similar response patterns. During wakefulness both reflexes were smaller than during quiet sleep, while during quiet sleep both reflexes were smaller than during active sleep (Figs. 5, 6). Thus, the pattern of response was one of increasing amplitude as the animal passed from wakefulness through quiet sleep into active sleep. During the brief periods of arousal which accompanied wakefulness, both reflexes were further suppressed. A similar reduction in amplitude occurred during active sleep in conjunction with rapid ocular movements or muscular twitches.

Kittens Three Weeks of Age

In kittens about 3 weeks old, both reflexes exhibited state-dependent responses whose amplitudes were between those of the immature and adult animal (Figs. 5, 6, 8). There was a relative decrease in the amplitude of the masseteric reflex during active sleep and an increase during the alert state. If one pictures a balance beam with quiet sleep as the fulcrum, and at one end the alert state, and at the other the active sleep state, then sometime around the third week of life the amplitude of the reflex during the alert and active sleep states shift and the beam becomes horizontal. This led to a curious phenomenon, that is, no change in reflex amplitude was observed as the animal passed from the alert state to active sleep (Figs. 7, 8). Although this critical period lasts for only a few days, it is quite dramatic when observed.

At about 3 weeks of age the amplitude of the digastric reflex has almost reached its adult values (Figs. 6, 8). As in younger kittens, it is suppressed during the alert state when compared with quiet sleep. There is a slight increase or no change in amplitude when quiet sleep is compared with active sleep. If the animal is relatively mature at this age, then a decrease in amplitude is observed when the active sleep state is compared with either quiet sleep or the alert state. This adult pattern appears to occur slightly earlier for the digastric than for the masseteric reflex.

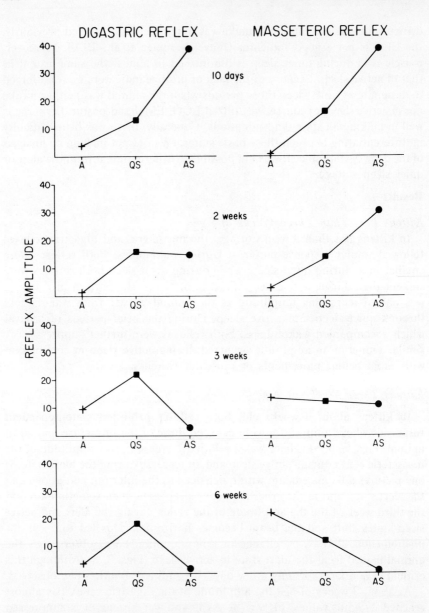

Fig.8.The mean amplitudes of 100 consecutively induced reflex responses (evoked at the rate of 0.5/sec) are plotted in this figure on an arbitrary but relative scale for each animal in each age group. The adult pattern for the digastric reflex appeared to be achieved by a gradual reduction in amplitude during active sleep and an increase during quiet sleep. As the kitten grew older this reflex remained relatively reduced during the awake state. The pattern of masseteric reflex activity during wakefulness and active sleep in the first two postnatal weeks was the opposite from that which occurred at four weeks of age, when the responses were similar to those repoted in the mature cat. (From Chase (1971).)

Kittens Older Than Three Weeks of Age

The state-dependent amplitude variations for both the masseteric and digastric reflexes reach their adult configuration in kittens older than 3 weeks (Figs. 5, 6, 8), although the specific age varies from kitten to kitten. Occasionally, in a relatively immature kitten, the adult pattern will not be reached until four or five weeks of age. However, it was our observation that most kittens older than three weeks exhibited a similar pattern of reflex modulation during sleep and wakefulness to that observed in the adult. For the masseteric reflex, this pattern was one of decreasing amplitude as the animal progressed from the alert state through quiet sleep and into active sleep (Figs. 5, 8). For the digastric reflex, the amplitude increased in the progression from the alert state to quiet sleep, then decreased during active sleep even below the level observed during the alert state (Figs. 6, 8). The characteristics of the adult pattern of reflex response during periods of sleep and wakefulness will be discussed in detail in the following section.

In summary, during wakefulness in the immature animal, the masseteric and digastric reflexes exhibited their smallest amplitude. During quiet sleep the amplitude of both reflexes increased. During active sleep there was a further increase in amplitude.

Discussion

A discussion of the development of somatic reflexes might take many directions. In previous articles, for example, I have described the modulation of state-dependent reflex activity in the immature organism as it reflects immaturity of the reflex arc and/or immaturity of descending suprasegmental influences (Chase, 1970, 1971, 1972b). The relationship between the development of sleep and waking patterns and the development of somatic reflex activity has also been discussed (Chase, 1972b). One observation in the present study not previously examined is that during the waking state in the immature animal, when muscle tone is greatest, there was suppression of both the masseteric and digastric reflexes. On the other hand, during active sleep, when muscle tone is suppressed, both reflexes were at their highest amplitude. This anomalous situation of increased reflex activity in conjunction with decreased tone (during active sleep) and increased tone in conjunction with decreased reflex activity (during wakefulness) does not occur in the adult (Giaquinto et al., 1963; Baldissera, et al., 1964; Gassel et al., 1964; Pompeiano, 1967b; Chase et al, 1968; Chase, 1970) and reflects an entirely unexpected organization of the somatomotor system.

We also observed in our youngest animals, as contrasted with adult cats, that the neck musculature was suppressed during quiet as well as active sleep. In addition, the reflexes were suppressed during quiet sleep, as they were during awake behavior. Thus, tone was reduced during quiet sleep and active sleep and during active sleep the reflexes exhibited their largest amplitude responses.

It is evident that reflex amplitude can be large or small even without a comparable change in the activity of the somatic musculature and it is therefore probable that the factors which regulate somatic reflex activity and muscle tone are different and not necessarily related. There is evidence that even in the adult animal the level of reflex excitability may not bear a strict relationship to the level of tonic EMG activity, for it has been demonstrated that, in certain cases, a decrease in motor neuron discharge may take place in conjunction with an increase in a somatic reflex response (Henatsch and Schulte, 1958). Indeed, in our own studies of the masseteric reflex in the adult, during wakefulness we observed that periods of heightened arousal occasionally occurred together with a brief decrease in reflex activity. This was true in spite of an increase in the tonic neck activity and level of arousal. Possible bases for atonia of somatic musculature in conjunction with heightened reflex responsiveness in the kitten were discussed in previous papers (Chase, 1971, 1972b).

> One often hears that ontogenetic research is carried out in order to study a system in its simplest form, the assumption being that knowledge of a presumably "simple" system will clarify many of the more complex interactions present in the adult. If, however, one examines the development of a relatively simple physiologic process, such as the mono- or polysynaptic reflex, these beliefs are quickly shattered. The modulation of a "simple" reflex in the developing animal is anything but "simple". On the contrary, our studies have revealed a complex pattern, which probably reflects a balance of influence between the development of the anatomical and physiological components of the segmental reflex and the anatomical and physiological processes of supersegmental origin. The fact is that a more complex system exists in immature animals than in adults, for in adults there is no change over time in the various factors which influence the final muscle twitch which we record as the reflex response. Therefore, it seems, that in order to understand more fully the development of somatic activity, we must turn to an analysis of reflex modulation in the adult.

REFLEX ACTIVITY IN THE ADULT CAT

Introduction

One can have a scientific field day developing hypotheses to explain the complex development of somatic reflex activity in the maturing kitten. One can invoke wonderfully complex combinations of inhibition or disinhibition and facilitation or defacilitation, either presynaptic or postsynaptic, of segmental or extrasegmental origin, to explain any specific reflex response. However, there is no basis at the present time for any substantive hypotheses to account for the modulation of somatic reflex activity in the developing animal. Luckily, in the adult, there is no such problem. Studies of mechanisms underlying the modulation of spinal cord somatic reflex activity during sleep and wakefulness have been successfully carried out and the rather clear-cut story of a descending pattern of activity of brainstem origin has emerged which describes the pre- and postsynaptic processes governing state-dependent changes in reflex amplitude (Pompeiano, 1967a,b).

There is a gradual suppression of spinal cord somatic reflex activity as adult cats progress from wakefulness to quiet sleep to active sleep (Pompeiano, 1967a,b). During quiet sleep the depression is primarily due to decreased excitability of gamma motor neurons. During active sleep there is a further reduction of gamma motor neuron excitability as well as postsynaptic inhibition of alpha motor neurons. During the active sleep state there are phasic periods of inhibition accompanied by phasic periods of facilitation. The phasic inhibitory phenomena are probably presynaptic. Facilitation is most likely postsynaptic—working directly upon the alpha motor neurons and overcoming for brief periods the ongoing period of pre- and postsynaptic inhibition. Since there are no a priori reasons to assume that the origin of modulation of brainstem somatic reflex activity is any different from that previously described for spinal cord somatic reflexes, we assume that the mechanisms are similar. A further assumption, made on shakier ground, is that any variation in brainstem reflex activity which is different from that already described for the spinal cord reflects a difference in the structure and function of the brainstem reflex itself rather than in the mechanisms responsible for its modulation. In order to gain an appreciation for the extrasegmental factors which govern the modulation of brain-stem somatic reflexes, we studied their variation in activity during sleep and waking states in adult cats. (Chase et al, 1968; Chase, 1970, in press.).

Methods

Adult cats were used in these experiments (Chase et al, 1968; Chase, 1970; Chase and McGinty, 1970b). Procedures for inducing and recording the masseteric and digastric reflexes were identical to those previously described for investigating spontaneous variations in reflex activity in the kitten (see preceding section).

Results

The Masseteric Reflex

A description of masseteric reflex variability during sleep and wakefulness is straightforward and can be stated without qualifications. The mean amplitude of the masseteric reflex was largest during wakefulness (Fig. 9). The mean amplitude decreased during quiet sleep, while during active sleep it was minimal (Fig. 9). During wakefulness and active sleep futher variations in reflex amplitude occurred in conjunction with variability in the level of arousal. During wakefulness, in conjunction with ocular activity or increased somatic movement, the reflex amplitude increased. During the rapid eye movements of active sleep the reflex amplitude decreased with respect to control conditions—periods of adjacent active sleep lacking eye movements.

The data presented in Figure 9 are results of a statistical analysis of the amplitude of the masseteric reflex during four states utilizing planned comparison tests based upon an analysis of variance. Each change in state, (that is waking compared with drowsiness, drowsiness with quiet sleep, and quiet sleep with active sleep) was marked by a statistically significant reduction in the amplitude of the reflex response (p less than 0.05).

In a related experiment we stimulated the mesencephalic nucleus at levels slightly below those sufficient to maintain a response during all states of sleep and wakefulness. The lack of a response to excitation of the mesencephalic nucleus is shown in Figure 10. In this analysis we did not observe state-dependent variations in activity during short episodes of a given state. However, the gradual reduction in reflex amplitude reported previously was mirrored by an increase in the *lack* of response as the animal passed from the alert state to quiet sleep to active sleep (Fig. 10). Thus, the reflex occurred

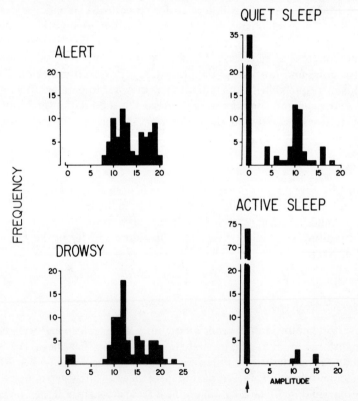

Fig. 9. Adult cat: Frequency histograms of the amplitudes of 80 consecutive masseteric reflex responses. These potentials were obtained during the alert, drowsy, quiet sleep, and active sleep states. The amplitude of the motor responses are plotted on an arbitrary scale as a function of the frequency of their occurrence. High amplitude potentials are reduced and then almost totally abolished as the animal progresses from wakefulness, through drowsiness and quiet sleep, into active sleep. (From Chase et al. (1968).)

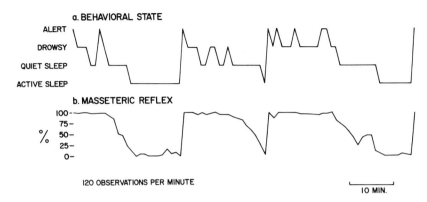

Fig. 10. This figure illustrates the % occurrence of the masseteric reflex (B) during consecutive sleep cycles (A). In this analysis the reflex responses were counted as either present or absent. Note the gradual decrease in the % response during the periods of quiet sleep preceding active sleep. (From Chase et al. (1968).)

always during the alert state, less frequently during quiet sleep and least frequently during active sleep.

The Digastric Reflex

The amplitude variations of the digastric reflex during sleep and wakefulness were as consistent as those reported above for the masseteric reflex (Fig.11), although the direction of response during the various states was different. During wakefulness the reflex was smaller than during quiet sleep, and during active sleep the reflex was smaller than during wakefulness (Fig.11). Thus, in a progression from wakefulness to quiet sleep to active sleep, the reflex first increased in amplitude and then decreased below the level observed during wakefulness (Fig.11).

The response was further suppressed during wakefulness and active sleep as the degree of arousal increased. Thus, during wakefulness, in conjunction with rapid eye movements and/or general behavioral arousal, the reflex decreased below the mean level for this state. During active sleep in conjunction with rapid eye movements, the reflex decreased below the level observed during those periods of active sleep which lacked rapid eye movements or muscular twitches.

Discussion

As previously noted, many studies have demonstrated a consistent pattern for modulation of spinal cord somatic reflexes, namely, a gradual reduction in reflex amplitude as the animal passes from wakefulness to quiet sleep to active sleep (Pompeiano, 1967a,b). A similar pattern was observed for the modulation of the masseteric reflex. However, an entirely different pattern was found for the digastric reflex, which increased in amplitude during quiet

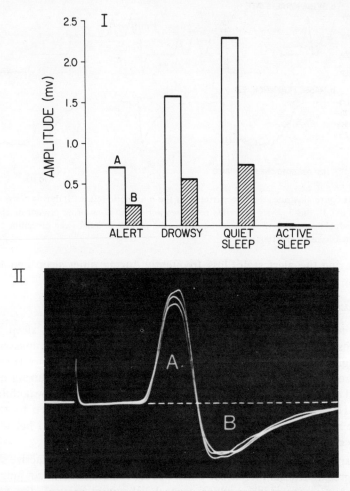

Fig. 11. Digastric reflex responses during states of sleep and wakefulness. Adult cat: Mean amplitude of 50 consecutive responses. Each wave of the reflex (II: A, B) was measured separately as the extent of its excursion from the base-line level (II: dotted line). As the animal changed state the amplitude of both waves varied in a parallel fashion (I: A, B). An increase in amplitude occurred when the drowsy state was compared with the alert state and when quiet sleep was compared with the drowsy state. During active sleep the reflex response decreased below the level obtained during the quiet alert state. Inferior dental nerve: 1.5 V, 0.1 msec, 1/sec. Calibration (II): 200μV, 2 msec. (From Chase (1970).)

sleep and then exhibited a reduction in amplitude during active sleep to a level below that observed during wakefulness. This state-dependent modulation of digastric reflex activity appears to be unique, and it is hoped that a comparison of its structure and function with that of other reflexes may provide relevant data as to the basis for its paradoxical pattern of activity.

It requires little explanation to account for the increased reactivity of masseteric and spinal cord reflexes during wakefulness, since there are antigravity and postural functions which must be maintained during this state. During quiet sleep, evidently because there is no need for such a high degree of motor activity, one observes a decrease in tone and reflex responsiveness. A further reduction in muscle tone and reflex amplitude occurs during active sleep. If we assume that the maintenance of the active sleep state is important, then the functional significance of profound motor inhibition is obvious. Without such inhibition, the facilitatory motor discharges (evidenced by muscular twitches), as well as the intense activity found in almost every part of the brain, would surely arouse the animal, thus disrupting the ongoing active sleep state. Of course, we leave unmentioned the functional basis for motor facilitation during active sleep, which is unknown.

Explaining the paradoxical pattern of digastric reflex activity is more complicated. Since this reflex is not involved in either postural or antigravity mechanisms, it is probable that its function emerges during quiet sleep when its amplitude is greatest. What possible reason might there be for an increase in the reactivity of this reflex during quiet sleep? To answer this question we must first ask, "What are the 'stimuli' adequate to initiate this reflex?" Various investigators have suggested that this reflex; a) transmits nociceptive or touch sensation (Pfaffman, 1939; Hugelin, 1955; Dumont, 1964); b) is involved in proprioceptive functions (Pfaffman, 1939; Hoffman and Tonnies, 1948); c) plays a role in mastication (Sherrington, 1917); and d) influences the digestion of food (Wyrwicka and Chase, 1969). While it is certainly possible that this reflex plays a part in the preceding activities, studies indicating its involvement in respiratory processes (Cardot et al, 1923; Pinotti and Granata, 1953) may be more relevant to the discussion of its function during all states, especially that of quiet sleep. It is important during quiet sleep for the mouth to be maintained in a open position or that it be able to open easily for purposes of providing uninterrupted respiration. One commonly observes in animals that a lowering of the mandible accompanies the quiet sleep state. One explanation for the increased reactivity of this musculature and the reflex which initiates its contraction is the need for an alternative airway to the nasal passage which would come into play without the need for the animal to become aroused. During quiet sleep, if other respiratory reflexes exhibit similar increased responsivity, this hypothesis would tend to be supported. During active sleep, when there is nonreciprocal inhibition of both the masseteric and digastric reflexes, atonia of the lower jaw musculature is probably sufficient to allow the mouth to open in accord with the demands of gravity.

It is also possible that primary digastric reflex functions are not specifically related to its reactivity during quiet sleep. Perhaps its response is strictly dependent on the *structural* features of its muscle and is not related to any functional goal. In support of this hypothesis, it should be noted that the anterior belly of the digastric muscle is unlike the trunk, limb, and masseteric musculature in that it lacks muscle spindles (Hosokawa, 1961; Smith and Marcarian, 1967). The absence of spindles precludes the presence of gamma motor neurons, whose modulation we know is responsible for variations in the amplitude of reflexes during sleep and wakefulness (Pompeiano, 1967a,b). At the level of the spinal cord, it is inhibition of gamma discharge which promotes the reflex inhibition observed during this state (Gassel and Pompeiano, 1965). The maintenance of the level of the digastric reflex during quiet sleep may, in this interpretation, be due to the lack of inhibition of gamma efferents, since they are not present in the reflex arc. Following this reasoning, one might be led to conclude that the baseline state of the digastric reflex occurs during quiet sleep. During the alert and active sleep states there may be inhibitory processes which are responsible for the decrease in activity. Since there is nonreciprocal inhibition of all somatic reflexes in active sleep and inhibition only of the digastric reflex during wakefulness, we might as easily draw the conclusion that the function of the digastric reflex is expressed during wakefulness or active sleep rather than during quiet sleep.

At present, our investigations have not explored the functional significance of masseteric and digastric reflex modulation. Rather, we have concentrated on analyzing the neural systems responsible for their variations in activity during sleep and wakefulness, which will be described in the following sections.

VAGAL CONTROL OF EEG AND REFLEX ACTIVITY

Introduction

A number of studies have demonstrated that central vagal excitation is capable not only of modifying central neural activity but also of producing an array of behaviors as different as sleep and sham rage (Kaada, 1951; Baccelli et al., 1963; Penaloza-Rojas, 1964; Guazzi et al., 1968). Since EEG patterns are correlated with ongoing behavior and since ongoing behavior is related to motor processes, we examined the influence of vagal afferent activity upon a fundamental component of motor behavior, the somatic reflex.

The study of the influence of afferent vagal stimulation upon brainstem somatic reflex activity arose initially from our investigations of vagal modulation of EEG activity (Chase et al., 1966; Chase and Nakamura, 1968). We had observed that EEG synchronization and desynchronization could be induced by stimulation of the cut central end of the cervical vagus nerve. The differentiating factor in the EEG pattern of response was related to the excitation of specific afferents within the vagus nerve. We determined that the large diameter fiber groups with rapid conduction velocities (20 meters per second or faster) were associated with EEG synchronization, while the smaller diameter fiber groups with slow conduction times (10 to 15 meters per second) were correlated with EEG desynchronization. We concluded that the afferent cervical vagal fiber system was comprised of specific groups which could initiate and maintain either a synchronized or desynchronized EEG pattern. We postulated that these fiber groups were both functionally and structurally discrete (Chase and Nakamura, 1968b). A brief description of these findings is presented in this section.

Methods

Our studies of the influence of vagal afferent excitation upon electro-encephalographic and reflex activity were carried out in immobilized adult cats (Chase and Nakamura, 1968a,b; Chase et al., 1970 a,b). The following surgical procedures were performed under ether anesthesia: a) transection of the spinal cord at C1: b) bilateral transection of the vagal and sympathetic trunks at a low cervical level; c) isolation and separation of the right or left cervical vagus nerve from the surrounding fasciae and sympathetic trunk; d) isolation and transection of the right masseteric nerve and the right mylohyoid nerve (i.e., the digastric branch to the anterior belly of the digastric muscle). Stimulating electrodes included: a)a bipolar electrode placed in the mesencephalic nucleus of the fifth nerve (for the induction of the masseteric reflex); b) bipolar screw electrodes placed in the mandibular canal (to induce the digastric reflex); and c) bipolar stimulating electrodes placed upon the cut central end of the cervical vagus nerve.

Recording electrodes were placed around the masseteric, mylohyoid and vagus nerves. Screw electrodes were placed in the calvarium to record EEG

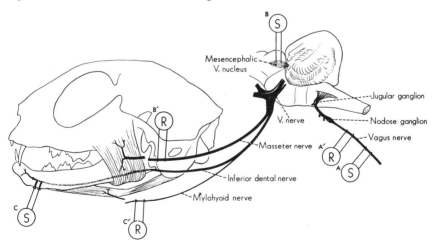

Fig. 12. Stimulation and recording paradigm for vagal-reflex studies. The masseteric reflex was induced by delivering an electrical stimulus to the mesencephalic trigeminal nucleus (B) and was monitored along the cut central end of the ipsilateral masseter nerve (B´). The digastric reflex was induced by stimulation of the inferior dental nerve (C) and was recorded along the cut central end of the ipsilateral mylohyoid (digastric) nerve (C´). A recording electrode was placed on the cervical vagus nerve (A´) approximately 5 cm central to the stimulating electrode (A) in order to monitor the induced afferent vagal activity. (From Chase et al. (1970a).

activity. The general pattern of stimulation and recording is shown diagramatically in Figure 12. (The cortical recording electrodes are not shown.) After all surgical procedures were completed, anesthesia was discontinued and gallamine triethiodide (Flaxedil) was administered. The animals were subsequently maintained by artificial respiration. This experimental arrangement allowed us to test the influence of afferent vagal fiber activity upon the masseteric reflex, the digastric reflex, and EEG activity. By placing a recording electrode on the vagus nerve between the point of stimulation and the brain, we were able to correlate the excitation of specific fiber groups within the vagus nerve with corresponding changes in reflex and EEG activity.

Results

Cortical and Subcortical Patterns of Response

Electrical stimulation of the cut central end of the cervical vagus nerve induced patterns of synchronization and desynchronization in cortical and

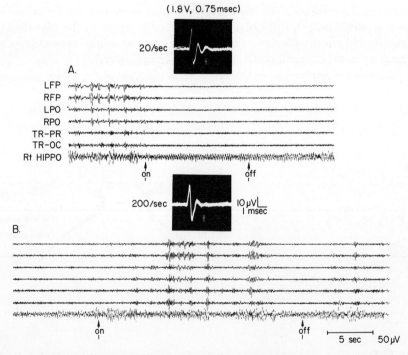

Fig. 13. Central vagal stimulation. Neurographic, EEG, and hippocampal responses to high and low frequencies of vagal stimulation demonstrate the relationship between EEG desynchronization and the neurographic potential indicated by the arrow in A, and EEG synchronization (B) which was correlated with the absence of this slow potential. (Neurographic records: superimposed traces; bipolar recording; left vagus.) Distance between stimulating and recording electrodes, 4.2 cm. (From Chase et al. (1967).)

subcortical structures (Fig. 13). The direction of response was found to be dependent upon the parameters of stimulation. High frequency, low voltage stimulation induced synchronization in the frontal and parietal areas of the cerebral cortex (Fig. 13). High amplitude slow waves were also observed in the central medianum, central lateralis, medialis dorsalis, ventralis posterior lateralis, and the lateral geniculate. The hippocampal response was one of high frequency discharge superimposed upon a background of intermittent high voltage spikes—a pattern normally seen in conjunction with cortical and subcortical patterns of synchronization (Fig. 13).

High voltage, high frequency stimulation resulted in cortical and thalamic patterns of low voltage fast activity, i.e., desynchronization. The hippocampal pattern showed pronounced theta activity (Fig. 13), while the cortical, thalamic, and hippocampal responses were those normally observed in conjunction with behavioral arousal.

Fiber groups excited by high frequency, low voltage stimulation were the ones with a conduction velocity greater than 20 meters per second (Fig. 13). High voltage, high frequency stimulation induced activity in fibers conducting at rates of less than 15 meters per second (Fig. 13).

Brainstem Somatic Reflex Modulation

Two analyses were performed on the response of the masseteric and digastric reflexes to afferent vagal stimulation. One analysis consisted of single pulse or pulse train stimulation of the vagus nerve in conjunction with the induction of the reflex at various conditioning-test latencies. The other was the repetitive induction of the masseteric reflex during high frequency vagal stimulation.

Single pulse or pulse train vagal stimulation led to a complex pattern of reflex response (Chase et al., 1910a). The masseteric reflex was facilitated when the conditioning-test latency was between 2 and 5 milliseconds. This period was followed by reflex suppression when the latency was between 10 and 35 milliseconds (Fig. 14). At conditioning-test latencies greater than 35 milliseconds, a relatively long period of facilitation occurred. The digastric reflex response was facilitated at short conditioning latencies (less than 5 milliseconds), but from approximately 10 to 100 milliseconds only suppression was observed.

Repetitive stimulation of the cut central end of the vagus nerve, in conjunction with the continuous induction of either test reflex at the rate of 1 per second, led to a consistent response pattern in which the digastric reflex was suppressed and the masseteric reflex was facilitated (Chase and Nakamura, 1968a; Chase et al., 1970a,b). All these responses were dependent upon the excitation of a single group of afferent vagal fibers whose conduction velocity was between 10 and 15 meters per second (Chase et al., 1970b). When fiber groups conducting at greater velocities were excited, no response was observed.

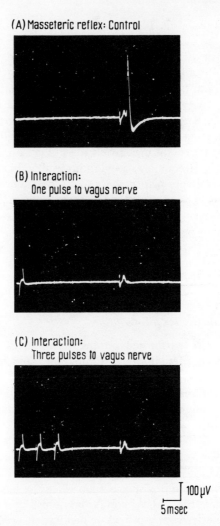

Fig. 14. Inhibition of the masseteric monosynaptic reflex by afferent vagal stimulation. In (A) the control reflex was elicited by stimulation of the mesencephalic nucleus of the fifth nerve. The reflex is completely abolished when preceded by either single (B) or multiple (C) vagal pulses. The antidromic potential persists unchanged. (3 superimposed traces—Mesen nuc. fifth: 4 V, 0.2 msec, 1/sec - Vagus: 10 V, 1 msec.) (From Chase and Nakamura (1968a).)

Discussion

In the previous section we reported that the masseteric reflex increased in amplitude during wakefulness as compared with quiet sleep, while the digastric reflex was found to be suppressed. A similar pattern of reciprocal response was induced by repetitive stimulation of an afferent vagal fiber group conducting between 10 and 15 meters per second. In previous studies we had found evidence that this fiber group has a thoracic origin and can induce cortical and subcortical desynchronization together with hippocampal theta activity, patterns normally seen in conjunction with behavioral arousal (Chase et al., 1967). Thus, activity in fibers of thoracic origin appears to be capable not only of modulating somatic reflex activity in a manner consistent with that observed in freely moving animals during wakefulness, but also of maintaining cortical and subcortical EEG patterns which normally occur during this state.

We did not observe the induction of vagal excitation of somatic reflex patterns typically seen during quiet sleep. Possibly this was due to the fact that our experiments were carried out with immobilized preparations which, by their very nature, are not prone to sleep. Also, repetitive vagal stimulation was maintained for only 10 to 30 seconds, probably an insufficient time to observe the motor suppression normally seen during EEG synchronization, since it is only in the more developed stages of quiet sleep that profound reflex depression occurs (Fig. 10).

It is evident that widespread changes in central neural and motor processes may result from vagal afferent discharge. Cortical, subcortical, and motor activity initiated by vagal input show a consistent pattern, one closely related in many aspects to that typically observed spontaneously during wakefulness and quiet sleep. The potential for the induction of these states clearly resides within fibers carrying impulses from visceral receptors. Stated another way, the changes in reflex amplitude and EEG activity induced by repetitive vagal stimulation are qualitatively similar to those variations which occur spontaneously in the freely moving unanesthetized animal during sleep and wakefulness.

Our studies of the vagal system led us to examine the orbital cortex because it is the primary cortical receiving area for vagal projections (Siegfried, 1961; Korn and Richard, 1963; Korn et al., 1966). In the cat, the orbital surface of the the cerebral cortex not only receives sensory information from the vagus nerve, but also from sensory systems including the visual, auditory, somesthetic, olfactory, and gustatory (see Chase and McGinty, 1970b). In turn, the orbital cortex influences a variety of somatic and visceral functions. Integrated processes such as directed attention, rage reactions, conditioned avoidance behavior, etc., are also modified by stimulation or destruction of the orbital cortex (see Chase and McGinty, 1970b). In addition to these sensory, motor, and integrative activities, repetitive stimulation of the orbital cortex has been shown to induce masticatory activity utilizing the musculature of the masseteric and digastric reflexes (Babkin and Van Buren, 1951; Hess et al., 1952). Therefore our studies of vagal modulation of central neural processes complement the following investigation of the modulation of brainstem reflexes exerted by the rostral projection area for vagal afferents, the orbital cortex.

CORTICAL CONTROL OF REFLEX ACTIVITY

Introduction

In the early years of sleep research almost all spontaneous changes in physiologic processes occurring as functions of sleep and wakefulness were examined extensively (Jouvet, 1970). The artificial excitation of the central nervous system in conjunction with an analysis of induced variations in physiologic activity has been examined in less detail (Jouvet, 1970) and only a few studies have been published which relate the effects of stimulation during sleep and wakefulness to peripheral motor responses (Tarchanoff, 1894; Hodes and Suzuki, 1965; Baldissera et al., 1966; Iwama and Kawamota, 1966). All these studies have dealt either with cortically or subcortically induced patterns of motor *excitation* even though an equally important function of corticofugal motor activity is *inhibition*. Indeed, there is a vast body of literature which postulates that the primary function of the cerebral cortex is related to the maintenance of inhibitory mechanisms in general and motor inhibition in particular (Sherrington, 1898; Preston and Whitlock, 1960, 1961; Lundberg and Voorhoeve, 1962; Agnew et al., 1963; Agnew and Preston, 1965; Hongo and Jankowska, 1967; Chase et al., in press). In the present study we examined both inhibitory and excitatory processes of cortical origin during sleep and wakefulness (Chase and McGinty, 1970a). We were fortunate to be able to obtain an effective measure of inhibition and excitation in the same preparation following stimulation of a discrete cortical area with a single stimulus. Our measure of motor inhibition was suppression of the masseteric reflex, while our measure of motor excitation was induction of evoked contraction of the digastric muscle.

The anatomical and physiological bases for induced orbital modulation of brain stem somatic reflex activity are based on studies in immobilized animals (Clemente et al., 1966; Nakamura et al., 1967; Sauerland et al., 1967; Wessolosky et al., 1968). Orbital stimulation induces hyperpolarization of masseter motor neurons and depolarization of motor neurons innervating the digastric muscle (Nakamura et al., 1967). An anatomical basis for these hyperpolarizing and depolarizing potentials may be found in the work of Mizuno et al. (1969). In order to relate this information to behavioral studies and to further our understanding of the role of the cortex in sleep and wakefulness, we examined the effectiveness of orbital stimulation in modulating brainstem reflex activity during various behavioral states (Chase and McGinty, 1970a,b). This investigation is outlined in the following section.

Methods

Animals were prepared under anesthesia for the placement of stimulating and recording electrodes. The procedures for the induction and recording of the masseteric and digastric reflexes were the same as those described in previous sections of this chapter. The cortex was stimulated with permanently placed bipolar electrodes resting on the orbital surface between the cerebral parenchyma and the dura mater (i.e., within the subarachnoid space). Additional electrodes were implanted to record the EEG, EOG, and neck EMG.

The reflex responses were displayed on an oscilloscope and an ink-writing polygraph. At the conclusion of the experimental procedures, the animals were dispatched and perfused for subsequent histologic verification of the cortical and mesencephalic electrodes.

Results

Both reflexes were examined during wakefulness at various conditioning-test latencies following single pulse or short pulse train stimulation of the orbital cortex. For the digastric reflex, facilitation followed inhibition, while for the masseteric inhibition followed facilitation (Fig. 15). The

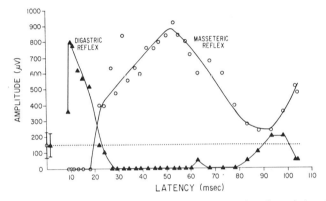

Fig. 15. Time course of modulation of the masseteric and digastric reflexes induced by orbital-cortical stimulation. Single pulse or short pulse-train stimulation of the orbital cortex gave rise to cyclic changes in the activity level of the masseteric and digastric reflexes. The masseteric reflex was initially inhibited, then facilitated, and subsequently passed through a second period of inhibition. During these periods reciprocal changes were induced in the activity level of the digastric reflex. The voltages for elicitation of the masseteric and digastric reflexes were adjusted so that the mean amplitude of the control responses were the same. The initial mean amplitude and the standard deviations are indicated by the dotted line and vertical bars. (Mesen. Vth nuc.: 5 V, 0.15 msec; Inf. Dent. Nuc. 1 V, 0.15 msec; Orbital Stim.: 10 V, 5 msec, 4 pulses, 250 pulses/sec.) Cortical conditioning test response interval was measured from onset of first cortical pulse to onset of the reflex pulse. (From Chase and McGinty (1970b).)

predominant response seemed to be one of masseteric inhibition and digastric facilitation, for an evoked digastric muscle potential was observed following orbital stimulation, while no response was observed in the masseter muscle (Fig. 16). We concentrated subsequent analyses on the orbitally induced response pattern which occurred at a conditioning-test latency of 10 to 20 milliseconds. These responses reflected the direct effect induced by orbital stimulation. Thus, two patterns of motor activity were examined following orbital cortical stimulation during sleep and wakefulness (Fig. 17). One was masseteric reflex inhibition, which occurred at latencies of 10 to 20 milliseconds. The other was a discrete stimulus-induced contraction of the digastric muscle, which arose in this same time period.

A. MASSETERIC MUSCLE   B. DIGASTRIC MUSCLE

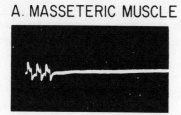
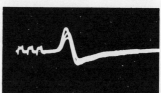

$$\underline{}\overline{\rule{0pt}{1em}}\ 500\mu V$$
5 msec

Fig. 16. Effect of orbital cortical stimulation upon the spontaneous activity of the masseter and digastric muscles. When the voltage of the orbital stimulus was increased above the level required to modify liminally induced masseteric or digastric reflexes, a discrete, stimulus time-locked contraction of the digastric muscle was observed. (Orbital Stim.: 8 V, 1 msec, 3 pulses, 500 pulses/sec.) (From Chase and McGinty (1970b).)

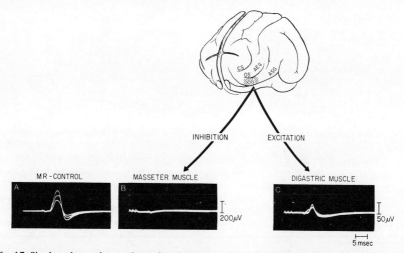

Fig. 17. Single pulse or short pulse-train stimulation of the orbital cortex (cross-hatched area) led to inhibition (B) of the masseteric reflex (MR). The same parameters of cortical stimulation initiated contraction of the digastric muscle (C). These two orbitofugal influences on somatomotor activity, i.e., inhibition of the masseteric reflex and contraction of the digastric muscle, were analyzed during sleep and waking states. Orbital stim.: 7 V, 0.5 msec, 3 pulses, (600 pulses/sec); Mesen. Vth nuc. stim.: 6 V, 0.8 msec. (From Chase and McGinty (1970a).)

Masseteric Reflex Inhibition During Sleep and Wakefulness

As described previously, the masseteric reflex is normally largest during wakefulness, decreasing in amplitude as the animal passes from quiet sleep into active sleep (Fig. 9). During wakefulness orbital cortical stimulation was capable of completely suppressing the masseteric reflex response (Fig. 18). The relative degree of inhibition was reduced during quiet sleep (Fig. 18).

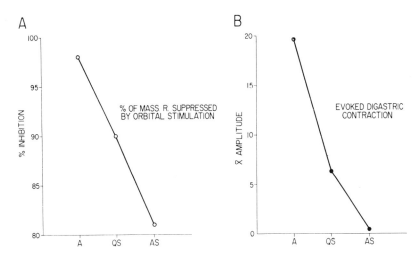

Fig. 18. Both the inhibition of the masseteric reflex (A) and the amplitude of the cortically-evoked digastric response (B) were greatest during the alert state and were least during active sleep. The amplitude of the evoked digastric contraction during sleep and wakefulness was, in general, parallel to the degree of inhibition of the masseteric reflex. The masseteric reflex was evoked at the rate of 1/sec and every fourth reflex elicitation was preceded by cortical stimulation (20 msec latency). The percent inhibition for each state was obtained by dividing the mean amplitude of 30 control reflexes by the amplitude of the intervening 100 reflexes which were preceded by orbital stimulation. The mean amplitude of the digastric response (20 trials) is plotted on an arbitrary, but relative scale. For each state the mean amplitude of 20 stimulation trials was obtained. A = Orbital stim.: 7 V, 0.75 msec, 3 pulses (500 pulses/sec); Mesen. Vth nuc. stim.: 6 V, 0.5 msec. B = Orbital stim.: 7 V, 0.75 msec. (From Chase and McGinty (1970a).)

During active sleep, with the same level and parameters of stimulation as had been employed during waking and quiet sleep episodes, a relatively minor degree of reflex suppression was observed (Fig. 18). Thus, as the animal passed from wakefulness to quiet sleep to active sleep, the degree of inhibition became less pronounced (Fig. 18).

We examined inhibition during sleep and wakefulness, both with fixed parameters of cortical and reflex excitation and with fixed parameters of reflex excitation and variable levels of orbital stimulation. We also examined the effect of orbital cortical inhibition of masseteric reflexes of different amplitudes. In all of these studies the same pattern was observed. Inhibition was most pronounced during wakefulness, decreased during quiet sleep, and became minimal during active sleep.

Evoked Digastric Contraction During Sleep and Wakefulness

The effectiveness of the orbital cortical stimulus in inducing contraction of the digastric muscle was examined during sleep and wakefulness. The amplitude of the evoked response was greatest during wakefulness, decreasing during quiet sleep, and becoming minimal during active sleep

(Fig. 18). Even at the highest levels of orbital stimulation it was difficult to induce contraction during active sleep, whereas only minimal levels of orbital stimulation were required to evoke a potential in the digastric musculature during wakefulness. Thus, a parallel relationship of decreased masseteric reflex inhibition and evoked digastric contraction was found as the cat passed from wakefulness to quiet sleep to active sleep (Fig. 18).

Discussion

Since it was evident that orbital stimulation was most effective in promoting motor inhibition *and* excitation during wakefulness and least effective in promoting these functions during active sleep, we conclude that the orbital cortex is, in a sense, "turned off" during active sleep and "turned on" during wakefulness. We are therefore persuaded that it is during the waking state that the physiological functions of the orbital cortex in motor modulation are expressed.

We should add a cautionary note to the interpretation of these results: it is possible that we have observed not two motor functions of the orbital cortex, but rather one response fluctuating purely as a dependent variable of the other. This possibility must be considered, since the masseter and digastric musculature are antagonistic, and since contraction of the digastric muscle is accompanied by inhibition of the masseter. However, even if one reflex was suppressed or facilitated as a result of induced activity in the complimentary musculature, we are still left with the observation that the orbital cortex is most effective in motor modulation (inhibition, excitation or both) during wakefulness and least effective during active sleep. Our studies in immobilized preparations and the studies of others who have examined intracellular variations in motor activity following orbital stimulation lead us to suspect that both patterns of motor response were induced *pari pasu,* and that each has an independent origin in the orbital cortex.

An extension of these findings leads to the hypothesis that other functions which rely upon corticofugal activity are decreased during the active sleep state and are most prominent during wakefulness. This hypothesis is supported by the fact that no current assessment of the role of the cerebral cortex in sleep implicates it in the *maintenance* of either active sleep or quiet sleep, or in any of the baseline physiological processes which attend these states.

> Our studies of the brainstem somatic reflex were designed so that each study related to the previous investigations and complemented the subsequent ones. By maintaining this systematic experimental approach, we were able to implement a comprehensive program designed to clarify the control of reflex activity during sleep and wakefulness.
>
> In previous sections we have described the development of somatic reflex activity during sleep and wakefulness, its spontaneous baseline variations in the adult and the modulation of this reflex by vagal and orbital cortical excitation. To these investigations we now add our most recent study of the reticular modulation of brainstem reflex activity during sleep and wakefulness.

RETICULAR CONTROL OF REFLEX ACTIVITY

Introduction

The reticular tegmentum of the brainstem has been the central neural system most persistently thought to be responsible for the initiation and maintenance of sleep and wakefulness (Jouvet, 1963; Menini, 1972; Moruzzi, 1972). The lesion experiments which have given rise to this hypothesis have been complemented by biochemical studies (Carli and Zanchetti, 1965; Jouvet, 1971, 1972; Pujol et al., 1971). An overview of the lesion studies indicates that quiet sleep is probably dependent upon the discharge of serotonergic neurons of the raphé complex and that active sleep is due to the activity of catecholaminergic cells of the locus coeruleus (Carli and Zanchetti, 1965; Jouvet, 1972). While these studies complement each other, electrical stimulation of the raphé and locus coeruleus have not been successful in inducing quiet and active sleep, respectively (Kostowski and Giacalone, 1969; Polc and Monnier, 1970; Gumulka et al., 1971; Jouvet, 1972).

It is interesting that this area of the brain, which is now related to sleep functions, has traditionally been considered part of or adjacent to the reticular activating system, which maintains the waking state and leads to a general pattern of motor facilitation (Menini, 1972) rather than sleep and motor inhibition. In an attempt to unravel the complex relationships between the brainstem structures responsible for either the maintenance or initiation of sleep and wakefulness and those which promote state-dependent patterns of physiological activity, we extended our previous studies to investigate the effect of electrical stimulation of the reticular tegmentum upon the masseteric and digastric reflexes during sleep and wakefulness (Chase and Babb, in press; Watanabe and Chase, in press).

Methods

The procedures previously· described for monitoring the masseteric and digastric reflexes in freely moving animals were employed once again in this study. The experimental paradigm was identical to that used in the study of orbital cortical modulation of the masseteric and digastric reflexes. In addition, bipolar strut electrodes were placed in the reticular tegmentum.

The incredible array of fiber tracts and nuclear groups which constitute the reticular tegmentum in the area of the pontomidbrain junction prohibit our designating, at this point in our studies, the responsive reticular area. A comprehensive examination of the effective sites is, however, currently in progress. In general, our electrodes were placed in the reticular tegmentum in the vicinity of the anterior raphé, bordering upon the locus coeruleus.

Results

Masseteric Reflex Response During Sleep and Wakefulness

Reticular stimulation facilitated the masseteric reflex during wakefulness and quiet sleep, and inhibited it during active sleep (Figs. 19, 20). This pattern of activity, induced at a conditioning-test latency of 20 milliseconds, was observed with single pulse or short pulse train stimulation of the reticular tegmentum.

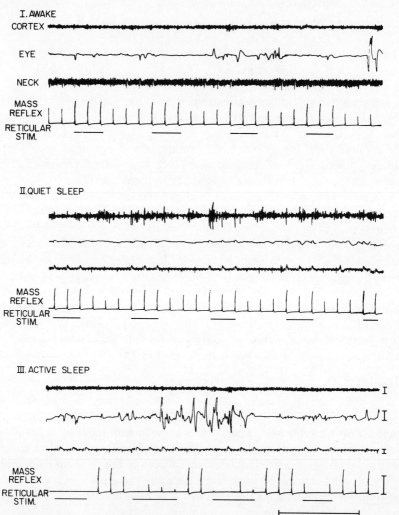

Fig. 19. Polygraph recordings of the amplitude of the masseteric reflex and the activity of the sensorimotor cortex, eyes and neck musculature. The reflex was recorded, on-line, by employing a window circuit to isolate the reflex and a peak-amplitude pulse-lengthening circuit to deflect the polygraphic pen commensurate with the reflex amplitude. Note the consistency of the reticular effects between states and within states, especially during periods of phasic activity such as ocular movements and spindle bursts. Mesen. 5th nuc. I-5 V, 0.5 msec; II-6 V, 0.5 msec; III-7 V, 0.5 msec. Reticular tegmentum: 5 V, 0.9 msec, 3 pulses. Calibration: cortex, eye, neck, 50μV; Reflex, 500μV; Time, 5 sec. (From Chase and Babb (in press).

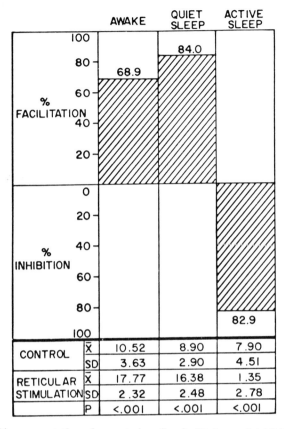

Fig. 20. Graphic representation of masseteric reflex facilitation and inhibition induced by reticular stimulation: statistical evaluation of data (T-test). Each data point is based on an amplitude comparison of 40 control reflexes with 40 reticular-modified reflexes. Amplitude measurements were calculated on an arbitrary but relative scale. All parameters of reflex and reticular stimulation were held constant. Note the normal decrease in spontaneous amplitude (awake—quite-sleep—active sleep) reported previously (Ausubel, 1966). Mesen. 5th Nucl.: 5 V, 0.5 msec. Reticular tegmentum: 4 V, 0.75 msec, 3 pulses. (From Chase and Babb (in press).)

A pattern of reflex facilitation during wakefulness and quiet sleep and inhibition during active sleep was observed in every animal (Figs. 19, 20). The direction of reticular effect remained constant although the degree of inhibition and facilitation depended both upon the amplitude of the control reflex and upon the parameters of reticular stimulation. The effectiveness of reticular stimulation in promoting facilitation or inhibition became greater as the degree of reticular excitation was augmented (by increasing voltage, duration, number of pulses, etc.). When the amplitude of the control masseteric reflex was increased, the degree of reticularly induced reflex modulation was reduced.

The preceding pattern of masseteric reflex response to reticular stimulation was observed throughout the states of sleep and wakefulness. No qualitative variations in response occurred during the rapid eye movements of wakefulness or active sleep or during the spindle activity of quiet sleep.

The level of reticular stimulation sufficient to induce modulation of the masseteric reflex produced, by itself, no behavioral or EEG response during any state. The animals' EEG activity and behavior appeared to be uninfluenced by the intermittent but continuous pattern of reticular excitation.

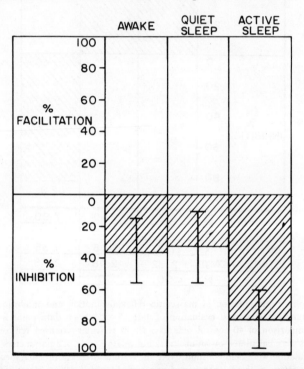

Fig. 21. Graphical representation of digastric reflex inhibition induced by reticular stimulation. Each bar indicates % inhibition. The amplitude of the digastric reflex immediately preceding reticular stimulation was used as the base-line control amplitude. The standard deviation is indicated by the vertical line in the middle of each bar. The data for each state were based upon the amplitudes of 40 control reflexes and 40 reflexes preceded by reticular stimulation. (From Watanabe and Chase (in press).)

Digastric Reflex Response During Sleep and Wakefulness

The digastric reflex was also modified in a consistent fashion during sleep and wakefulness by short pulse train or single pulse excitation of the reticular tegmentum (conditioning-test latency: 20ms). The reticular effect upon the digastric reflex was one of inhibition during wakefulness, quiet sleep, and active sleep (Fig. 21). As with the masseteric reflex response, this pattern was consistent and observed in every animal examined throughout all sessions. Also, as with the masseteric reflex, there were no qualitative variations in the direction of effect during intrastate variations in activity. No response was observed in the digastric muscle when reticular stimulation alone was employed. Moreover, the level of reticular excitation necessary to induce digastric inhibition resulted neither in behavioral or electroencephalographic responses nor in any variations in the animals' general pattern of sleep and wakefulness.

Discussion

In our previous study of the effect of orbital cortical stimulation upon brainstem reflex and evoked digastric activity we found a consistent pattern of decreasing cortical effectiveness as the animals passed from wakefulness to quiet sleep to active sleep (Chase and McGinty, 1970a). This is not surprising, since specific brain areas such as the orbital cortex have traditionally been assumed to exert a single function. However, we did not expect to find that different functions would appear related to the same area of the brain and yet emerge only during different states. Surprisingly, this was the case with the masseteric pattern of reflex modulation exerted by the reticular pontomidbrain tegmentum. Identical stimulation of the reticular locus led to masseteric reflex facilitation both during wakefulness and quiet sleep, but when the animal's state changed to active sleep, the direction of masseteric reflex response became one of inhibition rather than facilitation. On the other hand, digastric reflex activity was consistently inhibited by reticular stimulation throughout all states of sleep and wakefulness. A functional explanation for these patterns of state-dependent modulation is proposed below.

Let us examine the spontaneous variations in masseteric and digastric reflex activity and then add to them the variations induced by reticular stimulation. We will use as our baseline values the spontaneous amplitude of both reflexes during *quiet sleep*. Thus, relative to quiet sleep, during wakefulness the masseteric reflex is facilited while the digastric reflex is inhibited. Reticular stimulation during wakefulness facilitates the masseteric reflex and inhibits the digastric reflex. During active sleep, when both reflexes are spontaneously reduced in amplitude, reticular stimulation again induces a pattern of activity similar to that which occurs spontaneously. Thus, during both wakefulness and active sleep reticular stimulation promotes the same direction of reflex response as occurs spontaneously during these states. The function of the reticular tegmentum may therefore be expressed during both wakefulness and active sleep.

The reflex responses during wakefulness and active sleep may be the result of the excitation of a single system with dual functions. For example, when it appears that reticular stimulation mimics and promotes the spontaneous variations in activity which occur during wakefulness and active sleep, perhaps we are in actuality exciting a single neuronal group or fiber tract that exerts one function during wakefulness and another during active sleep. Indeed, a single system with dual functions may be what Michel Jouvet (1972) has in mind when he postulates that "the neural structures which trigger PS may be very close to those which are related to waking." Biochemical evidence supporting this view is cited by Barbara Jones (1972) who finds evidence to "suggest the implication of NA in the mediation of waking and of deaminated metabolites of NA in the generation of PGO spiking and PS." If we are, in fact, inducing activity in neurons which have the potential for producing both excitation and inhibition, we would have discovered a situation unique in the vertebrate nervous system, although such patterns of activity have been described in invertebrates (Tauc and Gerschenfeld, 1961; Gardner and Kandel, 1972). There are numerous other explanations for our finding of a response reversal of the masseteric reflex during the active sleep state as compared with wakefulness or quiet sleep. These may be found in a previous publication, which is concerned with the masseteric reflex response to reticular stimulation (Chase and Babb, in press).

Since this area of the brainstem is probably responsible for promoting motor functions during wakefulness and active sleep, we might examine the possibility that a disruption of its function would result in an abnormal pattern of state-dependent motor activity. For example, certain patterns of motor inhibition during wakefulness are clinically termed cataplexy, a condition included in the class of sleep disorders known as narcolepsy. In cataplectic patients abnormal discharge of this area of the reticular tegmentum may initiate motor inhibition while at the same time maintaining wakefulness. Indeed, concurrent discharge of inhibitory and excitatory mechanisms would explain the rather paradoxical findings of motor inhibition in alert patients during a cataplectic attack.

Until a more specific analysis of the extent of the effective reticular areas is obtained, credible hypotheses of the functional significance of the findings are limited. The fact remains, however, that this brain area *is* capable of promoting diametrically opposite patterns of response whose direction of effect is strictly dependent upon the state of the animal. The organization of central neuronal systems, therefore, is quite dynamic, for it is possible that a function observed and correlated with a specific brain area during one state may not be expressed by that same area during another state.

While our studies of the modulation of brainstem reflex activity by neural stimulation were being carried out, a complementary examination of these reflexes was undertaken during wakefulness in conjunction with the conditioned generation of a specific rhythm localized to the sensorimotor cortex (SMR, 12 to 14 cycles per sec). This rhythm has been implicated in various behaviors involved with internal inhibition and a cessation of somatic movements, which in turn have been related to the initiation of quiet sleep (Chase, 1971, in press, b; Babb and Chase, in press).

CONDITIONED SMR: SOMATIC AND VISCERAL CORRELATES

Introduction

The present investigation was an attempt to determine the relationship between the behavioral state of internal inhibition, which can lead to sleep, and its correlated somatomotor and visceromotor processes. We obtained experimental control over this state by operantly conditioning cats to maintain a specific cortical pattern which occurs spontaneously during wakefulness and is correlated with the state of internal inhibition (Roth et al., 1967). This cortical pattern is one localized to the sensorimotor cortex and is therefore called the sensorimotor rhythm, SMR (Roth et al., 1967). It consists of a synchronized pattern of electrical activity with a dominant frequency of 12 to 14 cycles per second. During periods of operantly conditioned SMR, variations in somatomotor and visceromotor activity, as well as correlated changes in brainstem reflex activity, were observed (Chase, 1971, in press, b; Babb and Chase, in press).

Methods

Adult freely moving cats were utilized in this study. According to techniques previously described, stimulating and recording electrodes were placed to monitor the respiratory and heart rate patterns and to induce and record the masseteric and digastric reflexes (Chase, 1971, in press, b; Babb and Chase in press). After the animals had recovered from the effects of the surgical implantations, they were placed within an environmental chamber and conditioned in a free operant paradigm to generate 12 to 14 cycle per second activity of the anterior and posterior sigmoid gyri. Reinforcement consisted either of the presentation of 0.2 milliliters of milk from an automatic dispenser or the application of reinforcing electrical stimulation to the brain via a depth electrode implanted in the hypothalamus (Chase, 1971, in press, b; Babb and Chase, in press). Cardiac and respiratory activity were monitored by electrodes placed in the fasciae overlying the thoracic cage. Respiratory activity was also monitored as a change in the temperature of a thermister applied to the external nares.

The integrated electromyographic activity of the neck was plotted in an analog pattern. Consecutive 1 second control periods of behavioral quiescence were compared statistically (Mann-Whitney U test) with periods of conditioned 12 to 14 cycle per second SMR activity. The slope of the respiratory wave at the onset and termination of conditioned SMR activity was analyzed statistically by calculating the frequency probability at which inspiration, expiration or null breathing occurred coincident with the onset and termination of SMR. The EKG was analyzed by comparing the interbeat interval for the 6 second period immediately preceding SMR with the interval during the conditioned rhythm. The amplitude variations in masseteric and digastric reflex activity were compared statistically (t-test) with contiguous periods.

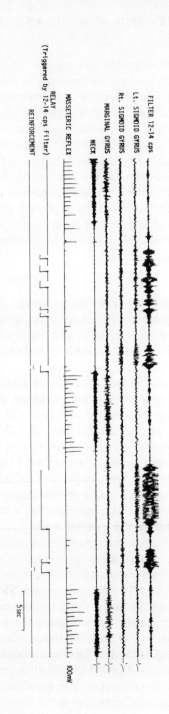

Fig. 22. Inhibition of masseteric reflex and neck tone during conditioned SMR. The top channel shows the filtered (left) coronal EEG. The relay was triggered every time the amplitude of SMR reached criterion and the feeder was operated when the required duration was accomplished. Generally, the marginal cortex was desynchronized during SMR but synchronized after reinforcement (post-reinforcement synchronization or PRS). Mesen. Vth nucl.: 5 V, 0.15 msec. (From Babb and Chase (in press).)

Results

A coherent pattern of somatomotor activity was found to occur in conjunction with the presence of the sensorimotor rhythm. During conditioned SMR a complete cessation of movement (except respiratory) occurred in all animals examined. Eye movements also ceased during periods of conditioned SMR, and the tonic electrical activity of the neck musculature decreased (Fig. 22). While the masseteric reflex was suppressed (Fig. 22), the digastric reflex showed no variations in amplitude during the control periods which were compared with contiguous periods of conditioned SMR activity (Fig. 23).

A shift in visceromotor processes toward the parasympathetic end of the spectrum was observed. The heart rate was reduced as much as 30% during periods of conditioned EEG activity (Fig. 24) as compared with control conditions ($P < 0.001$ for all animals). At the onset of each epoch of SMR the respiratory pattern was one of inspiration ($P < 0.005$) and the termination of SMR occurred during expiration ($P < 0.005$) (Fig. 25). In conjunction with long trains of SMR the respiratory pattern was regular and exhibited relatively few variations in amplitude or frequency.

Discussion

During quiet sleep there are specific changes in behavior, as well as in somatomotor and visceral processes. When our cats produced SMR, their behavior and their somatomotor and visceromotor processes changed to a pattern which occurs spontaneously during quiet sleep (Jouvet, 1967; Chase, 1971; in press, b; Babb and Chase, in press). For example, the animals' movements ceased, muscle tone decreased, and the masseteric reflex decreased in amplitude. Cardiac rate also decreased, while the pattern of respiration became more regular. Although there was no change in digastric reflex amplitude, this does not negate the basic hypothesis relating SMR to quiet sleep (see Chase (1971) and previous section).

We do not know whether the sensorimotor rhythm is an integral part of the process of internal inhibition or whether it is a relatively uninvolved correlate. Since animals simply conditioned to remain still also generate SMR (Howe and Sterman, 1972), we suspect that this rhythm is one linked primarily to the cessation of movement, whether or not internal inhibition is present.

The cessation of movement and correlated reductions in somatomotor and visceromotor activity may indeed predispose an animal toward the quiet sleep state. Alternatively, the underlying mechanism responsible for generating this behavior and its motor correlates may be similar to or identical with the mechanisms which promote the state of sleep. In any event, it is apparent that a behavioral modification during wakefulness can lead to variations in internal processes which are similar to those occurring during quiet sleep. We can therefore view SMR activity as an important neural pattern which influences somatic reflex activity, and may be one of the factors which predispose an animal to enter the state of quiet sleep.

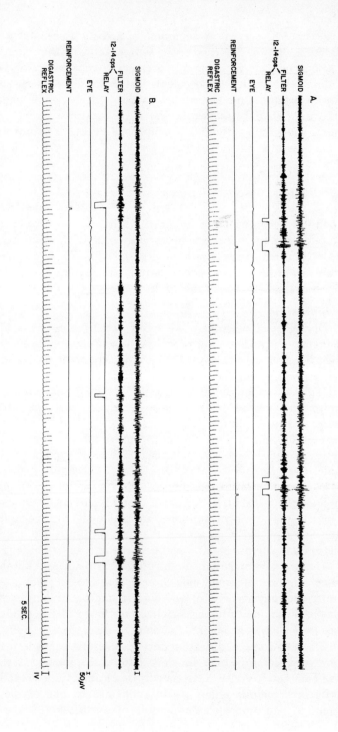

Fig. 23. Behavior of the digastric reflex during conditioned SMR episodes. Although reflex amplitude varied, it bore no relation to SMR episodes. Reflex suppression was often seen during movement, as indicated by fluctuations in the eye channel. Inferior dental nerve: 2 V, 0.01 msec. (From Babb and Chase (in press).)

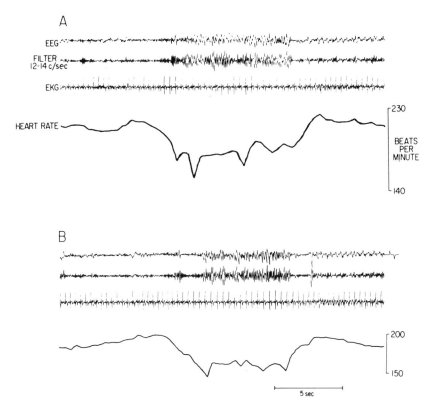

Fig. 24. Heart rate associated with conditioned 12-14 H$_2$ activity of the sensorimotor cortex. In most instances, before the onset of the conditioned EEG pattern, the heart rate increased for a brief period. During conditioned EEG activity, the heart rate decreased rapidly to a level that was maintained for the duration of the synchronized episode. In the absence of movement, heart rate was the same before and after episodes of the conditioned rhythm. Calibration: 50 μV. (From Chase (1971).)

SUMMATION

This summation will be concerned with a brief overview of the preceding studies of the central neural modulation of brainstem reflex activity which occurs during sleep and wakefulness. To recap, the studies of brainstem reflex activity which were described include: 1) spontaneous variations in the developing kitten and adult cat; 2) variations following vagal stimulation; 3) variations following orbital cortical stimulation; 4) variations following reticular stimulation; and 5) variations during conditioned SMR activity. Each of these studies brings information to bear upon the systems which

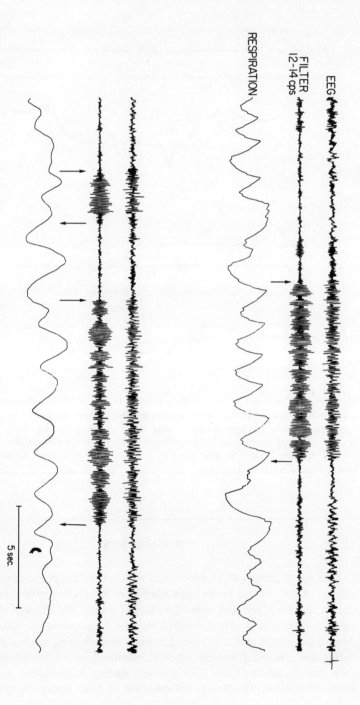

Fig. 25. Respiratory activity associated with conditioned 12-14 c/sec activity of the sensorimotor cortex. A regular pattern of respiration occurred during conditioned EEG activity. Short and long episodes began during inspiration (upward deflection) and were terminated during expiration (downward deflection). Calibration: 50μV. (From Chase (1971).)

control the amplitude of the masseteric and digastric reflexes during sleep and wakefulness.

The story of the central neural control of brainstem reflex activity is built on a foundation which consists of the spontaneous variations in the amplitude of these reflexes which occur (in the adult) during the natural states of sleep and wakefulness. During wakefulness compared with quiet sleep, the amplitude of the masseteric reflex is greatest while the amplitude of the digastric reflex is suppressed. During active sleep both reflexes are reduced to levels below those observed during any other state of sleep or wakefulness. Now, which experimental manipulations induce a pattern of reflex modulation similar to that observed spontaneously during these states of sleep and wakefulness?

First, we note that the early, direct, predominant effect of vagal and orbital cortical stimulation is to yield a pattern of reflex response during wakefulness which is exactly opposite from that observed *spontaneously* during this state. In addition, the effect of orbital cortical stimulation is greatest during wakefulness, indicating that orbital cortical reflex control functions are carried out primarily during wakefulness. It therefore appears that neither the orbital cortex nor the vagal system are responsible for the production of a spontaneous pattern of reflex activity, but rather for one related to mediating reflex activity during certain behaviors which accompany the waking state.

SMR conditioning promotes a pattern of masseteric activity similar to that found during quiet sleep, although the digastric reflex is not modified at all. Other physiological processes are modified in a fashion similar to that which occurs during quiet sleep. Therefore, the mechanisms responsible for SMR are probably related either to waking functions or to the initiation of quiet sleep.

The reticular system, on the other hand, appears to promote a pattern of reflex activity not only during wakefulness, but also during active sleep, which mimics the precise pattern that occurs spontaneously during these states. On the basis of the evidence previously cited, we propose that the pontomidbrain reticular tegmentum is responsible for the maintenance of the spontaneous patterns of brainstem reflex activity which accompany the states of sleep and wakefulness. It is likely that this brain area may also be responsible for the initiation and maintenance of the states themselves, as well as their physiological correlates, including the state-dependent modulation of the masseteric and digastric reflexes.

This research was supported by NIH grants NS-09999 and MH-10083. Bibliographic assistance was provided by the Brain Information Service (NINDS contract 70-2063). This paper represents the cumulated efforts of a number of investigators including: Margaret Babb, Carmine Clemente, Ronald Harper, Lorraine MacDonald, Dennis McGinty, Yoshio Nakamura, M.B. Sterman, Shizuo Torii, and Kyozo Watanabe.

REFERENCES

Agnew, R.F., Preston, J.B., and Whitlock, D.G. Patterns of motor cortex effects on ankle flexor and extensor motoneurons in the 'pyramidal' cat preparation.*Exp. Neurol. 8,* 248-263 (1963).

Agnew, R.F., and Preston, J.B. Motor cortex-pyramidal effects on single ankle flexor and extensor motoneurons of the cat *Exp. Neurol. 12,* 384-398 (1965).

Ausubel, D.P. A critique of Piaget's theory of the ontogenesis of motor behavior. *J. Genet. Psychol. 109,* 119-122 (1966).

Babb, M. and Chase, M.H. Reflex modulation during conditioned sensorimotor cortical activity. *EEG Clin. Neurophysiol.* in press.

Babkin, B.P., and Van Buren, J.M., Mechanism and cortical representation of feeding pattern. *Arch. Neurol. Psychiat. (Chicago) 66,* 1-19 (1951).

Baldissera, F., Broggi, G., and Mancia, M. Spinal reflexes in normal unrestrained cats during sleep and wakefulness.*Experientia 20,* 577 (1964).

Baldissera, F., Ettore, G., Infuso, L., Mancia, M., et Pagni, C.A. Etude comparative des réponses évoquées par stimulation des voies corticospinales pendant le sommeil et la veille, chez l'homme et chez l'animal. *Rev. neurol. 115,* 82-84 (1966).

Baccelli, G., Guazzi, M., Libretti, A., and Zanchetti, A. Effects of presso- and chemoceptive components of the cat's aortic nerve on sham rage behavior.*Experientia 19,* 534-535 (1963).

Bieber, I. Grasping and sucking.*J. Nerv. Ment. Dis. 91,* 31-36 (1940).

Cardot, H., Cherbuliez, A., et Laugier, H. Variations périodiques de l'excitabilité de l'arc reflexe linguo-maxillaire, en fonction de l'activité du centre respiratoire.*C.R. Soc. Biol., Paris 88,* 1088-1090 (1923).

Carli, G. and Zanchetti, A. A study of pontine lesions suppressing deep sleep in the cat. *Arch. Ital. Biol. 103,* 751-789 (1965).

Chase, M.H. The digastric reflex in the kitten and adult cat: Paradoxical amplitude fluctuations during sleep and wakefulness *Arch Ital. Biol. 108,* 403-422 (1970).

Chase, M.H. Brain stem somatic reflex activity in neonatal kittens during sleep and wakefulness. *Physiol. Behav. 7,* 165-172 (1971).

Chase, M.H. Cycles of inhibition and excitation and a short discourse on nomenclature. in, *The Sleeping Brain Perspectives in the Brain Sciences,* Vol. 1. M.H. Chase, Ed. Brain Information Service/Brain Research Institute, UCLA, Los Angeles, 1972a, pp. 493-501.

Chase, M.H. Patterns of reflex excitability during the ontogenesis of sleep and wakefulness. in, *Maturation of Brain Mechanisms Related to Sleep Behavior* C.D. Clemente, D.P. Purpura and F.E. Meyer, Eds. Academic Press, New York, 1972b, pp. 253-285.

Chase, M.H. Somatic reflex activity during sleep and wakefulness. in, *Basic Sleep Mechanisms,* O. Petre-Quadens and J. Schlag, Eds., Academic Press, New York, in press.

Chase, M.H. Research strategies in the study of EEG activity by operant conditioning techniques. in, *Operant Control of Brain Activity,* M.H. Chase, Ed., Brain Information Service/Brain Research Institute, UCLA, Los Angeles, in press.

Chase, M.H., Sterman, M.B., and Clemente, C.D. Cortical and subcortical patterns of response to afferent vagal stimulation. *Exp. Neurol. 16,*36-49 (1966).

Chase, M.H., Nakamura, Y., Clemente, C.D., and Sterman, M.B. Afferent vagal stimulation: Neurographic correlates of induced EEG synchronization and desynchronization. *Brain Res. 5,* 236-249 (1967).

Chase, M.H. and Sterman, M.B. Maturation of patterns of sleep and wakefulness in the kitten. *Brain Res. 5,* 319-329 (1967).

Chase, M.H., McGinty, D.J., and Sterman, M.B. Cyclic variations in the amplitude of a brain stem reflex during sleep and wakefulness. *Experientia 24,* 47-48 (1968).

Chase, M.H. and Nakamura, Y. Inhibition of the masseteric reflex by vagal afferents.*Experientia 24,* 918-919 (1968).

Chase, M.H. and Nakamura, Y. Cortical and subcortical EEG patterns of response to afferent abdominal vagal stimulation: Neurographic correlates. *Physiol. Behav. 3,* 605-610 (1968).

Chase, M.H. and McGinty, D.J. Somatomotor inhibition and excitation by forebrain stimulation during sleep and wakefulness: Orbital cortex. *Brain Res. 19*, 127-136 (1970).

Chase, M.H. and McGinty, D.J. Modulation of spontaneous and reflex activity of the jaw musculature by orbital cortical stimulation in the freely-moving cat. *Brain Res. 19*, 117-126 (1970).

Chase, M.H., Nakamura, Y., and Torii, S. Afferent vagal modulation of brain stem somatic reflex activity. *Exp. Neurol. 27*, 534-544 (1970).

Chase, M.H., Torii, S., and Nakamura, Y. The influence of afferent vagal fiber activity of masticatory reflexes. *Exp. Neurol. 27*, 545-553 (1970b).

Chase, M.H. and Harper, R.M. Somatomotor and visceromotor correlates of operantly conditioned 12-14 cps sensorimotor cortical activity. *EEG Clin. Neurophysiol. 31*, 85-92 (1971).

Chase, M.H., and Babb, M. Masseteric reflex response to reticular stimulation reverses during active sleep compared with wakefulness or quiet sleep. *Brain Res., in press.*

Chase, M.H., Sterman, M.B., Kubota, K., and Clemente, C.D. Modulation of masseter and digastric neural activity by forebrain stimulation in the squirrel monkey: Dorsolateral cerebral cortex. *Exp. Neurol., in press.*

Clemente, C.D. Chase, M.H., Knauss, T.A., Sauerland, E.K., and Sterman, M.B. Inhibition of a monosynaptic reflex by electrical stimulation of the basal forebrain or the orbital gyrus in the cat. *Experientia (Basel) 22*, 844-848 (1966).

Dumont, S. Contribution à l'étude du contrôle réticulaire des intégrations sensori-motrices au cours de la vigilance. Faculté des Sciences de l'Université de Paris, 1964.

Eccles, R.M. and Willis, W.D. The effect of repetitive stimulation upon monosynaptic transmission in kittens. *J. Physiol. (London) 176*, 311-321 (1965).

Gardner, D. and Kandel, E.R. Diphasic postsynaptic potential: A chemical synapse capable of mediating conjoint excitation and inhibition. *Science 176*, 675-678 (1972).

Gassel, M.M., Marchiafava, P.L., and Pompeiano, O. Phasic changes in muscular activity during desynchronized sleep in unrestrained cats. An analysis of the pattern and organization of myoclonic twitches. *Arch. Ital. Biol. 102*, 449-470 (1964).

Gassel, M.M. and Pompeiano, O. Fusimotor function during sleep in unrestrained cats. An account of the modulation of the mechanically and electrically evoked monosynaptic reflexes. *Arch. Ital. Biol. 103*, 347-368 (1965).

Giaquinto, S., Pompeiano, O., e Somogyi, I. Reflex activity of extensor and flexor muscles following muscular afferent excitation during sleep and wakefulness. *Experientia 19*, 481 (1963).

Guazzi, M., Baccelli, G., and Zanchetti, A. Reflex chemoceptive regulation of arterial pressure during natural sleep in the cat. *Amer. J. Physiol. 214*, 969-978 (1968).

Gumulka, W., Samanin, R., Valzelli, L., and Consolo, S. Behavioral and biochemical effects following the stimulation of the nucleus raphis dorsalis on rats. *J. Neurochem. 10*, 533-535 (1971).

Harvey, W. *Exercitationes de Generatione Animalium* O. Pulleyn, London, 1651.

Henatsch, H.D. and Schulte, F.J. Reflexerregung und Eigenhemmung tonischer und phasischer Alpha-Motoneurone während chemischer Daverregung der Muskelspindeln. *Pfluegers Arch. Ges. Physiol. Menschen Tiere 268*, 134-147 (1958).

Hess, W.R., Akert, A., and McDonald, D.A. Functions of the orbital gyri of cats. *Brain 75*, 244-258 (1952).

Hodes, R. and Suzuki, J.I. Comparative thresholds of cortex, vestibular system and reticular formation in wakefulness, sleep and rapid eye movement periods *EEG Clin. Neurophysiol. 18*, 239-248 (1965).

Hoffman, P. and Tonnies, J.F. Nachweis des völlig konstanten Vorkommens des Zungen-Kieferreflexes beim Menschen. *Pfluegers Arch. Ges. Physiol. Menschen Tiere 250*, 103-108 (1948).

Hongo, T. and Jankowska, E. Effects from the sensorimotor cortex on the spinal cord in cats with transected pyramids. *Exp. Brain Res. 3*, 117-134 (1967).

Hosokawa, H. Proprioceptive innervation of striated muscles in the territory of cranial nerves. *Texas Rep. Biol. Med. 19*, 405-464 (1961).

Howe, R.C. and Sterman, M.B. Cortical-subcortical EEG correlates of suppressed motor behavior during sleep and waking in the cat. *EEG Clin. Neurophysiol. 32*, 681-695 (1972).

Hugelin, A. Analyse de l'inhibition d'un réflexe nociceptif (réflexe linguo-maxillaire) lors de l'activation du système réticulo-spinal dit "facilitateur". *C. R. Soc. Biol. Paris 149*, 1893-1898 (1955).

Iwama, K. and Kawamoto, T. Responsiveness of cat motor cortex to electrical stimulation in wakefulness. in, *Correlative Neurosciences, Part B. Clinical Studies, Progress in Brain Research*, Vol. 21B. T. Tokizane and J.P. Schade Eds. Elsevier, Amsterdam,1966, pp.54-63.

Jones, B.E. The respective involvement of noradrenaline and its deaminated metabolites in waking and paradoxical sleep: a neuropharmacological model. *Brain Res. 39* 121-136, (1972).

Jouvet, M. The rhombencephalic phase of sleep. in, *Brain Mechanisms, Progress in Brain Research*, Vol. I, G. Motuzzi et al., Eds., Elsevier, Amsterdam, 1963, pp. 406-424.

Jouvet, M., Neurophysiology of the states of sleep. *Physiol. Rev. 47*, 117-177 (1967).

Jouvet, M. Some monoaminergic mechanisms controlling sleep and waking. in, *Brain and Human Behavior*, A. Karczmar and J. Eccles, Eds., Springer, New York, 1971, pp. 131-162.

Jouvet, M. The role of monoamines and acetylcholine-containing neurons in the regulation of the sleep-waking cycle. *Ergebnisse Physiol. 64*, 166-307 (1972).

Jouvet-Mounier, D., Astic, L., and Lacote, D. Ontogenesis of the states of sleep in rat, cat, and guinea pig during the first postnatal month. *Develop. Psychobiol. 2*, 216-239 (1970).

Kaada, B.R. Somato-motor, autonomic and electroencephalographic responses to electrical stimulation of "rhinencephalic" and other structures in primates, cat and dog. *Acta Physiol. Scand. 24* (Suppl. 83), 1-285 (1951).

Korn, H. et Richard, P. Voies spinales transmettant les messages somatiques vers le cortex orbitaire du chat. *J. Physiol. [Paris] 56* 387 (1963).

Korn, H., Wendt, R., and Albe-Fessard, D. Somatic projection to the orbital cortex of the cat. *EEG Clin. Neurophysiol. 21* 209-226 (1966).

Kostowski, W. and Giacalone, E. Stimulation of various forebrain structures and brain 5HT, 5HIAA, and behaviour in rats. *Europ. J. Pharmacol. 7*, 176-180 (1969).

Langworthy, O.R. A correlated study of the development of reflex activity in fetal and young kittens and the myelinization of tracts in the nervous system. *Contrib. Embryol. Carnegie Inst. 20*, 127-172 (1924).

Lundberg, A. and Voorhoeve, P. Effects from the pyramidal tract on spinal reflex arcs. *Acta Physiol. Scand. 56*, 201-219 (1962).

Menini, C. La formation reticulaire. *Rev. Med. Toulouse 8*, 545-567 (1972).

Mizuno, N. Sauerland, E.K., and Clemente, C.D., Projections from the orbital gyrus in the cat. I: To brain stem structures. *J. Comp. Neurol. 133*, 463-476 (1969).

Moruzzi, G. The sleep-waking cycle. *Ergebnisse Physiol. 64*, 1-165 (1972).

Nakamura, Y., Goldberg, L.J., and Clemente, C.D. Nature of suppression of the masseteric monosynaptic reflex induced by stimulation of the orbital gyrus of the cat. *Brain Res. 6*. 184-198 (1967).

Penaloza-Rojas, J.H. Electroencephalographic synchronization resulting from direct current application to the vagus nerves. *Exp. Neurol. 9*, 367-371 (1964).

Pfaffmann, C. Afferent impulses from the teeth due to pressure and noxious stimulation. *J. Physiol. 97*, 207-219 (1939).

Pieron, H. *Le Problème Physiologique du Sommeil*. Masson, Paris 1913.

Pinotti, O. and Granata, L. Effetto della stimolazione dei chemocettori carotidei sul riflesso linguo-mandibolare. *Boll. Soc. Ital. Biol. Sper. 29*, 375-377 (1953).

Polc, P. and Monnier, M. An activating mechanism in the ponto-bulbar raphé system of the rabbit. *Brain Res. 22*, 47-63 (1970).

Pollock, L.J. and Davis, L. Studies in decerebration. VI. The effect of deafferentation upon decerebrate rigidity. *Amer. J. Physiol. 98*, 47-49 (1931).

Pompeiano, O. Sensory inhibition during motor activity in sleep. in, *Neurophysiological Basis of Normal and Abnormal Motor Activities*, M.D. Yahr and D.P. Purpura, Eds., Raven Press, New York, 1967a, pp. 323-375.

Pompeiano, O. The neurophysiological mechanisms of the postural and motor events during desynchronized sleep. in, *Sleep and Altered States of Consciousness*, S.S. Kety, E.V. Evarts, and H.L. Williams, Eds. *Res. Publ. Assoc. Nerv. Ment. Dis. 45* 351-423 (1967b).

Preston, J.B. and Whitlock, D.G. Precentral facilitation and inhibition of spinal motoneurons. *J. Neurophysiol. 23,* 154-170 (1960).

Pujol, J.F. Buguet, A., Froment, J.L., Jones, B., and Jouvet, M. The central metabolism of serotonin in the cat during insomnia: A neurophysiological and biochemical study after p-chlorophenylalanine or destruction of the raphé system. *Brain Res. 29,* 195-212 (1971).

Roffwarg, H.P., Muzio, J.N., and Dement, W.C. Ontogenetic development of the human sleep-dream cycle. *Science 152,* 604-619 (1966).

Roth, S.R., Sterman, M.B., and Clemente, C.D. Comparison of EEG correlates of reinforcement, internal inhibition and sleep. *EEG Clin. Neurophysiol. 23,* 509-520 (1967).

Sauerland, E.K., Nakamura, Y., and Clemente, C.D. The role of the lower brain stem in cortically induced inhibition of somatic reflexes in the cat. *Brain Res. 6,* 164-180 (1967).

Scheibel, A.B. Neural correlates of psychophysiological developments in the young organism. *Recent Advan. Biol. Psychiat. 4,* 313-328 (1961).

Scheibel, M. and Scheibel, A. Some structural and functional substrates of development in young cats. in, *The Developing Brain, Progress in Brain Research*, Vol. 9, W.A. Himwich and H.E. Himwich, Eds., Elsevier, Amsterdam, 1964, pp. 6-25.

Schulte, F.J. and Schwenzel, W. Motor control and muscle tone in the newborn period. Electromyographic studies. *Biol. Neonatorum 8,* 198-215 (1965).

Sherrington, C.S. Decerebrate rigidity and reflex coordination of movements. *J. Physiol. [Lond] 22,* 319-332 (1898).

Sherrington, C.S. Reflexes elicitable in the cat from pinna, vibrissae and jaws. *J. Physiol. 51,* 404-431 (1917).

Siegfried, J. Topographie des projections corticales du nerf vague chez le chat. *Helv. Physiol. Pharmacol. Acta 19,* 269-278 (1961).

Skoglund, S. Central connections and functions of muscle nerves in the kitten. *Acta physiol. Scand. 50,* 222-237 (1960a).

Skoglund, S. On the postnatal development of postural mechanisms as revealed by electromyography and myography in decerebrate kittens. *Acta Physiol. Scand. 49,* 299-317 (1960b).

Skoglund, S. The reactions to tetanic stimulation of the two-neuron arc in the kitten. *Acta Physiol. Scand. 50,* 238-253 (1960c).

Skoglund, S. Muscle afferents and motor control in the kitten. in, *Muscle Afferents and Motor Control*, R. Granit, Ed., Almquist and Wiksells, Stockholm, pp. 245-259 (1966)

Smith, R.D. and Marcarian, H.Q. The neuromuscular spindles of the lateral pterygoid muscle. *Anat. Anz. 120,* 47-53 (1967).

Sterman, M.B., Knauss, T., Lehmann, D., and Clemente, C.D. Circadian sleep and waking patterns in the laboratory cat. *EEG Clin. Neurophysiol. 19,* 509-517 (1965).

Tarchanoff, J. Quelques observations sur le sommeil normal. *Arch. Ital. Biol. 21,* 318-321 (1894).

Tauc, L. and Gerschenfeld, H.M. Cholinergic transmission mechanisms for both excitation and inhibition in molluscan central synapses. *Nature 192,* 366-367 (1961).

Valatx, J.L., Jouvet, D., et Jouvet, M. Évolution électroencéphalographique des différents états de sommeil chez le chaton. *EEG Clin. Neurophysiol. 17,* 218-233 (1964).

Vlach, V. Some exteroceptive skin reflexes in the limbs and trunk in newborns. in, *Studies in Infancy*, M.C. Bax and R.C. MacKeith, Eds., Heinemann, London, 1968, pp. 41-54.

Wessolosky, J., Mizuno, N., and Clemente, C.D. Effect of orbital cortical stimulation upon the facial motoneurons of the cat. *Fed. Proc. 27* 451 (1968).

Watanabe, K., and Chase, M.H. Reticular control of digastric reflex activity during sleep and wakefulness. *Experentia*, in press.

Wyrwicka, W. and Chase, M.H. Projections from the inferior dental nerve to the dien- and mesencephalic areas related to feedings. *Physiologist 12*, 401 (1969).

Advances in Sleep Research, Vol. 1
© 1974, Spectrum Publications, Inc.

CHAPTER 6

Ultradian Rhythms in Sleep and Wakefulness

DANIEL F. KRIPKE

In trying to understand human feelings and behavior, the psychiatrist often finds himself using models and techniques which emulate ideas from physical and economic sciences. For example, mechanical models are imitated in attempts to explain behavior in terms of brain structure or to describe psychodynamics topographically. Images originating from hydraulics or chemistry may be represented in neuropharmacologic theories, for example, the hypotheses that depression is caused by diminished concentrations of noradrenalin in the brain, and that sleep results from filling and discharge of serotonin reservoirs (Wyatt, 1972). As our fellow scientists gain more sophisticated understanding, biologists also develop new models to describe the complexity of living systems. The investigator of biological rhythms mimics 20th Century engineering and economics, modeling his ideas after gasoline motors, oscillating electronic circuits, and economic feedback loops. We are now trying to understand the behavioral functions of oscillatory mechanisms.

Circadian† behavioral rhythms are well known and most prominently in the 24-hour sleep-wakefulness patterns (Luce, 1970). Circadian behaviors may be readily understood as adaptations to ecological niches which themselves vary with the terrestial light-dark cycle (Webb, 1971). Slower "infradian" †† rhythms in sexual behaviors have obvious adaptational relations to oestrus rhythms. Circannual rhythms of behavior, e.g., winter migrations south, are also clearly functional adaptations. The "ultradian"†† rhythms, those with frequencies greater than 1/day, are less known and less well understood.

---

†*Circadian* rhythms have a frequency of about 1 cycle per day, roughly 1 cycle/20-28 hr.

††*Infradian* rhythms have frequencies slower than 1 cycle/28 hr while *ultradian* rhythms have frequencies greater than 1 cycle/20 hr (Halberg, 1967).

This article will concern itself with ultradian oscillations having both physiological and behavior expression; the ultradian rhythm was first recognized in the EEG sleep stages. That this oscillatory complex modulates a variety of brain functions, physiological systems, and behaviors, shall be shown and the theory that these oscillations have functional significance shall be explored.

ULTRADIAN RHYTHMS IN SLEEP

In their earliest descriptions of the sleep stages, Dement and Kleitman (1957) reported that the sleep stages are cyclic phenomena. Excited by the discovery of the rapid eye movement (REM) sleep stage and its correlation with subjective dreaming, Dement and Kleitman were impressed by the rhythmic pattern with which Stage REM sleep recurs throughout the night, on the average every 90-100 min. The other sleep stages, for example, Stages 3-4, also appear cyclically at opposite phases from Stage REM in the same cycle, and these other stages may equally be considered cyclic in occurrence (Fig. 1). To be sure, sleep stage cycles usually lack the sinusoidal regularity

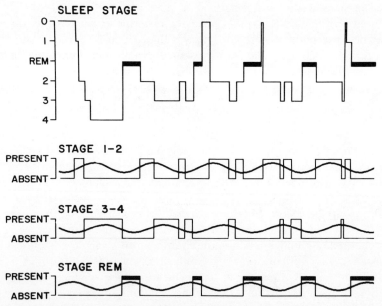

Fig. 1. A single night's sleep plot is analyzed into several sleep stage components. Sinusoids are fitted to each sleep stage component to illustrate the complementary phases.

we have learned to expect from electronic or astronomical oscillators. Dement and Kleitman reported that as the night progresses, Stage REM periods become longer in duration and also closer together. Thus, durations of the cycles and their amplitudes vary during the night. More recent data confirm that REM periods become longer (Verdone, 1968) and closer together (Kripke et al., 1968) as the night progresses. Similarly, Stage 3-4 periods become shorter or absent as the night progresses (Webb, 1971). The likelihood of occurrence of sleep stages, and perhaps also the frequency of their cycling, varies in daytime naps, as well, according to the time of day, so that part of the variability in ultradian cycles may be conceived as indicating circadian amplitude and frequency modulation of an ultradian rhythm (Webb, 1971) (Fig. 2). However, there is more variability in the timing and

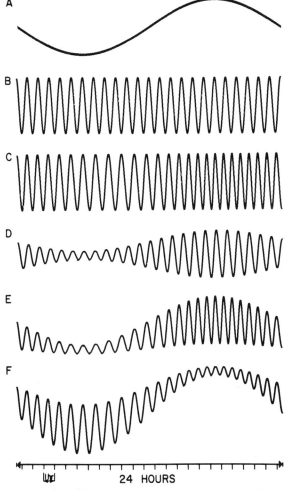

Fig. 2. Several model sinusoids are presented to demonstrate the possibilities for interrelationship of circadian and ultradian rhythm systems. (A) circadian rhythm; (B) ultradian rhythm (24 cycle/day); (C) ultradian rhythm with circadian frequency modulation; (D) ultradian rhythm with circadian amplitude modulation; (E) and (F) circadian rhythms with superimposed ultradian rhythms combining circadian frequency modulation and circadian amplitude modulation—the phase of frequency modulation is held constant but the phase of amplitude modulation is varied 180 degrees.

durations of the sleep stages than we can account for in terms of circadian amplitude or frequency modulation (Globus et al., 1972; Moses et al., 1972; Lewis, in press). The sleep cycle is less regular than circadian rhythms and probably less regular than respiratory and menstrual rhythms. Some observers have expressed doubt that these are rhythms at all, but if we define rhythmicity as a statistically reliable tendency for particular physiological patterns to repeat at certain intervals, and look not at a single night but at a statistical average of several recordings, there is little doubt that the sleep stages are rhythmic. With a variety of computational methods, many studies have replicated the statistical tendency for the sleep stages to repeat about every 90-100 min. (Kripke et al., 1968; Globus, 1972; Kripke, 1972). The null hypothesis, that is, random recurrence, has been consistently rejected, and some sort of oscillatory process must clearly underlie sleep stage progression.

Admitting that the occurrences of Stage REM (and the other sleep stages) are rhythmic, we must then ask what are the emotional, behavioral, or physiological functions in which this biological rhythm is expressed? At present, a comprehensive summary is not possible. The sleep stages themselves, both as originally defined by Dement and Kleitman, (1957) and in current usage (Rechtschaffen and Kales, 1968) are not defined by a single function but rather by patterns of function defined by the multivariate concurrence of several physiological states. It became popular for a time, because of the great quantitative usefulness of the sleep staging method, to reify the sleep stages and measure their durations as if the duration of a sleep "stage" was a discrete stoichiometrically measurable substance, rather than a loose mixture of functions. Much of the impetus to reify Stage REM came from the exciting discovery that when Stage REM is suppressed in some fashion, a "deprivation" syndrome usually appears, characterized by increasing tendency (decreasing threshold) for Stage REM to return. Stage REM rebounds to increased durations when REM recovery is permitted. REM deprivation experiments therefore suggest that Stage REM—and the REM cycle—are somehow needed functions. Neither interventions which suppress Stage REM nor the rebound which enhances it, however, greatly alter its pattern of cyclic occurrence. According to Hartmann's review (1968), the cyclic frequency of REM is much more stable that its duration-defined quantity. Moruzzi (1969) has argued that when the neurophysiological data concerning sleep mechanisms were reviewed, Stage REM could best be conceived not in terms of brain homeostatic mechanisms but as a consummatory state. It may readily be appreciated that ideas of waxing appetite, lowering threshold for release, and finally, consummatory satisfaction resemble the phenomenology of Stage REM very well and imply functionally a relaxation oscillator. Nevertheless, the REM sleep stage cannot be the essence of such a consummatory cycle.

Stage REM itself is not essential for ultradian oscillations to be expressed.

One hint of this was reported in the early study of Dement and Kleitman (1957), who noted that sometimes a "missed" REM period could be appreciated. In these instances, observed by everyone who does much sleep recording, the EEG amplitude decreases at that time of night when the first REM period might be expected, but the frank Stage REM pattern including eye movement fails to occur. Nevertheless, as viewed in the EEG or the remaining sleep stages, the underlying biological cycling continues to be obvious. Similar cycling is reflected in the genitals. Penile erections usually accompany Stage REM periods, but when a REM period is "missed," the penile cycle may be maintained, as it is also during Stage REM deprivation (Karacan, 1966; Karacan et al, 1966, 1972). Maintenance of the underlying cyclicity has also been noticed after administration of REM-suppressing drugs (Baekeland, 1966, 1967) (it is important to recognize that REM-suppressing drugs may not be cycle suppressing). Another hint that Stage REM is not the only form of ultradian consummatory state came from Dement's studies of PGO spikes (Dement et al., 1969). The PGO spikes, although usually a concomitant of Stage REM in the cat, do occur outside of Stage REM, and Dement found that suppression of PGO spikes was much better related to spike rebound than Stage REM suppression was related to Stage REM rebound. Unfortunately, these studies were not reported from the point of view of cyclicity, but they do reveal that Stage REM-like functions may take place outside of frank Stage REM. Cartwright's interesting experiments with REM deprivation lead toward a similar inference (Cartwright, 1969; Cartwright et al., 1967, 1972). Subjects who were permitted to fantasise on awakening from REM periods, or who were able to report dreams from non-REM sleep, showed less Stage REM rebound than those subjects who fantasised little outside of Stage REM. These results indicate that either sleep dreaming or waking fantasy, occurring outside of Stage REM, may replace the consummatory functions otherwise fulfilled within Stage REM. Thus whether the consummatory aspects of the Stage REM cycle involve the EEG sleep states, the genitals, PGO spikes, or fantasies, or some unidentified functions, the REM sleep stage is certainly not a crucial requirement for the cycle to operate.

There are many physiological systems which display rhythmic variation correlated with the sleep cycle. Kripke (1972) demonstrated with formal spectra that 10-20 cycle/day rhythms were present during sleep in a variety of separately measured but correlated variables including Stage REM, non-REM sleep, Stage 4, eye movement, and several EEG frequency bands (Fig. 3). Similarly, Hilbert and Naitoh (1972), Lubin et al. (1973), Sinha et al. (1972), Kripke et al. (1968), and others have reported equivalent cyclicity in EEG frequencies or sleep stages, using a variety of methods. Nocturnal ultradian rhythms have been demonstrated less formally but with equal confidence in many other physiological systems, for example, brain temperature (Kawamura et al., 1966; Reite and Pegram, 1968), blood pressure

(Coccagna et al., 1971), metabolism (Brebbia and Altshuler, 1968), arousal threshold (Pollak et al., 1967), gastric acid secretion (Kales and Tan, 1969), and genital engorgement (Karacan et al., 1972). 'At present, there is little evidence that the function of any single organ is the teleologic purpose of the biorhythmicity we have recognized during sleep, whether it be the brain, the eyes, the stomach, the penis, or some as yet unrecognized locus. Rather, oscillatory fluctuations in the functioning of all these organs are correlated. Neuroanatomic studies localizing nuclei originating Stage REM have rarely included any methodologically reliable analysis of biorhythmicity. Since Stage REM is not essential to the oscillations we are discussing, studies localizing Stage REM may not apply to the governing ultradian oscillator.

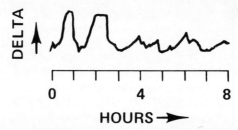

Fig. 3. EEG delta frequency band amplitude modulation is shown over an 8 hr sleep recording. The 90 min sinusoidal rhythm is obvious.

ENDOCRINE CORRELATES OF
NOCTURNAL ULTRADIAN RHYTHMS

During sleep, ultradian rhythms are seen in endocrine measures. When Weitzman began to measure plasma cortisol in sleeping subjects (Weitzman et al., 1966), he discovered that the plasma cortisol concentration was far from steady during the night, but instead underwent a series of 4-5 ups and downs, rising to the highest peak levels in the early morning hours at the same times that Stage REM was most prevalent. Weitzman's presumption that cortisol excretion might be specifically linked to REM periods was supported by Mandell and Mandell (Mandell et al., 1966), who measured urinary cortisol output in catheterized urology patients, and reported an apparent relationship between cortisol and REM periods. Later, it was shown that nocturnal cortisol pulses persist during sleep deprivation, or when the circadian sleep-wakefulness rhythm is reversed in phase (Weitzman et al, 1970), so it is certain that Stage REM is not obligatory to cortisol pulses. It has become clear that cortisol, as well as a variety of other neurally regulated hormones, is secreted in brief episodic pulses both during sleep and wakefulness (Weitzman et al., 1971). More careful statistical analyses have failed to confirm a correlation between Stage REM and plasma cortisol, when time-of-night effects are controlled. Believing there could be a consistent phase relationship between cortisol pulses and Stage REM at the peak ultradian frequency, even if a time lag between the events obscured linear correlations, I computed cross-spectra from some plasma cortisol data of Weitzman et al. (1970). Unfortunately, the computed phase relations of these two ultradian rhythms were randomly distributed.

Despite these disappointing findings with cortisol, clear evidence has been gathered that other endocrine measures are tied to the sleep cycle. There are abundant data that growth hormone secretion is linked to Stages 3-4 (Parker et al., 1969; Quabbe et al., 1966, 1971), and many published illustrations of nocturnal growth hormone levels suggest a 90-100 min cycle at the beginning of the night, although rhythm statistics for growth hormone have not been reported. Pulsatile secretion of luteinizing hormone is probably time-locked to the REM-non-REM cycle but may occur before the REM period (Boyer et al., 1972 a,b; Rubin et al., 1972). Mandell and Mandell reported that urine output decreases markedly with Stage REM (Mandell et al., 1966 b), a suggestion that ADH is secreted differentially during REM periods. VMA (Mandell et al., 1966) and dehydroisoandrosterone (Rosenfeld et al., 1971) may also have ultradian secretion patterns.

In conclusion, a variety of hormones subject to neural influence display ultradian rhythms during sleep. Some of these hormones may also display ultradian rhythms during wakefulness (Weitzman et al., 1971), although the rhythmicity of waking secretion, oddly, has been less studied. Much work needs to be done to survey a wider variety of hormones, to establish statistically which hormonal levels are governed by ultradian rhythmic systems, and to explore whether hormonal rhythms are phase-coupled to the sleep-stage cycles. The analyses should control for time-of-night effects and consider episodic secretion out of phase with Stage REM as well as in phase. While the ultradian rhythmicity of Stage REM sleep was the first aspect of the nocturnal rhythm complex to become widely recognized, there is no rationale for considering Stage REM a *sine qua non* of rhythmic phenomena in physiologic or endocrine measures, and there are abundant data that oscillatory phenomena may persist without Stage REM itself. Hypothalmic and pituitary endocrine systems may play as large a role as sleep physiology in the ultradian rhythm complex.

ULTRADIAN RHYTHMS OUTSIDE OF SLEEP: PROBLEMS OF DEFINITION

The extraordinary interest of Stage REM, a tendency to reify the sleep stages conceptually, the historic predominance of the sleep staging method in quantifying physiological recordings, all have contributed to a habit of mind in which the ultradian rhythms exemplified by Stage REM were conceptualized as unique to sleep or dependent on Stage REM's occurrence. Berger (1969) argued that if one talks of a "Stage REM" cycle, by definition this cannot occur except when REM sleep occurs, certainly not in waking states. Berger's argument is purely semantic, but it does point out that to avoid confusion, we must call these rhythms by some name which does not imply they are restricted to sleep. How then can we define ultradian rhythms in a way which is both precise and more general?

Kleitman (1963, 1967, 1969) hypothesized a "Basic Rest Activity Cycle," or BRAC, on the assumption that what was seen during sleep was a "basic" rhythm modulating rest and activity throughout the 24 hr from infancy to old age. The name BRAC was inspired by studies of cycles in infants, in whom Stage REM is accompaned by very substantial visible motor activity. Kleitman feels that BRAC in infants is subharmonically coupled to feedings. In neonates, a cycle of this type is expressed through most of the 24 hr. Certain laboratory species also fit the model. Unfortunately, the BRAC concept seems less appropriate for adult humans, who may sleep without interruption and then remain active for long periods and where arousability and muscle tone are greatly decreased during Stage REM, so that "activity" is confined largely to the eyes and the EEG. It would seem confusing to use "BRAC" for a cycle which is accompanied by alternating rest and activity neither at night nor during the day. The BRAC concept also becomes paradoxical for narcoleptics, some of whom have daytime Stage REM sleep attacks at regular 90-120 min intervals (Passouant et al., 1969). It seems obvious that for the narcoleptics, Stage REM is not a phase of activity, but a phase of inactivity, the matter of "rest" being harder to define. Speaking of "rest-activity" cycles in hormonal functions seems even less appropriate but carries along an unsupported teleological surmise. Nevertheless, Kleitman's contribution in suggesting there may be a generalized oscillatory system modulating behavioral functions throughout the 24 hr has inspired an extremely fruitful area of inquiry.

The most formally acceptable way of conceptualizing a generalized oscillator seems to be to discuss an "ultradian" oscillator, without denoting it in terms of any particular variable (Kripke, 1972). As Halberg defines "ultradian rhythms," these may include any cyclic phenomena ranging from 1 cycle/19 hr up to many cycles per second, a vast frequency range including respiratory, cardiac, and EEG rhythms as well as many others less explored. We cannot include just any ultradian rhythm but must narrow our definition to those particular ultradian frequencies which are exemplified by their effect on sleep stage cycles. In a particular preparation, we might define an ultradian rhythm explicity by frequency, restricting our definition to oscillations with the frequency of Stage REM cycles in that preparation. Unfortunately, since the Stage REM rhythm varies in frequency even within a single night (Kripke et al., 1968; Verdone, 1968; Webb, 1971; Globus et al., 1972), this kind of definition is certain to be inexact. More serious, there is a substantial intersubject variation, with night-to-night variation in sleep cycle frequency (Moses et al., 1972), as well as lengthening during development (Sterman, 1972) and interspecies variability, apparently in relation to metabolic rate (Hartmann, 1968). Thus, there is such variability in the frequency of the sleep-cycle-related oscillator that definitions solely in terms of ultradian frequency may lead to confusion.

For these reasons, I believe the investigator of ultradian oscillators cannot rest safely on semantic definitions. We will have to describe particular oscillatory phenomena in terms of their frequency, amplitude, and qualitative aspects, and we must also provide evidence that the oscillations described are related to the oscillatory system governing Stage REM, if this is our implication. Clumsy though it seems, this approach is the only one which separates fact from speculation.

ULTRADIAN RHYTHMS OUTSIDE OF SLEEP:
HUMAN STUDIES

Kleitman (1963) cites Wada's (1922) description of gastric motility cycles as among the first reports suggesting 90 min cycles in wakefulness. It is interesting that in the last two decades, more emphasis has been placed on continuous polygraphic recordings during sleep than during wakefulness, and relatively few attempts have been made to search for phenomena in wakefulness similar to those being uncovered in sleep. For example, in a confinement study focusing on circadian rhythms, Schaefer et al. (1967) demonstrated clear cycles of about 2 hr duration, both graphically and spectrally, but did not comment on the relationship of these cycles either to the sleep stages or to wakefulness.

Dr. Gordon Globus was one of the first to explore the concept of an ultradian rhythm persisting throughout the 24 hr. He first sought to imply continuous rhythmicity by demonstrating an influence on the onset of Stage REM in naps apart from the time of going to sleep (Globus, 1966). This study will be considered below in our discussion of ultradian rhythm phase synchronizers. Globus (1968) also examined Rorschach responses obtained serially, and reported briefly some evidence for an ultradian rhythm in these responses. More recently he has studied waking subjects with highly objective automated measures. In a study of continuous visual performance in an isolation model, equivocal evidence for an about 100 min ultradian rhythm was obtained by correlating sinusoids iteratively to performance curves (Globus et al., 1971). In another study, subjects were isolated, and activity was studied using telemetry. Again, correlating sinusoids to the activity recordings yielded dubious evidence of an about 90 min ultradian (Globus et al., in press). The spectral techniques Globus used, as will be discussed later, may have underestimated the ultradian rhythm intensities in an attempt to obtain unnecessary frequency resolution.

In 1967, Friedman and Fisher (1967) reported a study of "orality" in waking humans confined in an observation chamber. They measured "orality" by observing when their subjects ate sandwiches, drank beverages, smoked, etc., and scored these observations according to special formulae. Cyclic oscillations in oral behavior were found. Friedman and Fisher reported an average cycle duration of 96 min (method unstated), but published a peak-synchronized average curve suggesting 4 cycles in 8 hr, a 2 hr. cycle. Friedman and Fisher interpreted their findings in terms of psychoanalytic concepts of oral drive, which they felt they were measuring. Although their study was subject to a number of criticisms on methodologic grounds, it has since been replicated by Oswald et al. (1970) using a more satisfactory design. Friedman has also described orality cycles in schizophrenics (Friedman, 1968) and in obese patients whose cycle frequency was correlated with weight (Friedman, 1972).

Kripke (1972) applied continuous EEG recording techniques to 5 experimental subjects studied in a perceptual isolation chamber. With automated objective recording techniques and spectral analyses, statistically significant 10-20 cycle/day rhythms were demonstrated while the subjects were awake in EEG delta band amplitude and certain other EEG frequencies, as well as operant lever presses for water. The ultradian rhythm in lever presses for water confirmed the idea of an "oral" behavioral rhythm with a completely automated and objective behavioral technique, and suggested a correlation of physiological and behavioral rhythms. As in the studies cited above, the waking cycles in these subjects tended to be somewhat longer than 90-100 min.

Considering that biological oscillations like those associated with Stage REM sleep appear to occur in waking humans, one wonders if discrete periods like the REM periods of sleep may be identified while we are awake. Although obviously the REM sleep state, as such, cannot be present during waking life, some analogous state in which consciousness is maintained might be. Othmer et al. (1969) studied subjects in several isolation models, and reported that periods of rapid eye movement occurred throughout the 24 hr, both when the subjects were asleep, and when they were awake. Othmer et al. stated that the REM intervals of wakefulness were associated with "dramaturgic" daydreams, however their descriptions were not supported by formalized controls or time series analyses.

More recently, D. Sonnenshein and I have attempted to measure waking fantasy, predicting a cycle in daydreaming analagous to nocturnal dreaming (Kripke and Sonnenshein, unpublished). Naive subjects were confined for 10 hr in a well lighted room in which they could move about, and in response to a whistle sounded every 5 min, they wrote summaries of their thoughts over the 5 min intervals. These responses were randomized and sorted independently on a daydream-like fantasy scale by both the subjects and an experimenter. The ratings of two raters were always highly correlated (average Rs=0.83). Variance spectra were computed from the fantasy ratings, revealing a very plain and highly significant 90 min rhythm in the reports of daydreams. Analyses of simultaneous physiological recordings are presently being made.

In summary, there are now a variety of reports, some with acceptable design and statistical methods, demonstrating that ultradian rhythms can be found in waking humans. Such cycles have been described in subjective fantasy, operant behavior (especially oral behavior), and physiological measures. In adult humans, the waking cycles may be closer to 1 cycle/120 min than 1 cycle/90 min. Each of the studies has employed an isolation model both for its technical simplicity and to exclude environmental interference in presumed endogenous cycles. There is a need for measurement of subjects in normal perceptual environments, a task begun by Friedman and Fisher with one subject observed at home (Friedman and Fisher, 1967).

A problem with each of the studies so far is that the measurement of ultradian frequency has been unsatisfactory, and it remains to be demonstrated whether waking ultradian rhythms differ in frequency from those of sleep, as might be expected from circadian frequency modulation. More evidence is needed to establish that the phenomena result from a common oscillatory system, an inference based presently only on the resemblance of the cycles described. While rhythms have been measured in a variety of functions, very little is known about whether there is a primary oscillator to which all of these subsystems are coupled, and if so, what the primary oscillator is.

ANIMAL STUDIES OF ULTRADIAN RHYTHMS

The exploration of waking ultradian rhythms in experimental animals has only just begun. Laboratory animals, like infant humans, are less likely to be awake or asleep for long periods, so that studies of prolonged periods of extended wakefulness (or sleep) are more difficult. On the other hand, the ease of collecting well controlled data from experimental animals suggests rich possibilities for this field of study.

My colleagues at Holloman Air Force Base recorded a series of rhesus monkeys for over 24 hr each after they had been carefully stabilized on a 12 hr light, 12 hr dark regime (Crowley et al., 1972). During the dark span, the monkeys slept 80% of the time, and least squares spectra indicated ultradian rhythms in Stage REM as well as other sleep stages and EEG measures (Kripke, 1970). During the light span, the monkeys were awake about 80% of the time, and spent less than 1% of the time in Stage REM. Nevertheless, it was possible to demonstrate statistically significant ultradian rhythms in physiological measures during lights-on (Fig. 4). More recently, these data have been reanalyzed with variance spectra, which indicate that the ultradian rhythms were considerably slower during the lights-on interval than at night (unpublished data). Iterative least-squares spectra based on 4 hr intervals suggested circadian frequency modulation, with slowing during lights-on.

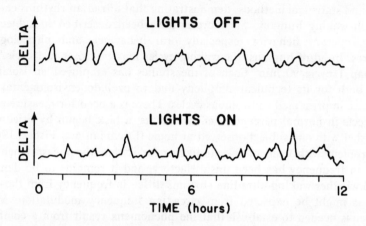

Fig. 4. EEG delta frequency band amplitude modulation in a monkey is shown for (A) 12 hr of lights-out when the monkey was largely asleep, and (B) 12 hr of lights-on when the monkey was largely awake. An about 1 hr cycle is obvious in both conditions.

Sterman and colleagues have reported an important series of studies of ultradian rhythms in cats (Lucas, 1972; Sterman, 1972; Sterman et al., 1972). They developed methods of reliably scoring the feline REM/non-REM cycle during sleep, and showed that there was an about 20 min ultradian rhythm in this measure, confirmed by spectral analyses. Sterman and Lucas then measured activity, EEG frequencies, and performance in waking cats under a variety of conditions. They found that operant EEG responses for a food reward, operant lever presses for food reward, and operant EEG responses for brain stimulation all displayed a 20 min ultradian rhythm which could be scored with methods similar to those used for scoring sleep stages. An interesting feature of the work of Sterman and Lucas was the clear demonstration in a formalized behavioristic model that ultradian rhythms may modulate a variety of appetitive performances, or to put it another way, consummatory behaviors occurred rhythmically. The cycles were similar from one performance to another. Not only the average intervals, but the interval histograms of sleep cycles and performance cycles were similar. When transitions from sleep to wakefulness or wakefulness to sleep were examined, there appeared to be a phase continuity between waking performance periods and REM periods in sleep. Finally, the duration of performance periods within the cycles was similar to the duration of REM periods, implying that during wakefulness as well as sleep, the ultradian cycles may be generated by a relaxation oscillator keyed by brief, intense consummatory states.

SYNCHRONIZATION OF ULTRADIAN RHYTHMS

For an oscillatory phenomenon to be defined as a biorhythm, it should display ongoing rhythmicity in the absence of known synchronizers, and it should also respond by being entrained to a known synchronizer. For the most part, synchronizers have been absent from studies of ultradian rhythms either in wakefulness or sleep. The ultradian cycles appear to be free-running, and the marked variability of these cycles—within single recordings, between recordings, between subjects, and between preparations— makes it difficult to conceive that an external synchronizer could be driving the rhythms. Thus, they seem to be endogenous. The response of the rhythms to synchronizers when they are presented is less well studied.

Globus (1966) reported data from the daytime naps of 2 subjects suggesting that the time of onset of REM periods within the naps was related to clock time. Globus operationally referenced the REM period onsets to actual clock times, but presented no data whether the relevant synchronizers were literally time pieces or some related circadian synchronizing reference such as luncheon. Further studies of naps have not been done. Lewis (in press) examined Globus's hypothesis as it applies to nocturnal sleep, arguing that since it is well known that the first REM period tends to occur 60-90 min. after sleep onset, the time of going to bed must have some influence on the phase of the REM cycle. If circadian references apart from the time of going to bed also influence when the first REM period occurs, then the time when the first REM period occurs should be less variable than the times of going to bed and of sleep onset. Lewis reported night sleep recordings which failed to support these predictions.

Crowley et al. studied the sleep cycles of a large group of monkeys whose circadian cycles had been rigidly synchronized by a controlled circadian lighting and feeding regime (Crowley et al., 1972). If light cycles entrain the phase of ultradian rhythms, the ultradian phases should certainly have been synchronized by these rigid conditions, and time-averaged curves of a group of animals should accentuate in-phase ultradian rhythms rather than averaging them out. We computed these curves and found that immediately after the lights-out events, the ultradian rhythms of these monkeys were indeed strongly synchronized (in preparation). Synchrony was rapidly lost during the night, disappearing after a few cycles. If the lights-off synchronizer did not completely set ultradian phase, we would expect averaged curves computed by aligning the first peaks of the ultradian rhythms to display additional rhythmicity. In fact, when the data from the monkeys was averaged in this manner, the ultradian cycle in the averaged curves was not only larger but also persisted through several more cycles. This seems to indicate that after the phase-resetting influence of the lights-off synchronizer diminished, an endogenous phase component was reasserted. Synchrony was lost in both forms of averaged curves before the end of the 12 hr dark intervals, no doubt because of slight variations in ultradian frequency between animals. The data confirm Globus's hypothesis, in the sense that a gross circadian synchronizer reset ultradian phases, but the implication that the phase is set in "real-time" apart from the obvious light-dark synchronizer was not confirmed, since the synchrony was lost late at night.

Some information is available concerning the effects of synchronizers on ultradian rhythms expressed under conditions of intermittent sleep. Passouant (in press) subjected narcoleptics to an experience where they were asked to recline briefly in a darkened room every 2 hr. In this environment, the patients fell asleep with a regular 2 hr rhythm, indicating that the experience acted as a synchronizer for daytime sleep attacks which were otherwise more variable. In addition, several studies have been performed presenting ultradian light/dark cycles to rodents. Whereas the usual Stage REM cycle in rats is around 12 min in duration, rats subjected to a cycle of 25 min light and 5 min dark (Lisk and Sawyer, 1966; Johnson et al., 1970), or 5 min light and 5 min dark displayed Stage REM almost wholly within the dark intervals, even though they are dark-active animals under circadian lighting cycles. Apparently, these experiments indicate that Stage REM can be entrained by light-dark cycles, but many issues involving the range of frequencies which entrain successfully, the time required for entrainment to occur, etc., remain to be resolved. It cannot be stated that the 30 min sleep-wake ultradian entrained was functionally the same rhythm as the free-running 12 min REM-non-REM sleep ultradian, for the question was not examined.

STATISTICAL DESCRIPTION OF ULTRADIAN RHYTHMS

There has been so little agreement among investigators in describing ultradian oscillators statistically, that a few comments concerning the problems involved may offer a useful perspective.

In reporting a biorhythm, one asserts that there is a substantial tendency for highs and lows in some measure to recur at regular intervals, and with a repeating waveform. Usually, there is unexplained "random" variance superimposed on the rhythm, so that a visual analysis of curve plots may leave the reader unsatisfied as to whether or not a rhythm is actually present. With a spectral analysis, one separates the total variance of the time series into its frequency components, and examines their relative amplitudes (Blackman and Tukey, 1958; Mercer, 1960; Halbert and Panofsky, 1961).

While random variance should yield a flat spectrum, a rhythm produces a sharp peak at its primary frequency. Nonsinusoidal rhythms will also produce peaks at harmonic frequencies, but often we can usefully assume a sinusoidal wave shape, and in some cases a sinusoidal ultradian frequency accounts for over 50% of the total variance of our data (Lubin et al., 1973). If we examine a group of subjects with spectra, a simple "T" test can demonstrate that variance at a predicted frequency exceeds variance in the adjacent frequencies at either side, so that the null hypothesis is rejected (A. Lubin, personal communication).

As has been mentioned, sleep stage cycles are very variable in amplitude and duration, even within a single night's recording. Amplitude trends, and probably frequency trends, have been well documented (Dement and Kleitman, 1957; Kripke et al., 1968; Verdone, 1968; Lubin et al., 1973). In addition, the amplitude of ultradian rhythms in particular variables certainly varies from sleep to wakefulness (Kripke et al., 1970), and there are many suggestions that waking ultradian frequencies are somewhat slower. In Figure 2, we illustrate how different curves might remain coupled in phase and undergo identical circadian frequency modulations but display opposite phases of circadian amplitude modulations.

Few investigators seem to have realized the consequences of frequency variability, both systematic and random, for analyses of ultradian rhythms. Statistical techniques derived from astronomy, electronics, or even circadian rhythm studies (where an astronomical synchronizer is present) are quite inappropriate when they assume phase and amplitude stationarity in the rhythms. For example, if one fits a sinusoid to nonstationary data (Fig. 5),

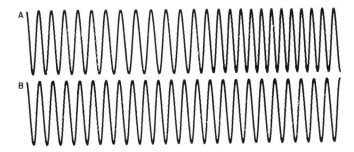

Fig. 5. The effect of fitting (A) a rhythm with frequency modulation to (B) a test sinusoid. The frequency modulated rhythm is at times in phase with the sinusoid and at times out of phase, so the effects cancel.

frequency shifting causes the data to shift in and out of phase with the test sinusoid, cancelling out an accurate estimate of the rhythm's amplitude. As I have learned from bitter experience, this is the case with any statistical method which effectively fits a sinusoid to the whole data interval, whether it be a least squares sinusoidal fit (Kripke et al., 1970; Kripke, 1972), a correlational sinusoidal fit (Globus et al., 1971), or the folded fast Fourier transform (Sterman et al., 1972). On the other hand, variance spectra derived from autocorrelation (Blackman and Tukey, 1958; Mercer, 1960; Halberg and Panofsky, 1961) are less sensitive to nonstationarity, providing that the maximum autocorrelation lag is only several cycle intervals. An illustration of the effects of non-stationarity is given in Figure 6, where variance spectra were computed both from short autocorrelations and from long ones (analogous in sensitivity to the least squares spectra, correlation spectra, or fast Fourier transform). The short autocorrelation spectra correctly display

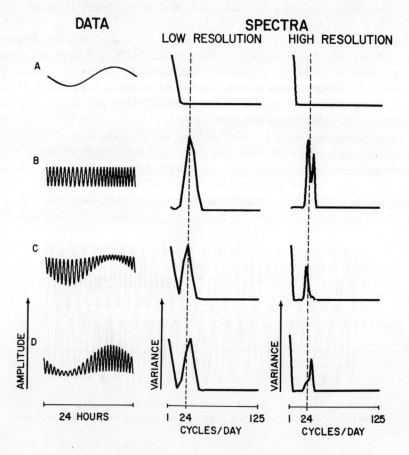

Fig. 6. (A) Circadian curve; (B) ultradian curve with circadian frequency modulation; (C) circadian rhythm with an ultradian rhythm superimposed having circadian frequency and amplitude modulation. The circadian and ultradian rhythms are of equal mean amplitude. (D) The same as (C) except the circadian amplitude modulation is out of phase, resulting in a shift in the high resolution ultradian spectral peak.

the average ultradian frequency in the curves as similar, even when circadian amplitude and frequency modulation are superimposed, and also, the short autocorrelation spectra correctly display the ultradian amplitude as comparable to the circadian amplitude. The high resolution spectra suggest that the ultradian rhythms in the two data curves differ substantially in frequency (which is misleading), and also, they severely underestimate the relative amplitude of the ultradian rhythm. Some investigators have avoided low resolution variance spectra because they wished very precise estimates of ultradian rhythm frequency. In actual fact, the spectral peak of ultradian rhythms is usually broad because of frequency modulation or variability, and little is gained from resolving beyond the consistency of the data. The higher the resolution of the spectral method, the poorer its reliability.

SPECULATIONS

The remarkable association of Stage REM with dreaming, the related proof that dreaming is part of everyone's normal function, and the discovery of extraordinary neurophysiologic and autonomic discharges during Stage REM have seemed to imply that Stage REM has something to do with emotion or appetency. Even from the neurophysiologist's viewpoint (Moruzzi, 1969), REM is seen as an instinctual consummatory process. Nevertheless, attempts to demonstrate direct relationships between the sleep stages and mental disturbances or the great passions have been discouraging. This has inspired a search for intervening variables, for example, the interest in PGO spikes and the turning of sleep physiologists to neuropharmacology. Our inquiry in ultradian rhythms has a similar motivation, for it would seem that if similar oscillatory systems can be identified in wakefulness and sleep, then a common function of waking states and REM sleep can be explored experimentally. Although Stage REM itself obviously does not occur during wakefulness, biorhythm measurement can give us a way of identifying when similar processes are occurring, and what influences their dynamics.

As expected from the association of ultradian oscillations with REM sleep, waking ultradian rhythms do appear to be related to appetitive functions. Consummatory behaviors such as "oral" ingestion, operant responses for rewarding brain stimulation, etc., have been among the most prominent indicators of waking ultradian rhythms, indeed, the behavioral measures may display the rhythms more clearly than physiological recordings. Although we need much more data to conclude that all "rhythms" are part of a unified system, it presently appears that eating, activity, fantasying, hormonal pulses, genital expressions, etc., may all be tied to the same oscillator, as if an ultradian oscillator modulates a polymorphous appetency similar to that hypothesized by Freud. Perhaps the oscillatory system serves to regulate the satisfaction of appetitive needs, which are more efficiently achieved through brief intense consummatory states. It seems almost obvious that brief consummatory experiences must—almost by necessity—express a relaxation oscillator, rather than the slow, steady "water over the dam" patterns of drive discharge more popular in metapsychologic modeling. The values of an oscillatory system gating an assortment of appetitive functions through a common mechanism must also be conceptualized. Certainly, mammals must display an adaptable range of behaviors and must satisfy various appetencies in a modulated sequence, rather than all at once. Stereotyped or uncoordinated goal-directed behaviors could endanger survival unless they could be deferred or redirected in response to environmental circumstances. Moruzzi (1969) argued that consummatory satisfactions may be accomplished through consummatory cerebral *sensations*, whether or not the teleological goal of the state is achieved through behavior—thus the sleep dream or waking fantasy and the waking behavior may equally relax a consummatory urge, but an opportunity is provided to modify the behavioral expression according to ecologic circumstances. Were it not possible to release appetency through varied modalities, they might build to an irresistable pressure—the very dangers the psychoanalysts warn against. Perhaps the ultradian oscillatory systems are those by which certain appetencies are modulated, directed or redirected, and discharged before building to dangerous levels. If this is the case, exploring ultradian oscillatory systems supplies us with an experimental approach to the motivational systems of human existence.

REFERENCES

Baekeland, F. The effect of methylphenidate on the sleep cycle in man. *Psychopharmacologia* 10, 179-183 (1966).

Baekeland, F. Pentobarbital and dextroamphetamine sulfate: Effects on the sleep cycle in man. *Psychopharmacologia 11*, 388-396 (1967).

Berger, R.J. Rapid eye movement sleep: A sleep-dependent process. *Science 166*, 530-531 (1969).

Blackman, R.B. and Tukey, J.W. *The Measurement of Power Spectra*, Dover Publications, New York, 1958.

Boyar, R., Finkelstein, J., Roffwarg, H. et al. Synchronization of augmented luteinizing hormone secretion with sleep during puberty. *New Engl. J. Med. 287*, 582-586 (1972a).

Boyar, R., Perlow, M., Hellman, L. et al. Twenty-four hour pattern of luteinizing hormone secretion in normal men with sleep stage recording. *J. Clin. Endocrinol. Metab. 35*, 73-81 (1972b).

Brebbia, D.R. and Altshuler, K.Z. Stage related patterns and nightly trends of energy exchange during sleep. in, *Computers and Electronic Devices in Psychiatry,* N. Kline and E. Laska, Eds., Grune & Stratton, 1968, New York, pp. 319-335.

Cartwright, R.D., Monroe, L.J., and Palmer, C. Individual differences in response to REM deprivation. *Arch. Gen. Psychiat. 16*, 297-303 (1967).

Cartwright, R.D. Dreams, reality, and fantasy. in, *The Meaning of Dreams: Recent Insights from the Laboratory.* J. Fisher and L. Breger, Eds., California Mental Health Research Symposium No. 3, California Department of Mental Hygiene, 1969, pp. 101-119.

Cartwright, R.D. and Ratzel, R.W. Effects of dream loss on waking behavior. *Arch. Gen. Psychiat.* 27, 227-280 (1972).

Coccagna, G., Mantovani, M., Brignani, F. et al. Arterial pressure changes during spontaneous sleep in man. *Electroenceph. Clin. Neurophysiol.* 31, 277-281 (1971).

Crowley, R.J., Kripke, D.F., Halberg, F. et al. Circadian rhythms of Macaca mulatta: Sleep, EEG, body and eye movement and temerature. *Primates* 12, 149-168 (1972).

Dement, W. and Kleitman, N. Cyclic variations in EEG during sleep and their relation to eye movements, body motility, and dreaming. *Electroenceph. Clin. Neurophysiol.* 9, 673-690 (1957).

Dement, W., Ferguson, J., Cohen, H. and Barchas, J. Nonchemical methods and data using a biochemical model: The REM quanta. in, *Methods and Theory in Psychochemical Research in Man,* A. Mandell and M. Mandell, Eds., Academic Press, New York, 1969, pp. 275-325.

Friedman, S. Oral activity cycles in mild chronic schizophrenia. *Amer. J. Psychiatry* 125, 743-751 (1968).

Friedman, S. On the presence of a variant form of instinctual regression: oral drive cycles in obesity-bulimia. *Psychoanalytic Quart.* 41, 364-383 (1972).

Friedman, S. and Fisher, C. On the presence of a rhythmic, diurnal, oral instinctual drive cycle in man: A preliminary report. *J. Amer. Psychoanal. Assoc.* 225, 959-960 (1967).

Globus, G.G. Observations on sub-circadian rhythms. *Psychophysiology* 4, 366 (1968).

Globus, G.G. Quantification of the sleep cycle as a rhythm. *Psychophysiology* 7, 244-253 (1970).

Globus, G.G. Rapid eye movement cycle in real time. *Arch. Gen. Psychiat.* 15, 654-659 (1966).

Globus, G.G., Drury, R.I., Phoebus, E.C., and Boyd, R. Ultradian rhythms in human performance. *Percept. Motor Skills* 33, 1171-1174 (1971).

Globus, G.G., Phoebus, E.C. and Boyd, R. Temporal organization of night workers' sleep. *Aerosp. Med.* 43, 266-8 (1972).

Globus, G.G., Phoebus, E.C., Humphries, J. et al. Ultradian rhythms in human telemetered gross motor activity, in press.

Halberg, F. and Panofsky, H. Thermovariance spectra: Method and clinical illustrations. *Exp. Med. Surg.* 19, 284-309 (1961); Thermovariance spectra: simplified computational example and other methodology. *ibid.,* 19, 323-338 (1961).

Halberg, F. Physiologic considerations underlying rhythmometry, with special reference to emotional illness. in, *Cycles Biologiques et Psychiatrie* (Symposium Bel-Air II), J. Ajuriaguerra, Ed., Geneve, 1967, pp. 73-126.

Hartmann, E. The 90-minute sleep-dream cycle. *Arch. Gen. Psychiat.* 18, 280-286 (1968).

Hilbert, R. and Naitoh, P. EOG and delta rhythmicity in human sleep EG. *Psychophysiology* 9, 533-538 (1972).

Johnson, J.H., Adler, N.T., and Sawyer, C.H. Effects of various photoperiods on the temporal distribution of paradoxical sleep in rats. *Exper. Neurol.* 27, 162-171 (1970).

Kales, A. and Tan, T.L. Sleep alterations associated with medical illnesses. in *Sleep Physiology and Pathology,* A. Kales, Ed., Lippincott, Philadelphia, 1969, pp. 148-157.

Karacan, I. The developmental aspect and the effect of certain clinical conditions upon penile erection during sleep. in, *Proc. Fourth World Congr. Psychiatry.* Excerpta Medica International Congress Series, No. 150, 1966, pp. 2356-2359.

Karacan, I., Goodenough, D.R., Shapiro, A. and Starker, S. Erection cycle during sleep in relation to dream anxiety. *Arch. Gen. Psychiat.* 15, 183-189 (1966).

Karacan, I., Hursch, C.J., Williams, R.L. and Thornby, J.I. Some characteristics of nocturnal penile tumescence in young adults. *Arch. 'Gen. Psychiat.* 26, 351-356 (1972).

Kawamura, H. Whitmoyer, D.I., and Sawyer, C.H. Temperature changes in the rabbit brain during paradoxical sleep. *Electroenceph. Clin. Neurophysiol* 21, 469-477 (1966).

Kleitman, N. *Sleep and Wakefulness.* University of Chicago Press, Chicago, 1963.

Kleitman, N. Phylogenetic, ontogenetic and environmental mental determinants in the evolution of sleep-wakefulness cycles. in, *Sleep and Altered States of Consciousness* (Research Publications of the Association for Research in Nervous and Mental Disease, Vol. 45), S.S. Kety, E.V. Evarts and H.L. Williams, Eds., Williams, and Wilkins, Baltimore, 1967, pp. 30-38.

Kleitman, N. Basic rest activity cycle in relation to sleep and wakefulness.in, *Sleep Physiology & Pathology*, A. Kales, Ed., Lippincott, Philadelphia, 1969, pp. 33-38.

Kripke, D.F., Reite, M.L., Pegram, G.V. et al. Nocturnal sleep in Rhesus monkeys. *Electroenceph. Clin. Neurophysiol. 24*, 582-586 (1968).

Kripke, D.F., Halberg, F., Crowley, T.J. and Pegram, G.V. Ultradian rhythms in Rhesus monkeys. *Psychophysiology 7*, 307-308 (1970).

Kripke, D.F. An ultradian biological rhythm associated with perceptual deprivation and REM sleep. *Psychosomatic Med. 34*, 221-234 (1972).

Kripke, D.F. and Sonnenshein, D. in preparation.

Lewis, S. The paradoxical sleep cycle revisited. in, *Chronobiology* (Proceedings of the International Society for the Study of Biological Rhythms, Little Rock, Ark.) L.E. Scheving, F. Halberg, and J.E. Pauly, Eds., Igaku Shoin, Ltd., Tokyo, in press.

Lisk, R.D. and Sawyer, C.H. Induction of paradoxical sleep by lights-off stimulation. *Proc. Soc. Exper. Biol. Med. 123*, 664-667 (1966).

Lubin, A., Nute, C., Naitoh, P. and Martin, W.B. EEG delta activity during human sleep as a damped ultradian rhythm. *Psychophysiology 10*, 27-35 (1973).

Lucas, E.A. Sleep-waking and rest activity cycles in the laboratory cat: Effects of behavioral conditioning and basal forebrain lesions. Thesis, UCLA, 1972 University Microfilms 72-18, 133.

Luce, G.G. *Biological Rhythms in Psychiatry and Medicine*. Public Health Service Publication No. 2088, 1970.

Mandell, A.J., Brill, P.L., Mandell, M.P. et al. Urinary excretion of 3-methoxy-4-hydroxymandelic acid during dreaming sleep in man. *Life Sci. 5*, 169-173 (1966a).

Mandell, A.J., Chaffey, B., Brill, P. et al. Dreaming sleep in man: Changes in urine volume and osmolality. *Science 151*, 1558-1560 (1966b).

Mandell, M.P., Mandell, A.J., Rubin, R.T. et al. Activation of the pituitary-adrenal axis during rapid eye movement sleep in man. *Life Sci. 5*, 583-587 (1966c).

Mercer, D.M.A. Analytical methods for the study of periodic phenomena obscured by random fluctations. *Biological Clocks. Cold Spring Harbor Symp. Quant. Biol. Vol. 25*, 73-84 (1960).

Moruzzi, G. Sleep and instinctual behavior. *Arch. Ital. Biol. 108*, 175-216 (1969).

Moses, J., Lubin, A., Naitoh, P. and Johnson, L.C. Reliability of sleep measures. *Psychophysiology 9*, 78-82 (1972).

Oswald, I., Merrington, J., and Lewis, H. Cyclical "on demand" oral intake by adults. *Nature 225*, 959-960 (1970).

Othmer, E., Hayden, M.P., and Segelbaum, R. Encephalic cycles during sleep and wakefulness in humans: A 24-hour pattern. *Science 164*, 447-449 (1969).

Parker, D.C., Sassin, J.F., Mace, J.W., et al. Human growth hormone release during sleep: Electroencephalographic correlation. *J. Clin. Endocrinol. Metab., 29*, 871-74 (1969).

Passouant, P. REM's ultradian rhythm during 24 hours in narcolepsy. in, *Chronobiology* (Proceedings of the International Society for the Study of Biological Rhythms, Little Rock, Ark.) L.W. Scheving, F. Halberg, and J.E. Pauly, Eds., Igaku Shoin, Ltd., Tokyo, in press.

Passouant, P., Halberg, F., Genicot, R. et al. La périodicité des accès narcoleptiques et le rythme ultradien du sommeil rapide. *Rev. Neurol. [Paris] 121*, 155-164 (1969).

Pollak, C.P., Weitzman, E.D., and Kripke, D.F. Arousal threshold ranges: Threshold ranges as determined by electrical stimulation of the brain during stages of sleep in the monkey (Macaca mulatta). *Arch. Neurol. [Chicago] 11*, 94-102 (1967).

Quabbe, H.J., Schilling, E., and Helge, H. Pattern of growth hormone secretion during a 24-hour fast in normal adults. *J. Clin. Endocrinol. Metab. 26*, 1173-1177 (1966).

Quabbe, H.J., Helge, H. and Kubicki, S. Nocturnal growth hormone secretion: Correlation with sleeping EEG in adults and pattern in children and adolescents with non-pituitary dwarfism, overgrowth, and with obesity. *Acta Endocrinol. 67*, 767-783 (1971).

Rechtschaffen, A. and Kales, A. *Manual of Standardized Terminology, Techniques, and Scoring System for Sleep Stages of Human Subjects.* National Institutes of Health Publication No. 204. Washington, Superintendent of Documents. Book 1-62, 1968.

Rechtschaffen, A., Dates, R., Tobias, M. and Whitehead, W.E. The effect of lights-off stimulation on the distribution of paradoxical sleep in the rat. *Commun. Behav. Biol. 3*, 93-99 (1969).

Reite, M.L. and Pegram, G.V. Cortical temperature during paradoxical sleep in the monkey. *Electroenceph. Clin. Neurophysiol. 25*, 36-41 (1968).

Rosenfeld, R.S., Hellman, L., Roffwarg, H. et al. Dehydroisoandrosterone is secreted episodically and synchronously with cortisol by normal man. *J. Clin. Endocrinol. Metab. 33*, 87-92 (1971).

Rubin, R.T., Kales, A., Adler, R. et al. Gonadotropin secretion during sleep in normal adult men. *Science 175*, 116-198 (1972).

Schaefer, K.E., Clegg, B.R., Carey, C.R. et al. Effect of isolation in a constant environment on periodicity of physiological functions and performance levels. *Aerosp. Med. 38*, 1002 1028 (1967).

Sinha, A.K., Smythe, H., Zarcone, V.P. et al. Human sleep-electroencephalogram:A damped oscillatory phenomenon. *J. Theoret. Biol. 35*, 387-393 (1972).

Sterman, M.B. The basic rest-activity cycle and sleep: Developmental considerations in man and cats. in, *Sleep and the Maturing Nervous System*, C.D. Clemente, D.P. Purpura, and F.E. Mayer, Eds., Academic Press, New York, 1972, pp. 175-197.

Sterman, M.B., Lucas, E.A. and Macdonald, L.R. Periodicity within sleep and operant performance in the cat. *Brain Res. 38*, 327-341 (1972).

Verdone, P. Sleep satiation: Extended sleep in normal subjects. *Electroenceph. Clin. Neurophysiol. 24*, 417-423 (1968).

Wada, T. An experimental study of hunger and its relation to activity. *Arch. Psychol. Monogr. 8*, 1 (1922).

Webb, W.B. Sleep behavior as a biorhythm. in, *Biological Rhythms and Human Performance*, W.P. Colquehoun. Ed., Academic Press, New York, 1971, pp. 149-178.

Weitzman, E.D., Schaumburg, H., and Fishbein, W. Plasma 11-hyroxycorticosteroid levels during sleep in man. *J. Clin. Endocrinol. Metab. 26*, 121-127 (1966).

Weitzman, E.D., Kripke, D.R., Kream, J. et al. The effect of a prolonged non-geographic 180-degree sleep-wake cycle shift on body temperature, plasma growth hormone, cortisol, and urinary 17-OHCS. *Psychophysiology 7*, 307 [1970].

Weitzman, E.D., Fukushima, D., Nogeire, C. et al. Twenty-four hour pattern of the episodic secretion of cortisol in normal subjects. *J. Clin. Endocrinol. Metab. 33*, 14-22 (1971).

Wyatt, R.J. The serotonin-catecholamine-dream bicycle: A clinical study. *Biol. Psychiat. 5*, 33-64 (1972).

Advances in Sleep Research, Vol. 1
© 1974, Spectrum Publications, Inc.

CHAPTER 7

Sleep and the Sudden Infant Death Syndrome: A New Hypothesis*

ELLIOT D. WEITZMAN
LEONARD GRAZIANI

INTRODUCTION

During the past 10 years, a series of epidemiologic studies, as well as in-depth analysis of the case histories of the Sudden Infant Death Syndrome (SIDS) have led to the following set of generally accepted conclusions (Bergman et al, 1970). The rate of occurrence (3 per 1000 live births or 10,000 deaths per year in the United States) makes it the greatest single cause of death during the first year after birth, excluding the first week of life. Since this syndrome has no code in the International Classification of Diseases, it has been suggested that this figure may be underestimated because of under-reporting and that the actual incidence may approach 18,000 deaths per year (Labor and Public Welfare Committee, 1972). The typical clinical syndrome is that of a generally healthy infant of 2-4 months of age who is put to sleep in his crib at night and is found dead shortly thereafter or in the morning, having died several hours before. Autopsy examination reveals no abnormalities recognized as cause for death.

Investigators have attempted to determine the cause of SIDS and have proposed a number of hypotheses. None of the following, however, has proved to be tenable when studied: stress, cortisol insufficiency, parathyroid inadequacy, bacterial infection, epidural hemorrhage, and infanticide. The recent series of workshops sponsored by the NICHD, have considered immunological mechanisms, cardio-respiratory, thermal and metabolic mechanisms, and epidemiological and behavioral aspects, have generated new hypotheses, and have reviewed evidence in support or against previously proposed hypotheses (Nat. Ins. Child Health and Develop., in press).

*This paper was derived in part from a report written by the authors for a workshop on neurophysiologic factors associated with the Sudden Infant Death Syndrome, sponsored by the U.S. Public Health Service, The National Institute of Child Health and Development.

An area of consideration notably overlooked until recently, has been the role of the central nervous system in the pathogenesis of SIDS. The following clinical observations strongly suggest that neuro-physiological events should be seriously considered as possible pathogenetic mechanisms in the cause of SIDS. In almost all cases carefully reviewed, the infant died during the sleeping period. For example, in a study carried out by Bergman et al., (1970) in Seattle, Washington, not one case out of 119 autopsied was observed while the infant was dying; all were discovered lifeless during or at the end of a sleeping period. A more recent report by Bergman (1972) on 170 cases confirms the previous findings. In a study carried out in Middle Bohemia, Czechoslovakia, 88 percent of 502 cases were *found* dead; only 7 percent died in the mother's arms and 5 percent died while being transported to a doctor or hospital (Bergman et al., 1970). In the Seattle study, 74 percent of the babies were found dead between 6 AM and noon, most between 7 AM and 9 AM, at the time the mother awoke in the morning and went in to tend the baby. Of the 14 percent found dead between 12 noon and 6 PM most were at the end of the afternoon nap. A similar pattern was noted in the Czechoslovakian study, with about 75 percent of the babies found dead between midnight and noon. Valdes-Dapena has made a careful analysis regarding the time of death in 90 babies; the great majority were found dead at night during the sleeping period (Valdes-Dapena et al., 1968). In addition, interviews with the parents indicate that the death was silent. That is, the baby was not heard to gasp, cough or have sounds of stridor. This has been reported by mothers who were in the same room, even next to the baby, both awake and asleep when death had occurred. There have been case reports of babies who stopped breathing either during or just after feeding—becoming cyanotic and dying. Autopsies of these infants revealed no specific cause of death; and no evidence of aspiration of the feeding fluid. There have been a number of case reports in which death occurred during a sleep period in a car bed while the parents were driving, again the death occurring silently (Labor and Public Welfare Committee, 1972).

The issues of prematurity, gestational age, and birth weight must be taken into account it appears, when considering possible CNS maturational factors. For babies born weighing 5.5 to 6.5 pounds (full term), the incidence is about 3 deaths per 1,000 live births; for those 3.5 to 4.5 pounds it is about 13 per 1,000. Because neonatal survivors with birth weights below 2.5 pounds are rare the incidence of SIDS is difficult to determine in the very low birth weight group. The postnatal age at death however is approximately the same for all groups. SIDS occurs more frequently in prematurely born infants, particularly those with gestational ages between 34 and 35 weeks (Dr. M. Duval, Labor and Public Welfare Committee, Senate Testimony January 25, 1972). If these figures are confirmed by subsequent studies, the incidence of SIDS will be significantly related to gestational age.

There is also evidence that the "aborted crib death" or "near miss" baby may be at a much higher risk level of subsequently dying of SIDS (Bergman et al, 1970, 1972). These are babies who are brought to the emergency room or to their doctor apneic and/or cyanotic and are resuscitated. Physical and laboratory examinations are normal and the infant is then taken home either immediately or after 1-2 days of hospital study. As many as 20 percent of them, however, may succumb to SIDS occurring within the next several weeks. These observations tend to support a concept that relates the occurrence of SIDS to a CNS maturational factor. If this is borne out by focused studies, the concept argues against a hypothesis of a specific exogenous factor(s) such as a particular infection or single environmental variable which occurs only once in the infant's life. Infants who have had a near-miss provide a unique and important study population. Steinschneider has studied heart rate and respiratory patterns in several of these infants (some from the same sib-ship) and his data are consistent with the theory that prolonged or excessive apneas occuring during sleep can result in SIDS if not reversed (Lipton et al., 1966; Steinschneider, 1972). On follow-up of some of these infants, prolonged apneas were noted during an upper respiratory infection. He found that a useful measurement during sleep is the ratio of apnea time to total sleep time with the frequency of apnea during REM sleep permitting quantitative comparisons between study and normal infants. For purposes of those studies, apnea was defined as cessation of respirations for 2 seconds or longer. In infants with a previous near-miss the ratio of apnea to sleep time was high and there were more episodes of prolonged apneas (15 sec or longer) compared to normal infants.

On the basis of the above evidence, a conceptual neurophysiological hypothesis related to the pathogenesis of SIDS can be formulated. The presumed critical event is a prolonged apneic episode occurring during sleep. If the prolonged cessation of breathing is not interrupted either by arousal and/or direct resuscitation, it will lead to progressive anoxia and cyanosis, elevation of blood CO_2, and cardiac arrest. If the baby is aroused or resuscitated in *time*, the situation is totally and immediately reversible and the baby appears to be quite healthy. This conceptual view presupposes that there is no pulmonary or cardiac disease, or bronchial or tracheal pathology severe enough to produce a cardio-respiratory cause of apnea. However, a relatively minor abnormality, such as upper respiratory viral infection might act as a contributing or initiating factor.

KNOWN DISORDERS IN MAN ASSOCIATED WITH APNEA DURING SLEEP

Three pathologic conditions are known to occur in man, in which apnea, associated with sleep, can lead to death. Such models might provide considerable insight into pathogenic mechanisms of CNS dysfunction and apply to SIDS.

1) A patient with early, mild, or chronic residual of bulbar poliomyelitis may develop periods of apnea lasting 4 to 12 seconds during sleep as an early manifestation of a deranged central respiratory regulation (Plum and Swanson, 1958). Arousal promptly reverses these abnormal respiratory patterns. Characteristically, breathing is entirely normal when the patient is awake. Irregular breathing during wakefulness is a more ominous sign in these patients, since sleep produces even longer periods of apnea. These patients often fear sleep. One patient studied by Plum and Swanson (1958), had complete cessation of respiration for 1 minute under supervision while asleep and had to be aroused to breathe. Many patients after acute poliomyelitis require artificial respiration for many months during their sleeping period, and show a significantly reduced responsiveness of the respiratory center to 5 percent CO_2 in the inspired air. Pathological studies in nonsurvivors demonstrate inflammatory changes and small areas of necrosis in the ventrolateral medullary reticular formation.

2) The so-called "Ondine's Curse Syndrome"* occurs occasionally in patients following high bilateral cervical cordotomy (Severinghaus and Mitchell, 1962; Mulland and Hasobuchi, 1968; Tenicella et al., 1968). A series of patients have been described in which sleep-induced apnea developed following high cervical or lower brainstem surgery. Several of these patients died of apnea during sleep. In a series of patients studied after percutaneous cervical cordotomy for the relief of chronic pain, the CO_2 response was significantly reduced (Kuperman et al., 1971). The lesions were made in the antero-lateral quadrants of the high cervical spinal cord.

3) A third condition which would fit a sleep-related apnea syndrome is the "Pickwickian Syndrome" (Gastaut et al., 1966, 1968). This is a condition in obese patients in which apnea occurs when the subject goes to sleep. Two groups of patients have been described—those in which periodic respirations during sleep result from intermittent upper-airway obstruction leading to chronic sleep deprivation, and those in which sleep-induced apnea occurs without obstruction (Walsh et al., 1972). Although the great majority of the patients with this syndrome are obese, not all are. They have also been found to be partially insensitive to inspired 5 percent CO_2. In a group of 15 patients with this syndrome studied over a 7 year period, five had sudden respiratory deaths during sleep (McGregor et al., 1970). Recent evidence has demonstrated that the somnolence and hypoventilation (apneic episodes) occur prior to elevation of $PaCO_2$ and that the $PaCO_2$ increase then is a consequence of the hypoventilation and apnea. Recent studies have demonstrated that a hypersomnia syndrome associated with sleep apnea may occur in patients who are not obese (Guilleminault et al., 1972; Lugaresi et al., 1972). (See also chapter by Guilleminault and Dement in this volume).

*Ondine's Curse—A German legend, in which a water nymph, Ondine, having been jilted by her mortal lover, puts a curse on him, requiring that he must voluntarily remember to breathe. He finally falls asleep and since the act of breathing is no longer automatic, he dies (Severinghaus and Mitchell, 1962).

One such patient spent 75 percent of his total sleep time in apnea, with the longest apneic period being 3 minutes. It is of considerable interest that the apnea was reduced with the drug chlorimipramine.

These findings support those of Gastaut et al. (1965), that associated with the sleep apnea there is a decrease in the tonus of the muscles of the larynx leading to a temporary airway obstruction. However, evidence supports the notion that the first event is a sleep apnea with no diaphragmatic movement. This is then followed by a loss of muscle tone in the oral pharynx and larynx, leading to the temporary obstruction. Diaphragmatic movement is then restored and since the airway is obstructed, the intrathoracic pressure can increase by 300 percent. At this point the patient arouses usually with a loud, snoring noise as the air moves through the partially obstructed upper airway and regular respiration resumes. Dr. Guilleminault and his group feel that such recurring episodes may induce right- and left-sided cardiac failure, arrhythmia, and perhaps myocardial damage. Of considerable interest is the fact that these patients are unaware of their abnormal respiratory patterns during sleep. They complain rather of a sleep disorder such as hypersomnia, insomnia or narcolepsy. A strong male predominance has been noted in this disorder, and an individual may have this abnormality for 20 to 25 years without its being recognized.

Recent studies have demonstrated that the syndrome of central alveolar hypoventilation, hypersomnia with periodic breathing, insomnia with periodic apnea, and the Pickwickian syndrome all have an important relationship with 24 hour sleep-waking functions. The results of these studies increasingly support the concept that a deranged CNS control mechanism underlies the pathophysiology of these sleep-respiratory disorders, rather than a primary respiratory etiologic mechanism (Symposium, 1972). One question is whether this group of patients with these functional sleep and respiratory disorders could be the near-misses of SIDS, that did not die in infancy.

Thus it is seen that several pathological conditions in an adult man may provide anatomical and physiological support for the hypothesis that SIDS may be due to a prolonged apneic episode occurring during sleep.

In a study carried out on 70 normal subjects, Bulow (1963) reported that periodic breathing was a normal and common phenomenon during sleep onset in two-thirds of the subjects. He had obtained continuous records of respiratory pattern during wakefulness and sleep for 3 to 6 hours, EEG activity, and alveolar CO_2 tension. The rate and degree of the initial fall in "level of wakefulness", was correlated with the degree of periodic breathing, and increase in $PaCO_2$. In several subjects, periods of total apnea occurred ranging from 20 seconds up to 1 minute. Some subjects showed "Biot's" type breathing (highly irregular respiratory pattern) during the onset of sleep. The change of ventilatory pattern in sleep was characteristic in a given subject. In addition ,the ventilatory response to CO_2 was invariably decreased during sleep. Among the 70 normal subjects, an "unstable" group could be identified in whom the change in CO_2 sensitivity was substantial during sleep onset, producing marked oscillations and also definite changes in respiration.

Aserinsky (1965) has also reported alterations in the rhythmic respiratory pattern of human adult subjects during REM sleep. He found that apnea would occur during short eye movement bursts and at the onset of a long train of eye movements during REM sleep. In some subjects, a Cheyne-Stokes-like pattern of respiration was present.

NEUROANATOMICAL CONSIDERATIONS

In man and in other animals, the medulla oblongata and lower pons contain the neuronal structures which control the automatic respiratory functions (Pitts et al., 1939). From pathological studies in man as well as those of the classical lesion recording and stimulating experiments in animals, it has been learned that lateral and paramedian regions of the medulla and lower third of the pons in the region of the obex, are critical areas for the maintenance of regular respiration (Plum, 1970). Recent studies in cats strongly suggest that the interaction between various groups of respiratory neurons in these areas, may be the origin of respiratory periodicity (Cohen, 1970). Different neurons having similar discharge patterns in relation to the respiratory cycle may have opposite responses to the same type of stimulus. In these studies, the condition of the animal in regard to level of consciousness was kept constant. In studies in which long term recordings of reticular neurons were made, or in which changes in depth of anesthesia were carried out, the pattern of responsiveness of individual neurons can change according to changes in CNS *"state"* (Schiebel and Schiebel, 1965; Bystrzycka et al., 1969, 1970). These medullopontine regions have also been shown to be intrinsically sensitive to CO_2 (Van Euler and Saderberg, 1952). The finding that partial lesions in the medulla and upper cervical spinal cord in man can, as outlined above, dissociate waking "voluntary" respiratory function from the "automatic" rhythm during sleep is of considerable interest in regard to SIDS, as well as our understanding of the changes in respiratory patterns which accompany the waking-sleep transitional period and specific sleep stages.

During the past 10 years, the anatomical organization of the brainstem catecholamine and indoleamine neurons and their pathways have been clearly defined. It is of considerable interest that the midline raphé nuclei in the medulla (nuclei raphé obscurus pallidus and magnus) are 5-HT (serotonin) cell groups. The catecholamine neurons of the lower brainstem are located in the ventrolateral part of the reticular formation in the caudal part of the medulla, as well as in the nucleus commisuralis in the dorsal paramedian region. These monoaminergic neurons send their fibers down the spinal cord in several bulbospinal pathways (Dahlstrom and Fuxe, 1965). The 5-HT neurons of the raphé obscurus and magnus almost exclusively send their fibers down in the superficial ventral-lateral portion of the cervical spinal cord. The noradrenergic (NA) fibers are more diffusely represented but also appear primarily in the ventral and lateral funiculus. Both of these fiber systems have terminals in the anterior horn cells throughout the length of the spinal cord, mainly the alpha-motoneurons of the skeletal musculature. In the thoracic spinal cord, the medial motor cell groups innervating the axial musculature receive large numbers of 5-HT and NA terminals. Dahlstrom and Fuxe (1965) suggest this might indicate "a more efficient supraspinal control over the part of the axial musculature involved in respiration".

Only recently with the studies of Golden (1972, 1973 in press) has there been a description of the maturation of the biogenic-amine neuronal system of the brainstem in fetal and newborn animals. In his studies of the fetal mouse (20 days gestation), no amines are seen through the 12th day of gestation. On the 13th day, however, NA cells appear in the locus coeruleus and 5 HT cells appear in the raphé system. By the 17th day, the raphé system can be recognized as a continuous line of 5 HT cells on either side of the median raphé of the myelencephalon in both the caudal and mesencephalic divisions. The catecholaminergic cells of the lateral reticular formation, however, are less well developed at the time of birth. These preliminary findings indicate that in an animal quite immature at birth (mouse) the monoaminergic systems are clearly present and may indeed be functionally organized at that time.

There is increasing evidence that the brainstem monoaminergic neurons are highly responsive to changes of sleep-waking states. Although apparently no one has studied the medullary midline and reticular "respiratory" neurons as a function of physiological sleep and waking state, studies of raphé dorsalis and lateral reticular pontine neurons show that marked changes in rate of firing occur in the transition and during defined sleep states in cats. McGinty and Harper (1972) have shown that during REM sleep in adult cats, the dorsal raphé serotinergic cells will almost completely stop firing whereas during non-REM sleep their rate of firing is much greater but still less than during wakefulness. Neurons recorded from the gigantocellular tegmental field of the pontine reticular formation, on the other hand show high rates of discharge in REM sleep as compared to non-REM sleep and the waking state (McCarley et al., 1972).

The above observations in concert with our knowledge of the epidemiology of SIDS suggests that the physiologic maturation of the sleep-wake cycle, and of cardio-respiratory function may be related to the pathogenesis of SIDS.

MATURATION OF SLEEP AND REST/ACTIVITY
CYCLES IN THE HUMAN

At 24 weeks postconception, sleep/wake cycles and sleep stages are poorly defined and cannot be distinguished (Dreyfus-Brisac, 1968). Between 33 and 35 weeks postconception, three sleep states, (active, quiet, and transitional) and a wake state can be identified from characteristic parameters obtained using behavioral observation, polygraphic recordings and evoked response measurements (Weitzman and Graziani, 1968; Dreyfus-Brisac, 1970). Transitional sleep may be variously defined but refers to the discordance among the parameters so that the state is neither clearly active nor clearly quiet sleep. With further maturation the baby obtains two highly specific and well organized sleep states, active and quiet, which are sustained for a variable period of time and alternate in a relatively fixed pattern. *Active sleep* is characterized by somatic activity, irregular respirations with short periods of apnea, rapid eye movements (REM), absence of muscle tone (measured by chin EMG), and a relatively variable cardiac rate. *Quiet sleep* is characterized by absence of phasic somatic activity except for occasional gross body movements, regular respirations (during which apneas may also occur), an absence of REM, a tonically active chin EMG, and a relatively regular heart rate.

In a full term infant, the EEG during quiet sleep characteristically shows a discontinuous type pattern and during active sleep a continuous pattern (Weitzman et al., 1965; Parmelee et al., 1968). In the premature infant, after 34 weeks an active-quiet sleep cycle is present but it is irregular and an ill defined active sleep state predominates. In the young premature, very little behavioral quiet sleep occurs and there is little or no concordance among the various parameters. At full term the sleep state cycles become more regular and consist of approximately equal amounts of active and quiet state with reliable concordance among the characteristic parameters within each state. By three months after term the sleep state cycles are quite regular and the baby spends twice as much time in quiet sleep as in active sleep. The lengthening of quiet sleep coincides with the development of the ability to sustain both prolonged periods of sleep and a wakeful state with visual attention and social behavior. This "basic rest-activity cycle" is continuous throughout the 24 hours, appears during very early life, and can be detected in utero (Sterman and Hoppenbrouwers, 1971). Importantly, maturation of sleep is a function of age postconception rather than extra-uterine experience, although environmental factors may influence maturation somewhat.

As the length of sustained sleep increases, it becomes entrained by environmental cues to the night period, such that after the fifth week of postnatal life, the longest sleep period occurs after 6:00 PM (Parmelee et al.,

1964). At 12 weeks of age 6-8 hours of sustained sleep occurs during the night in normal infants. Fussiness with crying which increases from birth and peaks at 4 to 6 weeks, is initially distributed throughout the 24 hour cycle but usually becomes concentrated in the early evening to midnight period. Waking activity is increasingly associated with the daytime, and sleep activity with night. After the first three months, suppression of crying and fussiness occurs, and wakefulness is used for other developmental phenomenon. Behaviorally indifferentiated REM states associated with fussiness, sucking, etc. decrease by 8-10 weeks and EEG sleep spindles rapidly mature by 3 to 4 months (Emde and Metcalf, 1970). The EEG patterns, which are not fully reliable predictors of sleep state in the premature (or even at term), are quite reliable in this regard by 3 months. Until 3 months of age an active state with REM occurs at sleep onset. The chin EMG reflecting muscle tonus in itself is not a reliable predictor of sleep state until 3 to 8 months of age (Parmelee and Stern, 1972). REM or active sleep periodicity in terms of average duration of cycle does not change markedly during the first year. However, the intensity of the somatic and autonomic manifestations of the REM sleep state is reduced during the first year, especially between 2 and 3 months.

In physiologic terms, quiet sleep may therefore be considered a more mature and more highly controlled state than active sleep. It has been suggested that each parameter of quiet sleep shows evidence of the development of inhibitory and feedback controlling mechanisms, originating in higher brain centers, and relates to the increasing complexity of the neural network and neurochemical development (Parmelee and Stern, 1972). The concordance of the various parameters for sustained quiet sleep periods and useful wakefulness requires a complex interaction of the brainstem and higher centers for a unity of control. With the development of higher nervous system influences, presumably forebrain modulation, as well as maturing lower central control, the basic rest/activity cycle becomes manifest as the REM-non-REM sleep cycle (Sterman and Hoppenbrouwers, 1971).

In summary, the infant's behavior in the 2 to 3 month age period reflects a rapid maturation of the ability to sustain longer periods of sleep, the development of a diurnal cycle, major changes in developmental psychology, the maturation of EEG patterns, and anatomic changes in the brain. More needs to be learned about the maturation of the basic rest/activity cycle, as well as the interaction and development of forebrain regulatory influences, and the relationships of these phenomena to respiratory and cardiac function since these factors may well be central to the problem of SIDS. Conceivably, a delay in the development of these behavioral inhibitory systems, or a premature loss or deficiency of protective postnatal mechanisms, may result in a vulnerable period (with increased risk of SIDS) at 2 to 3 months of age. Although sleep apnea associated with mild hypoxemia (Aserinsky, 1965) and an increase in variability of autonomic function occurs during REM sleep in adult subjects (Snyder et al, 1964; Coccogna et al., 1971), no harmful effects of these temporal events have been noted in normal individuals. In patients with physiologic abnormalities such as seizures (Broughton, 1971), nocturnal angina (Nowlin et al., 1965), peptic ulcers (Armstrong et al., 1965), and nocturnal migraine (Dexter and Weitzman, 1970), REM sleep may be correlated with these pathological conditions. Thus, dissociative physiologic conditions occurring during REM may be manifest in an increased risk of abnormalities in the susceptible individual, if not checked by regulatory influences.

SLEEP STUDIES IN ANIMALS

In studies of many maturational phenomenon related to sleep, animal research is of proven usefulness. There are similarities in the ontogenesis of the wakefulness-sleep cycle and the EEG correlates among mammals (Ellingson, 1972). In mammals, sleep is probably the most constant behavior available for comparative purposes. Sleep is more similar in the rat, man, and a variety of other mammals than most types of complex behavior. Although there are species differences in sleep related physiology, the in depth analysis of the association of many brainstem and spinal reflexes to sleep state can be studied only in nonhuman species. In the adult cat, as in man, spinal and brainstem reflexes are profoundly inhibited during the REM state whereas in the neonatal kitten they are facilitated (Iwamura, 1971). Facilitation of somatic activity during REM could be protective in the young organism to allow arousal if imbalance occurs. In the kitten at 3 weeks, which may be comparable to the human of 3 months, facilitation of certain brainstem reflexes (masseteric and digastric reflex) decreases during REM (Chase, 1972).

CENTRAL, PERIPHERAL AND MATURATIONAL FACTORS RELATED TO RESPIRATORY AND CARDIOVASCULAR FUNCTION

Responses of the autonomic nervous system, the central control of ventilation, and other brainstem neuronal activity, especially in relation to behavioral state and maturation, is relevant to the study of SIDS. The respiratory and ventilatory functions in the immature animal have been widely studied but information on the human infant in this area is incomplete. With maturation, higher nervous centers influence brainstem respiratory control and inhibition of regular respirations may occur. Periodic breathing may then develop, although shifts to regular respiration occurs. With maturation of the infant, longer periods of regular respiration associated with quiet sleep are noted, and irregular respirations (variations in the interval between breaths) are present during active sleep (Monod and Pajot, 1965; Prechtl et al., 1968). Thus, intrinsic rhythmic patterns under local brainstem control are influenced by higher centers resulting in a change in patterns of respirations (Parmelee and Stern, 1972). However, in the immature organism all centers are maturing such that their respiratory system is not entirely comparable to an adult with higher center pathology. There is some higher central control of respiration in term infants as illustrated by the change in respirations on the presentation of various stimuli including complex visual patters. Changes in heart rate patterns in response to stimuli are similar to respiratory changes. If tactile or other sensory stimuli are presented to sleeping full term infants, heart rate acceleration occurs: an initial pause is followed by an increase in rate (Lipton et al., 1966). With maturation, an initial drop in heart rate may occur followed by acceleration and subsequent deceleration. The prestimulus heart rate is related to the response. If high heart rate is present in the prestimulus state, the initial response to the stimulus may be deceleration, then acceleration.

The definition of respiratory irregularities varies with the age group studied. In the newborn period, two or more apneic episodes of 3 seconds or more within a 20 second epoch is termed periodic breathing, and a single nonbreathing interval of 6 seconds or more in a 20 second epoch has been called isolated apnea (Parmelee et al., 1972). Periodic breathing in which relatively short periods of nonbreathing recur without associated cyanosis or bradycardia and terminate spontaneously is commonly observed in premature infants during sleep (Sinclair, 1970); neonatal apnea may also be described as a nonbreathing interval associated with a fall in heart rate and cyanosis (Daily et al., 1969). Heart rate may decelerate at the beginning or end of the apnea (Deuel, 1973), and in the same infant bradycardia does not always occur in association with the apnea, suggesting a common (presumably vagal) as well as independent cause for both. Cardiac arrhythmias, other than bradycardia, have been noted during apnea in newborn infants (Valimaki and Tarlo, 1971). Daily and his group (1969) noted that regardless of the ultimate duration of apnea in premature infants, bradycardia was always present after 30 seconds of nonbreathing. It has also been reported that apneic episodes in premature infants were more commonly preceded by rising air temperatures of the isolette (Perlstein et al., 1970). In neonatal infants, apnea with or without bradycardia occurs in both REM and non-REM states and Deuel (1973) reported that intermediate length apneic pauses were more common in quiet than in active sleep.

Major neuropathological findings especially intracranial hemorrhage has been noted in autopsies of neonatal infants who had refractory apneic episodes, suggesting that cerebral hypoxia secondary to the apnea may have resulted in the brain pathology (Towbin, 1969). In some instances, apnea of the newborn may be due to seizures, hypoglycemia, sepsis, other systemic disorders, and neuromuscular diseases. Apneic episodes usually occur after expiration in both infants and adults.

Full term and premature infants at term have similar respiratory patterns (Parmelee and Stern, 1972; Parmelee et al., 1972), so that maturation of respiratory patterns is related primarily to age postconception rather than postnatal age. In premature infants, the absence of body activity or REM does not become closely associated with regular respiration until after 36 weeks. Not until 3 months after term does this association between regular respirations and quiet sleep mature completely (Parmelee and Stern, 1972).

Steinschneider (1972) has recently studied 5 infants with cyanotic episodes at about one month of age. His observations support the hypothesis that prolonged apnea during sleep may be part of the final pathway resulting in SIDS. In addition, he suggested that infants at risk might be identified prior to a terminal episode. In that study, apnea occurred in both REM and NREM sleep, although more commonly in the former. Also, prolonged apnea most often occurred in conjunction with an upper respiratory tract infection.

The relationships existing between respiratory metabolism and sleep state, including oxygen uptake and CO_2 excretion rates of the respiratory gases, have been studied in human adult subjects (Birchfield et al., 1958). As nighttime sleep progresses, there is an overall decline in O_2 uptake and a decline in CO_2 excretion rate. During REM sleep, and sometimes during stage 2, periodic increases in metabolism occur, superimposed on the continually descending trend during the night. CO_2 production appears to be at its lowest level during stage 3, accumulating in the body during stages 3 and 2. The amount of CO_2 discharged in expired air is greater during the REM period. O_2 uptake is greatest during REM, but variability is marked (Brebbia and Altshuler, 1965). In normal adults, if CO_2 is added to inspired air during sleep, the ventilatory response varies from absent to marked depending on the individual and concentration used (Bulow, 1963). Similar or modified studies in the human infant would be of considerable importance, especially in helping to identify a population possibly at risk for SIDS. The feasibility of such studies needs to be explored.

Lower brainstem motor neuron activities have characteristics of both somatic and autonomic function. The process involved in the integration of the separate motor neuron clusters is not well understood. Stimulation experiments of these brainstem neurons in animals have been reported but their relationship to respiratory function has yet to be defined. The possible role of the cerebellum as a regulatory system is of interest since autonomic function and somatic respiration is influenced by cerebellar stimulation.

In summary a respiratory and cardiovascular model of central regulation possibly influenced by peripheral factors, brainstem neuronal activity, and other regulatory phenomenon may be useful in determining the pathogenesis of SIDS.

PROPOSED HYPOTHESIS FOR THE PATHOGENESIS
OF SIDS AND PROPOSED STUDIES

On the basis of the preceding data and concepts, the following hypothesis is proposed for the pathogenesis of the Sudden Infant Death Syndrome. A small number of newborn infants may have a functional abnormality of the respiratory centers in the lower brainstem regions (ponto-medullary respiratory center). It might affect 2-4 per 1000 live full-term infants and up to 20 per 1000 live premature infants depending on the degree of prematurity. This functional abnormality would be such that during sleep, either at the onset of sleep, in transitional periods between sleep stages, or during a specific sleep stage, the automatic inspiratory-expiratory rhythmic cycle is disrupted by recurrent periods of apnea. Although recurrent tran sient apneic periods during sleep is a normal phenomenon in infants as well as in adults (especially in REM sleep and at transition of waking to sleep) in these susceptible infants, the sleep correlated apneic periods would be more frequent and prolonged and therefore constitute a significant threat to the infant's gas exchange needs. Certain contributory factors, especially a mild viral upper respiratory infection, might play a significant role in precipitating a prolonged apneic period in these susceptible infants. If the infant were sleep deprived either because of mild illness such as fever, URI, skin irritation, etc. or because of environmental disruptions of the regular sleep-waking schedule such as missed feeding period, physical dislocations, environmental air temperature differences (cold room), or forced wakefulness by parents, etc., the ensuing sleep period might have exaggerated physiologic and autonomic characteristics (such as seen during sleep recovery after partial sleep deprivation) and a prolonged apneic episode might result. This apneic episode might or might not be associated with the loss of tonus of the laryngeal and posterior pharyngeal muscles, laryngospasm, excessive vagal discharge or other autonomic responses which contribute to or increase hypoxia.

Since apnea occurs frequently during the transition from waking to sleep and has been shown to be more frequent in adults during non-REM sleep, it is suggested that non-REM sleep stages in the infant might be more prone to be correlated with a prolonged apnea than the REM sleep stage. Such a prolonged apneic episode during sleep would result in increased CO_2 retention and a fall in the arterial pO_2. The ability of the ponto-medullary respiratory centers to respond to such an increase in CO_2 might be significantly decreased during sleep in normal infants and infants with SIDS may be especially resistant because of the postulated abnormality of these neuronal centers. The prolonged turn-off (inhibition?) of the inspiratory synchronized neuronal drive could lead to severe anoxia, cyanosis, and cardiac failure with ultimate cardiac arrest. Such a sequence of events would therefore be fully reversible if arousal and/or resuscitative measures are instituted before cardiac arrest and/or CNS damage occurred. The evidence of near-misses with the repeated description of infants having full normal recovery and sent home from doctors' offices and hospital emergency rooms supports this concept. Although the specific pathology of the respiratory control centers cannot be postulated at the present time, it is suggested that the interrelationship of maturing brainstem neuronal systems may play an important role in such a functional disorder. It is possible that as CNS development proceeds, a maturational mismatch or lag develops within the central respiratory systems. The temporal relation of inhibitory-excitatory synaptic systems during certain critical periods of growth may conceivably be temporally misprogrammed, leading to a prolonged apnea. The maturation of the indole and catecholaminergic neuronal systems of the brainstem could be intimately related to such critical periods of functional organization.

This suggested hypothesis implies that with appropriate neurophysiologic and respiratory function tests, one could identify the specific high risk infant population. One could then institute special monitoring procedures to prevent or immediately reverse the prolonged apneic episode and its consequences thereby be averted. Physicians could advise parents of such susceptible infants about ideal sleep-waking habits and in the case of a minor illness what special precautions to follow. Specific drug therapy might eventually be developed to significantly reduce the possibility of a prolonged sleep related apnea. For example, if it were shown that it was due to a prolonged catecholaminergic inhibitory synaptic drive an effective drug might be one that would partially suppress noradrenergic release or synthesis. Finally, it is possible that the identification of the specific high risk infant group might permit the recognition of a genetic subgroup, thus leading to appropriate genetic counseling.

The usefulness of any proposed hypothesis depends on the formulation of scientific investigations which will allow its acceptance or rejection. Accordingly, the following experimental approaches are suggested: That study be undertaken to determine if there is in fact, a small percent of full-term and premature infants who have a consistent sleep-respiratory pattern abnormality with prolonged apneic episodes. The sample population should be drawn from the different risk groups implicated in epidemiological studies. If such a group emerges, a prospective study be undertaken to determine if this high risk group is the major source of near-misses and actual SIDS. These studies should be carried out in several centers. The development of improved and standardized polygraphic measurement techniques would permit telemetric or telephone recordings for 24 hour periods in both laboratory and home environments. The CO_2 respiratory responsiveness during waking and sleeping be evaluated in full term and premature infants to determine the normal differences, and also whether a rapid technique might identify a specific high risk infant group.

Studies with animals, including nonhuman primates, are needed to determine whether sleep-induced apnea can be produced at various ages by making appropriate small lesions in the lower brainstem and upper cervical cord regions. If so, such an animal model could then be used to test the effect of sleep deprivation, drugs, and other environmental stresses on the susceptibility to sleep-induced apnea. A study of central and autonomic control in relation to respiratory and cardiovascular physiology would be helpful in developing information to support or reject the proposed hypothesis. Relevant animal research recommended might include: 1) the measurement of brainstem neurophysiologic events and their fatigue in response to CO_2; 2) the influence of cerebellar ablation and stimulation on respiratory and cardiovascular responses; 3) the effects of sleep deprivation and fatigue on respiratory and other physiologic function during subsequent sleep; 4) the effects of local (brainstem) and systematic pharmacologic agents on sleep and respiratory physiology; 5) studies of the biogenic amine neuronal systems in immature animals; 6) neuroanatomic, neurochemical, and histochemical maturational studies of those brain structures related to sleep, respiration, and brainstem reflexes.

REFERENCES

Armstrong, R.H., Burnap, D., Jacobson, A., Kales, A., Ward, S., and Golden, J. Dreams and gastric secretions in duodenal ulcer patients. *New Physician 14*, 241-243 (1965).

Aserinsky, E. Periodic respiratory pattern occurring in conjunction with eye movements during sleep. *Science 150*, 763-766 (1965).

Bergman, A.B., Beckwith, J.B., and Roy, C.G., Eds. *Sudden Infant Death Syndrome, Proc, Int. Conf. on Causes of Sudden Death in Infants*, Univ. of Washington Press, Seattle, 1970.

Bergman, A.B., Roy, G.C., Pomeroy, M.A., Wahl, P.W. and Beckwith, J.B. Studies of Sudden Infant Death Syndrome in King County, Washington 3, Epidemiology. *Pediatrics 49*, 860-870 (1972).

Birchfield, R., Sieker, H. and Heyman, A. Alterations in blood gases during natural sleep and narcolepsy. *Neurology 8*, 107-112 (1958).

Brebbia, D.R. and Altshuler, K.Z. Oxygen consumption rate and electroencephalographic stage of sleep. *Science 150*, 1621-1623 (1965).

Broughton, R. Neurology and sleep research. *Canadian Psychiat. Assoc. J. 16*, 283-293 (1971).

Bulow, K. Respiration and wakefulness in man. *Acta Physiol. Sca. 59* (Suppl. 209) *1-110 (1963)*.

Bystrzycka, E., Gromysz, H., Huszczuk, A. and Karczewski, W. Influence de l'hyperventilation et de la Narcose sur l'activité bioeléctrique des neurons respiratoires chez les lapius. *Bull. Acad. Pal. Sci. 17*, 713-716 (1969).

Bystrzycka, E., Gromysz, H., Huszczuk, A. and Karczewski, W. Etude chez le lap de l'activité électrique des neurons respiratoires du trouc cerebral: Influence de la vagatomie et de l'injection d'histamine. *Electroenceph. Clin. Neurophysiol. 29*, 363-372 (1970).

Chase, M.H. Patterns of reflex excitability during ontogenesis of sleep and wakefulness. in, *Sleep and the Maturing Nervous System*, C. Clemente, D. Purpura, and F. Moyer, Eds. Academic Press, New York, 1972 pp 253-280.

Coccogna, G., Montovani, M., Brignani, F., Monzini, A. and Lugaresi, E. Arterial pressure changes during spontaneous sleep in man. *Electroenceph. Clin. Neurophysiol. 31,* 277-281 (1971).

Cohen, M.I. How respiratory rhythm originates: Evidence from discharge patterns of brainstem respiratory neurones. in, *Symposium on Breathing,* (Ciba Found. Symp.), J. & A. Churchill, London, 1970, pp. 125-157.

Dahlstrom, A. and Fuxe, K. Evidence for the existence of monoamine neurons in the central nervous system. *Acta Physiol Scan. 64* (suppl. 247) 1-85 (1965).

Daily, W.J., Klaus, M. and Meyer, H.B. Apnea in premature infants: Monitoring incidence, heart rate changes, and an effect of environmental temperature. *Pediatrics 43,* 510-518 (1969).

Deuel, R.K. Polygraphic monitoring of apneic spells. *Arch. Neurol. 28,* 71-76 (1973).

Dexter, J.D. and Weitzman, E.D. The relationship of nocturnal headaches to sleep stage patterns. *Neurology 20,* 513-518 (1970).

Dreyfus-Brisac, C. Sleep ontogenesis in early human prematurity from 24 to 27 weeks of conceptional age. *Develop. Psychobiol. 1,* 162-169 (1968).

Dreyfus-Brisac, C. Ontogenesis of human sleep in human prematures after 32 weeks of conceptional age. *Develop. Psychobiol. 3,* 91 (1970).

Ellingson, R.J. Development of wakefulness—Sleep cycles and associated EEG patterns in mammals. in, *Sleep and the Maturing Nervous System* Eds. C. Clemente, D. Purpura, and E. Moyer, Eds. Academic Press, New York, 1972.

Emde, R. and Metcalf, D.R. An electroencephalographic study of behavioral rapid eye movement states in the human newborn. *J. Nerv. Ment. Dis. 150,* 370-376 (1970).

Euler, U. van, and Soderberg, U. Medullary chemo-sensitive receptors. *J. Physiol. 118,* 545-554 (1952).

Gastaut. H., Tassinari, C,A, and Duron, B. Etude polygraphique des manifestations episodiques (hypniques et respiratoires) diurnes et nocturnes du syndrome de Pickwick. *Rev. Neurol. 112,* 568-578 (1965).

Gastaut, H., Tassinari, C.A. and Duron, B. Polygraphic study of the episodic diurnal and nocturnal (hypnic and respiratory) manifestations of the Pickwickian Syndrome. *Brain Res. 1,* 167-186 (1966).

Gastaut, H., Duron, B., Tassinari, C.A. et al. Mechanism of the respiratory pauses accompanying slumber in the Pickwickian syndrome. *Activ. Nerv. Sup.* [Praha] *11,* 209-215, (1969).

Golden, G.S. Embryologic demonstration of a nigro-striatal projection in the mouse. *Brain Res. 44,* 278-282 (1972).

Golden, G.S. Prenatal development of the biogenic amine systems of the mouse. *Brain, Develop. Bio.* (1973, in press).

Guilleminault, C., Eldridge, F. and Dement, W.C. Insomnia, narcolepsy and sleep apneas, *Bull. Physio-Patho. Respir. 8,* 1127-1138 (1972).

Iwamura, Y. Development of supraspinal modulation of motor activity during sleep and wakefulness. in, *Brain Development and Behavior,* M.B. Sterman, D.J. McGinty and A.M. Adinolfi, Eds. New York Academic Press, 1971, ch. 8, pp 129-143.

Kuperman, A.S., Krieger, A.J. and Rosomoff, H.L. Respiratory function after cervical cordotomy. *Chest 59,* 128-132 (1971).

Labor and Public Welfare Committee Hearing, United States Senate, on Examination of the Sudden Infant Death Syndrome. U.S. Government Printing Office, Washington, D.C., 1972.

Lipton, E.L., Steinschneider, A. and Richmond, J.B. Autonomic function in the neonate: VII Maturational changes in cardiac control. *Child Development 37,* 1-16 (1966).

Lugaresi, E., Coccagna, G., Montovani, M. Pathophysiological, clinical and nasographic considerations regarding hypersomnia with periodic breathing. Bull. Physio-Pathol. Respir. 8, 1249-1256 (1972).

McCarley, R.W., Hobson, J.A. and Pivik, R.T. Activity of individual brainstem neurons during repeated sleep-waking cycles. Presented at the APSS meeting, New York, 1972 (in press, abstract).

McGinty, D. and Harper, R.M. 5HT-containing neurons: Unit activity during sleep. Presented at the APSS meeting, New York, 1972 (in press, abstract).

McGregor, M.I., Block, A.J., and Ball, W.C., Jr. Serious complications and Sudden Death in the Pickwickian syndrome. *Johns Hopkins Med. J. 126,* 279-295 (1970).

Monod, N. and Pajot, N. Le sommeil du nouveau-ne et du premature. 1. Analyse des etudes polygraphiques (mouvements oculaires, respiration et EEG) chez le nouveau-ne a terme. *Biol. Neonat. 8,* 281-307 (1965).

Mullan, S. and Hasobuchi, Y. Respiratory hazards of high cervical percutaneous cordotomy. *J. Neurosurg. 29,* 291 (1968).

National Institute of Child Health and Development Planning Workshops on Sudden Infant Death Syndrome, U.S. Government Printing Office, in press (1974).

Nowlin, J.B., Troyer, W.G. Collins, W.S., Silverman, G., Nichols, C.R., McIntosh, H.D., Ester. E.H., Jr. and Bogdonoff, M.D. The association of nocturnal angina pectoris with dreaming. *Ann. Int. Med. 63,* 1040-1046 (1965).

Parmelee, A.H. Wenner, W.H. and Schulz, H.R. Infant sleep patterns from birth to 16 weeks of age. *J. Pediatrics 65,* 576-582 (1964).

Parmelee, A.H. Jr., Akiyama, Y., Schultz, M.A., Schulte, F.J., and Stern, E. The electroencephalogram in active and quiet sleep in infants. in, *Clinical Electroencephalography of Children,* Kellaway and I. Peterson, Eds., Grune and Stratton, New York, 1968, pp 77-88.

Parmelee, A.H. and Stern, E. Development of states in infants in sleep and the maturing nervous system. in, *Sleep and the Maturing Nervous System,* C. Clemente, D. Purpura, and F.E. Moyer, Eds. Academic Press, New York, 1972 pp 200-215.

Parmelee, A.H., Stern, E. and Harris, M.A. Maturation of respiration in prematures and young infants. *Neuropediatrics 3,* 294-364 (1972).

Perlstein, P.H., Edwards, N.K. and Sutherland, V.M. Apnea in premature infants and incubator-air temperature changes. *New Eng. J. Med. 282,* 461-466 (1970)

Pitts, R.F., Magoun, H.W. and Ranson, S.W. Localization of medullary respiratory centers in the cat. *Amer. J. Physiol. 126,* 673-688 (1939).

Plum, F. Neurological integration of behavioral and metabolic control of breathing. in, *Symposium on Breathing,* (Ciba Found. Symp.), J & A Churchill, London, 1970, pp 159-181.

Plum, F., and Swanson, A.G. Abnormalities in central regulation of respiration in acute and convalescent poliomyelitis. *Arch. Neurol. Psychiat. 80,* 267-285 (1958).

Prechtl, H.F.R., Akiyama, Y., Zinkin, P. and Grant, D.K. Polygraphic studies of the full-term newborn. in, *Studies in Infancy.* M.C.O. Box and R.C. MacKeith, Eds. Heinemann, London, 1968 (Clinic in Develop. Med. 27, pp. 1-40).

Schiebel, M.E. and Schiebel, A.B. Periodic sensory non-responsiveness in reticular neurons. *Arch. Ital. Biol. 103,* 300-316 (1965).

Severinghaus, J.W. and Mitchell, R.A. Ondine's curse—failure of respiratory automaticity while awake. *Clin. Res. 10,* 122 (1962).

Sinclair, J.C. The premature baby who "forgets to breathe." *New. Eng. J. Med. 282,* 508-509 (1970).

Snyder, F., Hobson, V.A., Morrison, D.F. and Goldfrank, F. Changes in respiration and heart rate and systolic blood pressure in human sleep. *J. Appl. Physiol. 19,* 417-422 (1964).

Steinschneider, A. Prolonged apnea and the sudden infant death syndrome: Clinical and laboratory observations. *Pediatrics 50,* 646-654 (1972).

Sterman, M.B. and Hoppenbrouwers, R. The development of sleep-waking and rest activity patterns from fetus to adult in man. in, *Brain Development and Behavior,* M.B. Sterman, D.J. McGinty and A.M. Adinolfi, Eds. Academic Press, New York, 1971, ch. 11, pp. 203-227.

Symposium: Hypersomnia with periodic breathing. *Bull. Physio-Pathol. Respir. 8,* 967-1288 (1972).

Tenicella, R., Rosomoff, H.L., Feist, J. et al. Pulmonary function following percutaneous cervical cordotomy. *Anesthesiology 29,* 7 (1968).

Towbin, A. Cerebral hypoxic damage in fetus and newborn. Basic patterns and their clinical significance. *Arch. Neurol. 20,* 35-43 (1969).

Valdes-Dapena et al. Sudden unexpected death in infancy: A statistical analysis of certain socio-economic factors. *J. Pediat 73,* 387-394 (1968).

Valimaki, I. and Tarlo, P.A. Heart rate patterns and apnea in newborn infants. *Amer J. Obste. and Gyncol. 110,* 343-349 (1971).

Walsh, R.E., Michaelson, E.D., Harkehood, L.E., Zighelboim, A. and Sackner, M.A. Upper airway obstruction in obese patients with sleep disturbance and somnolence. *Ann. Int. Med. 76,* 185-192 (1972).

Weitzman, E.D., Fishbein, W. and Graziani, L.J. Auditory evoked responses obtained from the scalp, electrocenphalogram of the full-term human neonate during sleep. *Pediatrics 35,* 458-562 (1965).

Weitzman, E.D. and Graziani, L.J. Maturation and topography of the auditory evoked response of the prematurely born infant. *Develop. Psychobiol. 1,* 79-89 (1968).

Advances in Sleep Research, Vol. 1
© 1974, Spectrum Publications, Inc.

CHAPTER 8

Pathologies of Excessive Sleep

CHRISTIAN GUILLEMINAULT
WILLIAM DEMENT

For ease of description, clinical sleep disorders may be divided into four general categories: 1) those in which patients complain that their *sleep is disturbed* (insomnia); 2) those in which patients complain that they sleep too much (hypersomnia); 3) those in which *others complain* because the patient's sleep problem is disturbing them (sleepwalking, bedwetting, nightmares, sleeptalking, etc.); and finally, 4) those conditions in which some *other illness secondarily affects sleep* (endocrine disorders, nocturnal asthma, nocturia, epilepsy, etc.). In this presentation we shall be primarily concerned with the second group.

However, we would like to emphasize that the distinctions between groups are neither as precise nor as simple as we have outlined above. Because certain conditions associated with hypersomnia were originally described and evaluated from the viewpoint of "too much sleep," it is appropriate for historical purposes to describe them in this chapter. Yet it must be remembered that several of these conditions may also be associated with the complaint of insomnia. The Sleep Apnea Syndrome is an excellent example of such complexity.

One may draw other analogies between hypersomnia and insomnia. Most obvious is the fact that both disorders are described with inferential reference to "normal" sleep. Thus it would be helpful to consider the question: "What is normal sleep?" By and large, the concept of normal sleep is statistical, just as is the concept of the "normal man". Yet we know that the sleep patterns of normal individuals are widely distributed around the statistically derived "normal". A dramatic case in point is the description of two "healthy insomniacs" (Jones and Oswald, 1968) both of whom regularly slept less than 3 hours out of 24. Thus the concept of "normal" sleep, while valuable in many instances, is presently of little use in evaluating sleep disorders. For example, we may have one patient who complains that he is more sleepy during the day than he feels he ought to be and another patient who says he does not sleep enough at night, yet in both instances, the objectively measured sleep times are 7 1/2 hours!

This touches on another problem area that is becoming quite serious; that is, controversies with regard to the objective evaluation of sleep. Should sleep be evaluated only in the home situation? or should it be done under laboratory conditions alone? How many 24-hour periods of recording constitute a valid sample? We must simply recognize that these controversies are completely appropriate for we are in the very beginning phases of an active clinical interest in these problems. Indeed, we may even be participating in the inauguration of an entirely new area of clinical medicine in which sleep disorders will be recognized as a legitimate clinical speciality.

In spite of the many difficulties inherent in staking out new clinical terrain, the effort must be made. The "sleepy" patient has often received short shrift at the hands of practicing physicians who are handicapped by lack of adequate diagnostic facilities, by lack of effective treatments, and, above all, by lack of up-to-date information. It is hoped that this latter group will constitute at least part of the readership of the following material wherein we will attempt a lucid and reasonably scholarly discussion of REM narcolepsy, sleep apnea, mixed hypersomnia, subwakefulness syndrome, and other hypersomnias and "sleepy" conditions. Some of these syndromes present us with a fascinating pathophysiology from the point of view of clinical sleep research, but we must never lose sight of the exquisite torture of being sleepy all the time and the urgent need to improve the lot of those who are thus afflicted.

In the following material, when data are presented without citation, the reader may assume that they are from our own clinical population of more than 250 patients.

NARCOLEPSY

For many years, the term narcolepsy was synonymous with hypersomnia. However, while narcolepsy is included as a *type* of hypersomnia in our general schema, it should be understood that the condition rarely, if ever, is characterized by excessive sleep within a 24-hour period.

Narcolepsy was initially reported by Westphal in 1877, but it was the French neurologist, Gelineau, who in 1880 first defined this syndrome as a "neurosis characterized by an imperative need to sleep of sudden onset and short duration, recurring at more or less close intervals." Daniels, in 1934, wrote an extensive monograph which is still among the best descriptions of the clinical symptomatology of narcolepsy.

This extensive historical background not withstanding, the pathogenic interpretation of the disease has long been controversial and some ambiguities still exist. Narcolepsy has been considered an epileptic equivalent by some physicians who have proposed phenobarbital for its treatment (Wilson, 1928; Serejski and Frumkin, 1930; Cohn and Cruvant, 1944; Roth, 1946). Others have taken the position that the condition is a direct psychiatric disorder. For example, Levin (1959) has stated that "cataplexy. . . is. . . a response to the guilt that attends aggression even when it is only unconscious."

Rechtschaffen et al. (1963)* were the first to suggest that narcolepsy with cataplexy might be a specific entity in which a disorder of rapid eye movement (REM) sleep might be involved. Their assumption was based on continuous polygraphic recordings during sleep and wakefulness which included not only EEG monitoring, but also EMG obtained from hyoidien muscles as well as EOG. Since that time, polygraphic monitoring has been a very useful tool, and the recent use of telemetry in narcoleptics (Cadilhac et al., 1971) has enabled researchers to have an even better understanding of the symptomatology and pathogenesis of the disease.

Narcolepsy characteristically begins at a point of maturational crisis such as puberty or pregnancy. The common age of onset is between 15 and 25 years, although approximately 5% of the cases seem to begin before the age of 10 and 18% after the age of 30 (Roth, 1957; Zarcone, 1973). It is very uncommon for "idiopathic" narcolepsy (i.e., unrelated to a primary neurologic disorder such as brain tumor, encephalitis or vetebral artery insufficiency) to begin after the age of 40. In addition, males and females seem to be similarly affected.

Daytime "sleep attacks" and daytime drowsiness appear to be the most frequent beginning symptoms, but cataplexy, sleep paralysis or hypnagogic hallucinations may precede the complaint of daytime drowsiness by as long as several years. Data compiled recently at Stanford University on 40 REM narcoleptics revealed that the first clinical symptom to appear in two cases was cataplexy which preceded the appearance of daytime sleepiness by 2 and 6 years; hypnagogic hallucinations were the first symptom in 1 case where they preceded the appearance of daytime sleepiness by approximately 3 years.

The incidence of narcolepsy in the general population is not known with certainty, but it is believed to range from 0.02% to 0.05% (Bruhova and Roth, 1972). Recent prevalence studies conducted in the San Francisco (Dement et al. 1972) and Los Angeles (Dement et al, in press) areas, showed that the incidence may be as high as nearly 0.1% (0.09%).

Characteristics of the Clinical Symptoms

In its most characteristic pattern, narcolepsy is associated with attacks of sleep, cataplexy, sleep paralysis, hypnagogic hallucinations, and disrupted nocturnal sleep.

*Probably the first "report" of sleep onset REM period was that of Vogel (1960) who used polygraphic techniques to aid in eliciting dream recall in a single narcoleptic patient. He recorded three naps and noted "the early appearance of dreaming" on two occasions.

Attacks of Sleep

Diurnal naps occurring in response to a more or less irresistible desire to sleep generally constitute, by reason of their frequency and persistence, the most troublesome manifestation of narcolepsy. This overwhelming desire to sleep generally recurs daily or several times daily. If the patient is in a comfortable position and if he is engaged in monotonous work, he will have a greater tendency to fall asleep. But if the patient tries to resist the drowsiness, he may be able to maintain alertness with some measure of success. However, during that time he will generally experience very brief and sudden sleep periods occurring each time his resistance is lowered. One of our patients has described occasions during driving when he would fall asleep while stopped for a red traffic light, but he was able to drive away when the green light appeared and to maintain his alertness until he reached his destination. In general, patients are aware of sudden, short microsleeps. For example, they will realize that they have not followed a conversation and will ask for a sentence to be repeated.

Occasionally, patients are unable to maintain sufficient alertness to react properly to the demands of the environment. One of our patients was severely burned while preparing a meal; she suddenly became drowsy and dropped her hand into a pan of hot oil. Several of our patients have had automobile accidents secondary to drowsiness while driving. However, patients are generally able to resist their sleepiness in dangerous situations and fall asleep only when the environment is not absolutely hostile. In most instances the patient is aware of a sudden and imperious desire for sleep prior to the "attack" of sleep and has accustomed himself to this warning signal. Postprandial periods tend to exacerbate the drowsiness and sleepiness; patients have tried without any great success to avoid the increased sleepiness by having small or high protein meals.

The sleepiness which precedes the sleep attack may be accompanied by a feeling of physical exhaustion. Usually, after a short nap, patients arouse fully alert and greatly refreshed. While drowsy, the patients may also complain of blurred vision, burning eyes, and sudden headache. These feelings may increase if the patient resists the sleep attack. Observers may notice slow rolling eye movements during this period and the patient may experience hypnagogic hallucinations.

Hypnagogic Hallucinations

Hypnagogic hallucinations can be very terrifying, particularly if they are the first symptom to appear in a young individual who is not aware of the disease. These experiences can be visual, auditory and tactile; in fact, they are usually very complex hallucinations. The patient may try to respond to the hallucinations, attempting to escape from the sudden terrifying image.

In general, patients usually realize the hallucinatory quality of the images fairly quickly. They are often aware of an association between the hallucinations and dreams. However, if hypnagogic hallucinations are not readily understood, serious difficulties may result. Acute schizophrenic psychosis can be the initial diagnosis in narcoleptics where this symptom is unsually prominent.

Another common problem is the reaction young adolescents, unaware of the origin of the hallucinations, may have to them. One of our young patients began refusing to go to bed and trying to resist his sleepiness as long as possible to avoid what he called his "daytime nightmares." He also began to question his sanity and refused to discuss this imagery with anyone, fearing that he would appear abnormal.

The unpleasant effect of hypnagogic hallucinations is sometimes greatly intensified if the patient also has the feeling of being unable to move. In other words, he effectively may experience a complete paralysis simultaneous with the hypnagogic hallucinations.

Sleep Paralysis

Sleep paralysis occurs in the transition between sleep and wakefulness. Although the individual feels awake, he is incapable of voluntary movement. The patient can be aroused from the disturbance by simply touching him; but, if undisturbed, the sleep paralysis may have a duration of as long as 20 minutes.

Cataplexy

Cataplexy is a symptom characterized by precipitous episodes of inability to perform voluntary movements secondary to a sudden drop of muscle tone. The severity and extent of the attack itself varies from a state of absolute powerlessness involving the entire voluntary musculature to limited involvement of certain groups of muscles or no more than a fleeting sensation of weakness more or less throughout the body. The extraocular muscles do not seem to be involved in the process, but the palpebral muscles may be affected. Sagging of the jaw, combined with inclination of the head, and sometimes associated with slight buckling of the knees seem to be the most common complaints. However, a sudden complete drop of muscle tone resulting in collapse in not uncommon in severe attacks. In general, patients are able to reach a chair or at least to break a dangerous fall, but sometimes the collapse is completely uncontrolled and potentially very dangerous. Speech may be impaired during an attack and the patient may also complain of blurred vision. Cataplexy may be elicited by emotion, stress, fatigue, or heavy meals. Laughter and anger seem to be the most common precipitants, but the attacks can also be induced by a feeling of elation while reading a book or watching a movie. Cataplexy can also be induced in some individuals by merely remembering a happy or funny situation. Finally, in rare instances, cataplectic attacks appear to be completely without precipitating emotions or acts.

Disturbed Nocturnal Sleep

Sleep attacks, cataplexy, hypnagogic hallucinations, and sleep paralysis represent the classical tetrad. But a fifth symptom reported by Daniels (1934) must be re-emphasized—the disturbed nocturnal sleep. That is, the narcoleptic's sleep is interrupted by frequent wakeful periods throughout the night. This symptom has been observed by several researchers during continuous polygraphic monitoring. Passouant et al. (1967) and Mouret et al. (1972) have insisted on the importance of such disturbance. In their most recent review, based on 6 patients continuously monitored for several 24-hour periods, Mouret et al. (1972) confirmed the term "dys-somnia" given by Passouant to characterize narcolepsy. Total sleep time is generally not greater than normal, but sleep appears at inappropriate times and REM sleep can be abnormally increased (Mouret et al., 1972).

One of the major problems in dealing with narcolepsy is that all these symptoms are not always seen in every so-called "narcoleptic" patient. In fact, the "auxiliary" symptoms (i.e., cataplexy, sleep paralysis, and hypnagogic hallucinations) may appear in a different combination for each patient. The case history studies of Roth (1957), Yoss and Daly (1960), Bowling and Richards (1961), Goode (1962), and Sours (1963) have shown that cataplexy is the most common of the auxiliary symptoms and is associated with daytime sleepiness in 70% of the cases. Sleep attacks, cataplexy, and sleep paralysis appear together in 30% of narcoleptic patients. Hypnagogic hallucinations associated with sleep attacks with or without cataplexy is noted in 25% of the cases (Zarcone, 1973). In 30% of the so-called narcoleptic patients, only the symptom of daytime sleep attacks is present. Thus, in several studies, the term "narcolepsy" is synonymous with daytime sleepiness or daytime sleep attacks alone.

REM Narcolepsy vs. Narcolepsy

Since their initial report based on nocturnal polygraphic recordings (Rechtschaffen et al., 1963), Rechtschaffen and Dement (1967, 1969; Dement et al., 1966; Dement and Rechtschaffen, 1968) have insisted on the importance of the REM sleep mechanism in the appearance and development of narcolepsy. However, controversy has subsequently developed over the question: Is narcolepsy a disease of REM sleep?

Rechtschaffen and Dement have suggested that there is a decreased inhibition by the wakefulness sytem in narcoleptic patients which allows REM sleep phenomena to erupt into waking life. Thus, the sleep attacks would represent the inappropriate appearance of REM sleep during wakefulness. This hypothesis was supported by the discovery reported in 1963 (Rechtschaffen et al.) that full-blown REM periods could occur at the onset of sleep in narcoleptic patients; this pattern presented a completely abnormal sleep structure (Fig. 1). During the past decade, this assumption has been

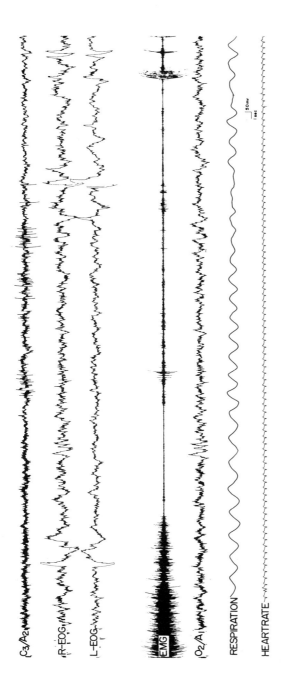

Fig. 1. Abnormal sleep onset in a REM narcoleptic patient. In less than 1 min the patient passed from wakefulness into a full-blown REM sleep period characterized by the complete muscle atonia, the low amplitude fast frequency EEG, and the rapid eye movements, which are very similar to those seen on the left of the figure when the patient was still very much awake. There was no transitional period; REM sleep developed instantaneously.

largely confirmed in neurophysiological studies conducted not only by Dement et al. (1966), but also by Hishikawa et al. (1963; 1968), Takahashi et al. (1963), Passouant et al. (1964), Suzuki (1966), Berti-Ceroni et al. (1967a), Roth et al. (1969), Nan'no et al. (1970), Mouret et al. (1972), and Wilson et al (1973).

Let us specify some of these findings which support the "REM narcolepsy" hypothesis as it is reflected in daytime sleep. First, a very systematic study was recently conducted at the Stanford University Sleep Disorders Clinic (Wilson et al., 1973) on 49 narcoleptic patients who complained of uncontrollable attacks of sleep with one or more auxiliary symptoms. The 49 patients had a total of 95 3-hour daytime nap recordings which represented from 1 to 4 naps per patient. In 90% of the patients, a sleep onset REM period was present in at least one nap recording. Five patients (10%) did not show a sleep onset REM period during any nap. However, two of these patients evidenced the sleep onset abnormality when recorded continuously for 24 hours; one patient was taking REM suppressant drugs while recorded; and the other 2 patients were in their early 20's and just developing the disease. Thus, we can confidently predict that if a continuous 24-hour polygraphic recording is performed on a patient who complains of narcolepsy and cataplexy and who has not taken any REM suppressant drug for at least 15 days, we will see an abnormal REM period at the onset of one of the sleep periods (either diurnal or nocturnal).

A second study that supports the REM narcolepsy hypothesis was reported by Hishikawa et al. in 1965. This group compared the electromyograms of the mental and hyoid muscles recorded during sleep in two populations: 1) control subjects with normal sleep; and 2) narcoleptic patients who presented sleep onset REM periods. When a normal subject fell asleep, the EMG did *not* disappear although the activity declined from original relatively high levels in the drowsy stage to lower levels as sleep progressed into NREM stages 3-4

The *only* state in which tonic EMG activity disappeared was REM sleep. During the sleep onset REM period observed in narcoleptics, the tonic EMG discharges of the mental and hyoid muscles disappeared completely, exactly as occurred during the REM periods recorded late in the nocturnal sleep of both the normal and narcoleptic subjects.

Hishikawa et al. (1965) also looked at H reflex in these subjects. This reflex is a very valuable neurophysiological tool for characterizing "REM narcolepsy." The H reflex is a monosynaptic reflex induced by percutaneous electrical stimulation of the calf muscle afferents in the tibial nerve at the popliteal fossa and observed as a reflex contraction of the same muscle. This reflex activity prominently decreases or cannot be recorded at all in control subjects during normal nocturnal REM sleep (Hodes and Dement, 1964; Hishikawa and Kaneko, 1965). In the study of Hishikawa and Kaneko (1965), they reported that during the sleep onset REM period of narcoleptics, the H reflex almost completely disappeared; an H reflex of low voltage only occasionally persisted in correlation with sudden phasic EMG discharge.

Sleep paralysis and hypnagogic hallucinations can also be easily explained according to the Rechtschaffen and Dement REM sleep hypothesis. These two events are interpreted most parsimoniously as sleep onset REM periods in which there is a very high degree of correspondence between the mental content of the REM period and the content of the immediately preceding period of wakefulness.

Cataplectic episodes are not so easily associated with the REM sleep hypothesis of narcolepsy. The cataplectic attack is clearly not a state of sleep in the conventional sense, but it may be considered as a fractional or dissociated manifestation of the REM process. This concept of cataplexy can be best understood by a closer examination of the motor inhibitory components of REM sleep.

Continuous 24-hour polygraphic recordings in both men and mammals have shown that the only normal condition in which nonreciprocal motor inhibition occurs spontaneously is during REM sleep period. However, narcoleptics evidence this same phenomenon during cataplectic attacks in which a total or near total abolition of EMG potentials occurs simultaneously in different muscle groups (Rechtschaffen and Dement, 1967; Guilleminault et al., 1973f; Dement et al., 1973a). The cataplectic attack is also associated with a complete abolition of tendon reflexes (Fig. 2).

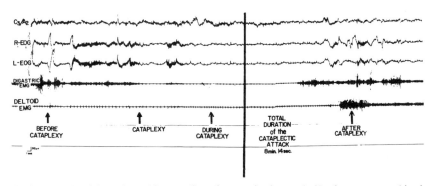

Fig. 2. Example of the polygraphic recording of a cataplectic attack. No change occurred in the EEG during this particular attack. The patient attempted to move several times without success. There is a complete drop of activity in the digastric and deltoid EMG during the entire length of the attack.

Another well-known peculiarity of the motor inhibition of REM sleep is the fact that it does not include the extraocular muscles. The same intriguing exception also applies to narcoleptic patients who may present paralysis and complete areflexia during cataplexy but are able to execute voluntary rapid fixation shifts of the eyeballs during the height of the paralytic episode and EMG suppression (Rechtschaffen and Dement, 1967; Guilleminault et al., 1973f).

Another compelling argument for the interpretation of cataplectic attacks as a dissociated manifestation of REM sleep processes is the fact that although the electroencephalographic recording does not usually change from the prior waking state, the patient may grade smoothly from cataplexy into a full-blown sleep period with the characteristic EEG changes and bursts of rapid eye movements (Rechtschaffen and Dement, 1967; Scolla-Lavizzari, 1970).

A further study of the cataplectic attack was recently conducted at Stanford University (Guilleminault et al., 1973f). Although it is quite difficult to induce cataplexy in a laboratory situation, patients with numerous completely disabling cataplectic attacks were specifically selected for an H reflex study. Complete H reflex inhibition, identical to that reported during normal REM periods and sleep onset REM periods (Hodes and Dement, 1964; Hishikawa and Kaneko, 1965), were observed during several cataplectic attacks in these patients (Fig. 3).

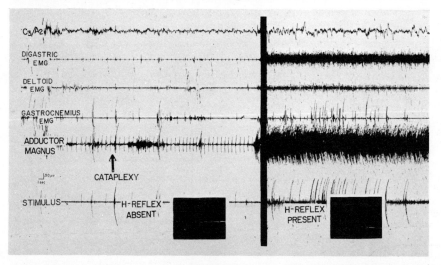

Fig. 3. Another example of polygraphic recording during a cataplectic attack (left) compared with the recording in the same subject 2 min after the end of the attack (right). During the cataplectic attack, there is a complete inhibition in the muscles (leads 2, 3, 4, and 5) and H reflex cannot be recorded. After the attack, EMG activity returns and H reflex was unchanged throughout the session; the intensity selected in this sample induced "H maximum."

The chief difficulty in accepting the hypothesis that cataplexy is a REM inhibitory process in the face of all the evidence we have marshalled, is the fact that cataplexy is very often elicited by strong emotion. As has been previously described, laughter and anger seem to be the most common precipitants of cataplexy, but an attack may also be induced by a feeling of elation while reading a book or watching a movie. Vizzioli (1964) has proposed a neurophysiological theory in which the limbic system and bulbar inhibitory formation could be responsible for cataplexy. The bulbar inhibitory formation is always involved in the motor inhibition which appears during REM sleep. Vizzioli postulates a defect in the REM sleep control system. Animal studies have shown the complex relationship between the ascending influence from the pons to the hypothalamus (and, for Vizzioli, the "Papez bundle") and the feedback circuit to the pontine sleep structures. Vizzioli hypothesizes that in narcoleptics an abnormal activation of this inhibitory system occurs secondary to emotion. This activation would not appear during wakefulness in non-narcoleptics since the wakefulness system normally has an inhibitory influence on the anatomic components of the REM system. However, even in normals, strong emotion can lead to a very short inhibitory discharge, and many people experience their knees "buckling" under great emotional stress; but the strong control of the wakefulness structures over these REM structures is overwhelmed for only a very short time, and the knee buckling is more a "feeling" than an objective "drop." Vizzioli postulates that in narcoleptic patients this control does not exist and the "REM system" partially or totally overcomes the "waking system."

Thus, as we have shown, although the REM hypothesis is somewhat incomplete as a neurophysiologic theory, there are some very convincing arguments in its favor. However, Roth et al. (1969) have questioned the term "REM narcolepsy." For these authors, this terminology is inappropriate because "in most cases of narcolepsy accompanied by cataplexy or sleep paralysis, the NREM sleep system is disturbed in addition to the REM system." They base their argument on 68 1-hour afternoon nap recordings performed on 50 patients who had narcolepsy with cataplexy or sleep paralysis. In 35 of these naps only NREM sleep was present.

On the other hand, Dement et al. (1973b) have argued that there are at least three important reasons for occasional failure to see sleep onset REM periods in patients who complain of sleepiness and cataplexy: 1) a recent drug treatment may still be exerting a REM suppressive effect; 2) NREM sleep is greatly potentiated during early stages of withdrawal from amphetamine or Ritalin which temporarily favors a NREM sleep onset in daytime sleep (this is not true for tricyclic drugs, such as imipramine or other derivatives, which favor sleep onset REM periods during the withdrawal); 3) a REM sleep episode may have already occurred inadvertently while the patient is waiting in the laboratory or even during the actual preparation while the patient is sitting in a chair having electrodes applied.

It seems that a refractory period of as long as a few hours may develop after a short REM nap. If a patient is recorded during this refractory period, he will, of course, present NREM sleep. The fact that "REM narcoleptics" occasionally go from wakefulness into NREM sleep in daytime naps probably reflects the temporary absence of the abnormal REM tendency and not the transient presence of an abnormal NREM tendency. Reports from Passouant et al. (1968) and from Cadilhac et al. (1971) also tend to support the latter assumption.

Cadilhac et al. (1971), using a telemetry system, continuously monitored 19 narcoleptic patients with cataplexy. Follow-up recordings were conducted on several of these patients during the ensuing months. In these recordings, it appeared that the narcoleptic symptomatology, without any treatment, may have a spontaneous tendency to fluctuate. In 8 patients, there were periods when the cataplexy and hypnagogic hallucinations decreased markedly in importance and frequency, but at other times the symptomatology increased for an unknown reason. If patients were recorded in the "latent" period, NREM sleep was nearly exclusively monitored; when cataplectic attacks and/or hypnagogic hallucinations reappeared or suddenly increased in frequency, sleep onset REM periods were almost exclusively recorded. Furthermore, these authors stated that daily variations were noted in the kind of sleep recorded in these patients. Unfortunately, they do not say whether or not the daily variations were associated with daily variations in the symptomatology (i.e., cataplexy, sleep paralysis, and hypnagogic hallucinations). On the other hand, three of the patients in this study repeatedly evidenced abnormal sleep onset REM periods without any fluctuation from month to month. Thus, it appears that the "REM drive" may oscillate in some patients, while at the same time the symptomatology will also have a tendency to fluctuate. Finally, a NREM sleep recording wll be seen more frequently when the so-called auxiliary symptoms are reduced in frequency and intensity.

Mouret et al. (1972) confirmed this general idea in a study which included several 24-hour polygraphic recordings of 31 patients with daytime sleepiness. A complex analysis of their data considered many sleep and wakefulness parameters as a function of the 24-hour period, the daytime hours and the nighttime hours. The findings isolated a REM narcolepsy in six patients. These patients were characterized by numerous sleep onset REM periods in the day, as well as by an abnormally high value of REM% (total REM sleep time/total sleep time) in the daytime and nighttime hours.

Mouret et al. (1972) also characterized 12 of their patients as "mixed hypersomnia," similar to patients reported by Passouant et al. (1968) and by Cadilhac et al. (1971). The "mixed hypersomnia" patients are described by an increased total sleep time during both the day and the night. In these patients, sleep onset could be either NREM or REM sleep. In addition, there is an increased amount of REM sleep similar to that seen in REM narcolepsy. However, in mixed hypersomnia, there is no dys-somnia; there is a harmonious distribution of sleep stages and nocturnal sleep is not disrupted (Fig. 4).

The new category of mixed hypersomnia, while descriptive, is not really helpful in explaining why patients may have sleep onset REM periods at certain times and not others. There are two approaches which may prove to be more helpful in interpreting the findings.

The first approach is based on several general principles associated with the REM sleep process. First, as Passouant et al. (1969; 1972) have shown, a diurnal rhythm of REM sleep becomes very obvious when certain narcoleptics are recorded in a laboratory situation. If a patient is asked to lie in bed, a sleep onset REM period can be recorded every 2 hours (mean value). We also know that the two states of sleep (slow-wave sleep and REM sleep) are not single, discrete phenomena, but each is a confluence of many variables locked together in a phase relationship. This relationship is particularly obvious in REM sleep where variables such as muscle inhibition,

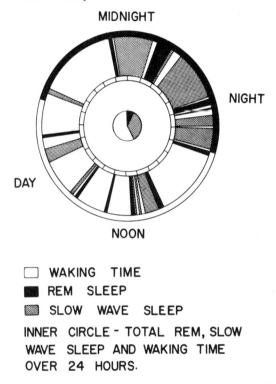

□ WAKING   TIME
■ REM   SLEEP
▓ SLOW   WAVE   SLEEP

INNER   CIRCLE – TOTAL   REM, SLOW
WAVE   SLEEP   AND   WAKING   TIME
OVER   24   HOURS.

Fig. 4. Schematic representation of "mixed hypersomnia." As shown in the figure, there is a nocturnal sleep disruption which is contrary to the report of Mouret et al. (1972) in such patients. This discrepancy leads one to question the usefulness of the distinction between REM narcolepsy and mixed hypersomnia.

rapid eye movements, PGO waves, and in humans, phasic integrated potentials (PIPs),* are closely associated. One may suppose that if one or more variables were no longer in this phase relationship secondary to any type of interference (such interference could even be the personal voluntary struggle of a patient against his sleepiness), the REM drive might still exist, but would not be permitted to develop. At this time, NREM sleep would be recorded. Finally, we know that in cats, certain components of

*Phasic integrated potentials (PIPs) are potentials recorded from the extraocular muscles and were first described by Rechtschaffen et al. (1971).

REM sleep, in particular PGO waves, normally appear in slow-wave sleep, and under certain pharmacologic manipulations, they can also be made to appear in wakefulness. It has also been shown (Pivik and Dement, 1970) that in man, whose plasticity is even greater than mammals, this dissociation of REM sleep phenomena also occurs. It would be of very great interest to study the so-called NREM sleep periods of "REM narcoleptics" and see if polygraphic recordings show some dissociated REM sleep components. In other words, do these NREM sleep periods show an abnormal amount of muscle tone inhibition, an abnormal sudden disappearance of H reflex, or an abnormal increase in the number of PIPs? Such studies may offer a solution to the problem.

Another very promising approach is genetic. Several studies (Krabbe and Magnussen, 1942; Daly and Yoss, 1959; Bruhova and Roth, 1972) have shown that narcolepsy is concentrated in families, and that relatives of a narcoleptic index case have approximately a 200-fold greater risk for narcolepsy than individuals in the general population. Imlah (1961) has reported a pair of monozygotic twins concordant for narcolepsy. All these findings suggest that narcolepsy may have a genetic basis. Kessler et al. (in press) have recently conducted a study on the families of 50 index cases of REM narcolepsy. The diagnosis of each index case was always confirmed by means of a polygraphic recording performed at the Stanford University Sleep Disorders Clinic. In 18% of the cases, a positive family history for daytime sleep attacks and cataplexy was found. In 34%, a positive family history of "disorders of excessive sleep" (DES) was present. An assessment of DES was made if daytime sleep attacks were reported without a positive history of symptoms related to narcolepsy with cataplexy. In 48% of the cases, there was a negative family history. The occurrence of the disorders among the relatives is too low to be compatible with a simple monogenic theory of transmission. A genetic model incorporating a threshold appears to be more applicable to the data. Several investigators (Krabbe and Magnussen, 1942; Yoss and Daly, 1960; Imlah, 1961; Yoss, 1970) have suggested that narcolepsy may be transmitted by means of a multifactorial system, and that isolated narcolepsy and hypersomnia may follow an antizonal dominant mode. Kessler et al. (in press) suggests, but do not prove conclusively, that different thresholds (at least two) may be present on a single continuous distribution of liability. Such an explanation may perhaps account for the different clinical findings.

To summarize, we are reasonably certain that REM narcolepsy, sleep attacks associated with cataplexy, can be individualized as a specific syndrome. It also appears that certain conditions, long reported as "narcolepsy" and synonymous with "daytime sleepiness," may in fact represent several different disorders. On the other hand, the presence of daytime sleep attacks alone may occasionally be associated with REM narcolepsy. This is particularly true in the developing phase of the syndrome when some patients may present sleep attacks as a unique symptom for as long as 15 years. In a recent study of 40 REM narcoleptics, 22 patients presented daytime sleep attacks as the only symptom for a mean value of 6 years and 2 months (Guilleminault et al. in press 1973). However, daytime sleepiness may also indicate the presence of other disorders of "excessive" sleep which have no relation at all with REM narcolepsy.

SLOW-WAVE SLEEP* HYPERSOMNIA OR SWS NARCOLEPSY

One entity has been variously classified as "independent narcolepsy," "essential narcolepsy," "narcolepsy with slow wave sleep," and "hypersomnia with normal sleep" (Berti-Ceroni et al., 1967 a, b; Passouant et al., 1967; Roth et al., 1969; Mouret et al., 1972). This condition seems to exist as a syndrome different from other hypersomnia syndromes. However, this type of "narcolepsy" can only be described when REM narcolepsy, sleep apnea-hypersomnia, and other syndromes with impairment of the waking system, such as the "subwakefulness syndrome" (Jouvet and Pujol, 1972) and the syndrome of "nonmaintenance of vigilance" (Guilleminault et al., 1973d, in press) have been ruled out. Thus several previous reports of this disorder are questionable because respiration and other variables necessary to characterize the above conditions have not been recorded. However, Berti-Ceroni et al. (1967, a,b), Passouant et al. (1968), and Mouret et al. (1972) have studied patients throughout the nycthemere quite extensively.

It appears that a SWS narcolepsy can be distinguished by the occurrence of a great amount of SWS during the 24 hours, a very low percentage of REM sleep (REMS/TST=5.1%), and a significant amount of stages 3 and 4 NREM during the daytime naps. Moreover, Berti-Ceroni et al. (1971) have demonstrated another distinctive feature of this condition. They conducted total sleep deprivation for 24 to 40 hours in patients with REM narcolepsy and in patients with independent or SWS narcolepsy. The two populations responded very differently during the postdeprivation recovery phase. In REM-type narcoleptics, total sleep time was very seldom higher than baseline values and the patients continued to present very significant nocturnal sleep disruption with several conscious arousals on the recovery night and with an abnormally short latency to the onset of the first REM period. The independent narcoleptics, on the other hand, had prolonged recovery sleep with a normal progression of NREM to REM sleep. Futhermore, if there were any nocturnal disruptions on baseline nights in these patients, none could be noted during the recovery phase.

Another interesting difference between the two populations seems to be the duration of each sleep period. It is well known that REM narcoleptics can be refreshed by very short naps (10 to 20 min). But in independent narcolepsy, the duration of each sleep period seems to be much longer (30 to 60 min), and the "refreshing" quality of sleep is not as clear as in REM narcolepsy.

*In this usage "Slow Wave Sleep" is roughly synonymous with NREM sleep: we use it because the term is used by other authors.

HYPERSOMNIA WITH "SLEEP DRUNKENNESS"

Roth et al. (1972) have individualized another clinical entity: hypersomnia with sleep drunkenness (HSD). This syndrome is characterized by diurnal sleep spells, and in that regard is similar to the "SWS hypersomnia" described by Berti-Ceroni et al. (1967 a,b) and by Mouret et al. (1972). However, these patients complain of a very peculiar symptomatology: when awakened in the morning, which seems to be very difficult to do, the patients appear to be confused, disoriented, very slow and unable to react adequately to external stimuli. Frequently, the movements of the patients are uncoordinated, particularly their gait. This symptomatology disappears progressively throughout the morning, but may return at intervals during the day. The patients also complain of very "deep" sleep at night. The daytime symptomatology seems very similar to that reported in children awakened during stage 4 slow-wave sleep, or to that noted by Fisher et al. (1970) in patients who arouse suddenly from a stage 2 or stage 4 nightmare.

For this reason, we might postulate that hypersomnia with sleep drunkenness involves an abnormal increase of stage 3 and stage 4 NREM sleep. However, the first report of the syndrome reported no information on the polygraphic aspect. More studies need to be conducted before an adequate description and definition of the HSD can be given.

Finally, the syndrome seems to occur quite infrequently. In our experience, we have been unable to find a single hypersomniac with sleep drunkenness in our clinic population of approximately 120 patients who complain of excessive sleep or sleepiness.

Two additional entities have been described in the past few years. One has not been well documented, the syndromes secondary to a dysfunction of the waking system; and the other has been much more extensively studied, the sleep apnea-hypersomnia syndromes.

DYSFUNCTION OF THE WAKING SYSTEM

In 1970, Petitjean and Jouvet showed that a stereotaxic lesion of the dorsal noradrenergic bundle at the level of the isthmus in the brainstem of the cat induced a true "hypersomnia" with an increase in both slow-wave sleep and REM sleep to well above baseline levels. In these cats, "an increase in telencephalic 5HIAA and tryptophane parallels the decrease in noradrenaline" (Jouvet, 1972).

Various biochemical and neurophysiologic studies have implicated two mechanisms involved in the maintenance of wakefulness in the cat. The first mechanism affected by the manipulation described above appears to be a noradrenergic system "issuing from the anterior part of the locus coeruleus complex, ascending through the dorsal noradrenergic bundle and also probably situated in group A8 of catecholamine-containing neurons of the mesencephalic tegmentum" (Jouvet, 1972). This system, it appears, is

"responsible for the tonic cortical activation which accompanies waking."
For Jouvet, the cat lesioned in this system is an animal model very closely
related to the so-called SWS hypersomnia of Mouret et al. (1972).

In describing the second system involved in maintaining wakefulness in the
cat, Jouvet (1972) reports that, if a lesion is performed on the catecholaminergic bundle rostral to the isthmus, a different syndrome can be observed in cats. In these animals, there is a "decrease in EEG desynchronization" (Jones et al., 1969) which appears to be directly related to a
decrease in NA in the rostral brain. Furthermore, no increase in NREM or in
REM sleep can be seen, but one can observe what Jouvet called a "de-
activated EEG" (Jouvet, 1972) or an "intermediate state" that appears when
wakefulness would normally occur. This intermediate state, different from
both wakefulness and sleep, is defined as a "nonwakefulness state" by Jouvet
(1972). In man, this intermediate state might appear as stage 1 or stage 2
NREM sleep (Jouvet and Pujol, 1972; Mouret et al., 1972).

Mouret et al. (1972) have reported six patients whom they classified as a
human analogue of the cat nonwakefulness syndrome. These patients
presented daytime drowsiness and daytime sleep spells. When recorded, the
sleep spells were always stage 1 or stages 1 and 2 sleep; they appeared in a
repetitive way; and deep slow-wave (stages 3, 4) sleep was never recorded. In
nocturnal sleep recordings, however, stages 3 and 4 developed harmoniously,
and a slight reduction of REM sleep was noted.

Mouret and his colleagues (1972) have attempted to correlate these
polygraphic findings with biochemical data. They have measured
cerebrospinal fluid (CSF) levels of one metabolite of the serotonergic system,
5 hydroxyindole-acetic acid (5HIAA), and one metabolite of the
catecholaminergic system, homovanillic acid (HVA). Measures were obtained
both before and after probenecid ingestion. The biochemical findings in
these patients tend to parallel those seen in cats. However, as the authors
have carefully emphasized, while biochemical data may suggest
neurotransmitter dysfunction, they can by no means be interpreted as
positive proof. On the other hand, the correlation between polygraphic and
biochemical findings in humans that parallel the animal findings is highly
suggestive of a possible relationship between the two syndromes.

Several questions arise when considering the data of Mouret et al. For
example, should stage 2 NREM sleep be considered "sleep"? For a number
of years, it has been conventional to assume that "sleep" was "well-
established" when sleep spindles and K complexes could be recorded. For
Mouret et al., however, there are two types of "stage 2" sleep depending upon
the underlying metabolic changes. In other words, the "metabolic
background" would define the "kind" of stage 2 sleep although EEG itself
might show an identical configuration. However, the acceptance of stage 1
NREM sleep and stage 2 as an intermediate state is far from unanimous.
Interpretation of the data of Mouret et al. is further complicated by the small
number of patients reported and the fact that the authors do not describe

their methodology. Thus, we are not told how many 24 hour recordings were performed, in what kind of environment the patients were recorded, whether the patients were in bed, in an armchair, on a stool, and so on.

However, in support of Mouret's findings, we have studied several patients who complained of daytime sleepiness in the Stanford Sleep Disorders Clinic and at least one grossly resembles Mouret's description. This patient was a medical student who had difficulty maintaining alertness in the daytime during his classes and who complained of "intellectual difficulty, with memory impairment secondary to his sleep problem." Continuous polygraphic monitoring of this patient was carried out for 5 nights and 4 days (a total of 105 hours). After one adaptation night, the patient was placed on a restricted sleep schedule of 8 1/2 hours nocturnal "time in bed" (from 11 pm to 7:30 am) for the first two days (Phase I). During Phase I, the patient was administered two different 1 hour performance tests (the Wilkinson Addition Test (WAT) and the Light Stimulus Vigilance Test (LSVT) three times during the day, a total of 6 hour-long sessions. On days 3 and 4 (Phase II) the patient was on an *ad libitum* sleep schedule and was allowed to lie down on his bed any time he felt drowsy. No performance tests were conducted in Phase II. On the last two days of the study (Phase III) biochemical data were gathered. A lumbar puncture was performed on day 5 followed by oral administration of probenecid (50 mg/kg) during the next 15 hours and a second lumbar puncture 20 hours after the first. HVA and 5HIAA levels in the CSF were measured with the following results: Baseline HVA $= 37.5$ ng/ml; baseline 5HIAA $= 33.8$ ng/ml; post-probenecid HVA $= 34.4$ ng/ml; post-probenecid 5HIAA$= 41.3$ ng/ml. An interesting finding seen here is that the HVA level did not increase after probenecid administration. (The probenecid level was also determined in the CSF). Finally, results of the polygraphic recordings during the *ad libitum* period were similar to those reported by Mouret et al. (1972) in their six "nonwakefulness syndrome" patients.

We have also utilized the above protocol to study four other patients in whom REM narcolepsy and sleep apnea syndrome had been previously ruled out (Guilleminault et al., 1973; Phillips et al., in press). All patients were males, ranging in age from 23 to 40 years, who complained of excessive daytime sleepiness. Two normal 26-year old male control subjects were also studied for Phase I of the same protocol.

The results of this study were quite surprising in several respects. No difference was seen in total sleep time between the patients and the normal controls during the Phase I restricted sleep period. One of the most striking findings was the fact that in 3 of the so-called hypersomniac patients, the total sleep time was *higher* during Phase I (fixed nocturnal time in bed) than in Phase II (*ad lib.* sleep and activity). The fourth patient showed no difference in total sleep time between the two phases. Another important finding was that the two control subjects had much greater amounts of stage 3 and stage 4 NREM sleep (mean $= 114$ min) than the hypersomniac patients (mean = 42 min) during Phase I. Conversely, the hypersomniacs had much more stage 2 sleep than the normals. These differences were unrelated to age (Fig. 5).

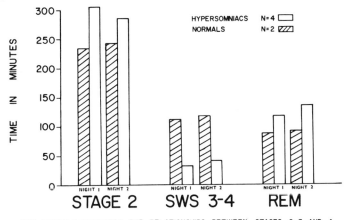

THIS FIGURE ILLUSTRATES THE RELATIONSHIPS BETWEEN STAGES 2, 3 AND 4, AND REM SLEEP. THE RANGE OF TIMES SPENT IN STAGE 2 AND STAGES 3 AND 4 FOR HYPERSOMNIACS AND NORMALS ARE MUTUALLY EXCLUSIVE.

Fig. 5. Total sleep time in hypersomniacs and normal controls.

The LSVT and WAT also demonstrated highly significant differences between the normal subjects and the patients. The control subjects *never* fell asleep during any of the LSVT sessions. In marked contrast, each patient showed EEG and behavioral signs of sleepiness or "microsleeps" in virtually every testing session. We defined these microsleeps as a burst of theta activity recorded from the EEG, slow rolling eye movements apparent in the EOG, and a response failure to the light stimulus. Occasionally, signs of stage 2 NREM sleep were also present during the LSVT in the patients.

The biochemical results were unremarkable. We were unable to find any abnormal HVA or 5HIAA values, either before or after probenecid administration, which would correlate with the findings of Mouret et al. (1972).

In conclusion, our admittedly small group of patients never presented an excessive amount of sleep, even when permitted to sleep as much as possible. In fact, during the *ad libitum* period, the patients' sleep time actually decreased and the structure of their sleep became disrupted. Moreover, the daytime performance of the patients decreased abnormally and this decrease could not be explained on the basis of a normal circadian variation.

Our studies, and those of Mouret et al. (1972), although performed on a very small number of patients, may nonetheless indicate that the complaints of "excessive" sleep, inappropriate sleep spells, or simply a loss of intellectual capacity (loss of memory, difficulty in performing at a high level, etc.) secondary to microsleeps, may be due to an inability to "maintain wakefulness" not necessarily associated with a disruption of the NREM sleep system. Thus, the hypothesis of an abnormality of the "waking system" must be considered in the presence of such a complaint. Finally, new approaches must be developed for a better understanding of these patients.

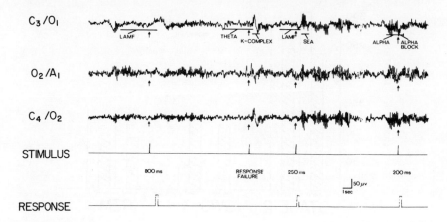

AN EXAMPLE OF BRAINWAVE STATE ALTERNATIONS IN A HYPERSOMNIAC DURING THE LSVT. THREE GENERAL BRAINWAVE STATES: ALPHA; LOW AMPLITUDE MIXED FREQUENCY (LAMF) AND THETA ARE SEEN WITH THEIR RESPECTIVE REACTION TIMES. FOUR LEVELS OF POST STIMULUS EEG ACTIVITY RELATED TO LEVEL OF AROUSAL ARE SEEN: ALPHA BLOCK; STIMULUS EVOKED ALPHA (SEA); NO CHANGE; K-COMPLEX.

Fig. 6. EEG changes and response failure in a hypersomniac patient during LSVT.

HYPERSOMNIA AND SLEEP APNEAS

Although the association of respiratory problems and the complaint of hypersomnia has been known for many years, extensive studies have not been conducted until the last decade. In 1810, Wadd noted that "excessive" obesity could be associated with periodic breathing and diurnal somnolence. In 1936, Kerr and Lagen added that a cardio-circulatory problem could develop in such patients. Burwell et al., in 1956, proposed to call the cardio-respiratory syndrome of obesity the "Pickwickian Syndrome," after the famous fictitious character described by Charles Dickens. The authors characterized this syndrome as diurnal hypersomnolence, obesity, cyanosis, polycythemia, and cardio-respiratory disorders with respiratory pauses. In 1965, Jung and Kuhlo reported a patient who had presented abnormal sleep apneic episodes for 10 years prior to the clinical appearance of a typical Pickwickian syndrome; and Gastaut et al. (1965; 1966) have shown that the sleep disturbance and hypersomnolent state were related to so-called "periodic breathing." Since that time, numerous nocturnal polygraphic studies have given a better understanding of the condition called "hypersomnia-hypoventilation syndrome" by Coccagna et al. (1970b), "hypersomnia with periodic breathing" by Lugaresi et al. (1972a), and which we prefer to call "sleep apnea-hypersomnia." Before describing this syndrome, however, it is necessary to review the relationship between cardio-respiratory functions and sleep in normal individuals.

Respiration and Sleep in Normal Adults

Several studies of respiratory function during physiologic sleep have been performed on normal adults using different techniques. Simple polygraphic recordings were conducted by Dement (1964), Snyder et al. (1964), Aserinsky (1965; 1967), and Bristow et al. (1969). Other investigators have used spirographic techniques (Robin et al., 1958; Bulow and Ingvar, 1961; Bulow, 1963; Duron et al., 1966). One of the most complete studies of respiration in normal sleep was recently conducted by Duron (1972), who obtained results from three different techniques applied successively to the same subjects and systematically included measurements during wakefulness. Respiratory irregularities during sleep were noted by all the above investigators. Several general areas of agreement were apparent. Minor apneic episodes and spirographic irregularities during REM periods are most frequently related to bursts of rapid eye movements although significant individual differences are present. Respiratory pauses in REM periods are seldom longer than 15 seconds. Periodic breathing may develop during NREM sleep, but respiratory pauses are exceptional, and if noted, never exceed 10 seconds.

Several investigators (Sieker et al., 1960; Bulow and Ingvar, 1961; Ingvar and Bulow, 1963) reported a relative hypercapnia during sleep. However, this seems to be a controversial point since Duron (1972) denies the development of any hypercapnia during normal sleep.

Arterial Pressure and Pulmonary Artery Pressure Changes During Normal Sleep

Using indirect methods, Snyder et al. (1963, 1964) and Richardson et al. (1964) have shown that significant hemodynamic changes occur during sleep in human volunteers. Khatri and Freis (1967), Bristow et al. (1969), and Coccagna et al. (1971) generally confirmed these earlier reports by cannulating the brachial artery for direct continuous recording of the arterial pressure during sleep. One description will illustrate the complexity of the technique: Coccagna et al. (1971) used a needle connected by Teflon tubing to a P23Db Statham transducer whiih was in turn connected to a Model Kemt-a electromanometer. Simultaneous continuous polygraphic recording of EEG, EOG, chin EMG, respiration, and EKG were also obtained by Coccagna et al. (1971) on 8 normal volunteers.

Khatri and Freis (1967), Bristow et al. (1969), and Coccagna et al. (1971) showed that the arterial pressure decreases rapidly during the first hours of sleep and gradually increases in the second part of the night. These authors agreed that there is a direct relationship between sleep stages and arterial pressure changes: the lowest systolic and diastolic values were noted in stages 3 and 4 NREM sleep. Bristow et al. (1969) also reported very low values in REM sleep, but this finding was not confirmed either by Khatri and Freis (1967) or by Coccagna et al. (1971). Snyder et al. (1963, 1964) found that the arterial pressure was higher in REM sleep than in stages 3 and 4, sometimes exceeding the highest values recorded in the same subject during the waking hours (confirmed by Coccagna et al., 1971). A general agreement seems to exist that there is an extreme variability of arterial pressure during REM sleep which is not correlated with any changes in heart rate or in arterial tone (Coccagna et al., 1971).

Another controversy exists between Khatri and Freis (1967) and Coccagna et al. (1971). The former have found that the decrease in arterial pressure during sleep shows no statistically significant difference from values obtained during wakefulness, while the findings of Coccagna et al. (1971) are contradictory. Finally, Coccagna et al. (1971) speculate that an ultradian variation may be superimposed on the pressure variations linked to the sleep stages.

There is only one study of pulmonary arterial pressure (PAP) changes during sleep in normals. Lugaresi et al. (1972b) continuously monitored PAP in three normal controls by means of a microcatheter positioned in the pulmonary artery using Grandjean's technique (1967). Polygraphic recording of EEG, EOG, EKG, chin EMG, and respiration was conducted simultaneously. Cyclic variations of PAP with a period of approximately 20 to 30 seconds were noted during stages 1 and 2 NREM sleep. The variations in PAP reach a maximum of 2 to 4 mm Hg above the baseline value obtained during wakefulness. Finally, stages 3 and 4 NREM sleep seem to be the most stable periods, with no significant PA pressure fluctuations (personal communication, 1973).

Pathologic Apneic Episodes in Sleep

Three types of sleep apnea have been described in the literature (Gastaut et al., 1965, 1966; Duron et al., 1966; Tassinari et al, 1972). In the first type, the diaphragm, the principal inspiratory muscle, may cease movement for an abnormal length of time, as long as 180 seconds (Guilleminault et al., 1972c; 1973b; in press). During this time, absolutely no diaphragmatic movements can be recorded, even with a catheter tip pressure transducer positioned in the lower esophagus (Guilleminault et al., 1972c). The chest and abdominal actograms are flat; and no muscle activity can be recorded in the inspiratory intercostal muscles (Smirne et al., 1971; Tassinari et al., 1972). Obviously, no air flow can be recorded either by means of buccal and nostril thermistors or by a tube positioned through the nostril in the nasopharyngeal junction (Guilleminault et al., 1973b). When the apneic episode terminates, air flows through the upper airway with one cycle delay due to the dead space. This type of apnea is classified as "central" apnea, or, as we prefer to designate it, "diaphragmatic" apnea. (Fig. 7).

Very different from the foregoing is the "obstructive" apnea. In obstructive apnea, despite the persistence of diaphragmatic contractions which progressively increase in strength during the "apneic" period, no air flows through the upper airway. Continuous recording performed with an esophageal catheter tip pressure transducer (as described by Petit and Milic-

Emili, 1958) shows an incredible rise of intrathoracic pressure during these episodes. Lugaresi et al. (1972a) have reported extremely high peak values of nearly 100 cm of water at the end of an obstructive apnea. Progressively increasing muscle activity can be recorded in the inspiratory intercostal muscles throughout the apneic period. Then, suddenly, the obstruction is lifted and, with a great cacaphonous snort and snore, the apnea is resolved. (Fig. 8).

The "mixed-type" or "complex" apnea was originally described by Gastaut et al. (1966) who characterized a short "central" (or diaphragmatic) apnea at the beginning followed by a prolonged obstructive apnea as described.

Data collected at the Stanford University Sleep Disorders Clinic has led us to question this classification. In our own experience with Dr. F. Eldridge, we

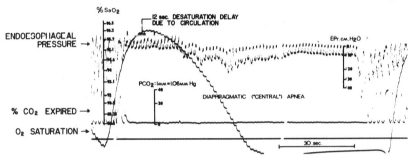

Figure 7. Diaphragmatic or central apneic episode. On the top line the diaphragmatic movements stopped for approximately 3 minutes. (EKG artifacts are superimposed during the apneic episode.) On the second line (percentage of CO_2 expired) no air flows through the upper airway during the entire apneic episode. The oxygen saturation (third line from the top) dropped dramatically during the apneic episode.

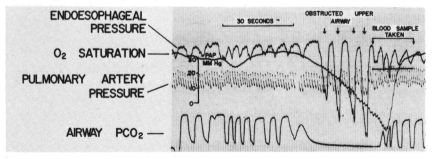

Fig. 8. Example of an "obstructive" or "peripheral" apnea in a 42-year-old male complaining of hypersomnia. No long diaphragmatic apnea is present, but one can see some diaphragmatic irregularity on the left side of the picture with no air flow for a short period through the upper airway (airway PCO_2 tracing). A long obstructive apneic episode is clearly seen on the right side of the picture. No air flows through the upper airway in spite of increasing diaphragmatic movements (endoesophageal pressure tracing). The endoesophageal pressure greatly increases and the oxygen saturation drops.

have diagnosed sleep apnea in 20 patients with different sleep complaints. We have performed very extensive cardio-respiratory studies during wakefulness and sleep in 10 of these patients to date. In this series of patients, we have always observed the mixed-type of apnea. Thus, in patients with predominantly "diaphragmatic" apneas, we have always been able to find some mild obstructive signs (usually very slight) when we have scrutinized the entire night of recording.

On the other hand, we have never seen a completely pure "obstructive" apneic syndrome during sleep—a diaphragmatic component is always present. In fact, all our patients, when a careful look was given to the entire recording, presented mixed or complex apneas; in some patients the obstructive component was predominant, and in others the diaphragmatic component predominated, but there was always at least a slight obstructive or diaphragmatic component. (Fig. 9).

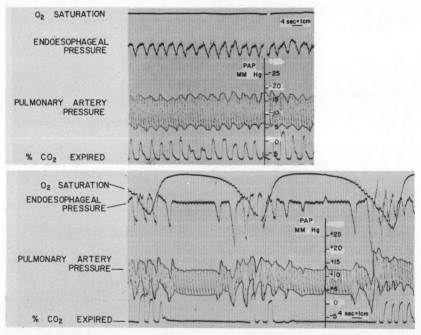

Fig. 9 (Upper). Example of a normal polygraphic recording in an awake 49-year-old narcoleptic male. (1) Oxygen saturation is obtained from an ear oxymeter. (2) Endoesophageal pressure is measured by an esophageal catheter-tip pressure transducer. (3) Pulmonary artery pressure is measured by means of a Swan-Ganz catheter. (4) Expired carbon dioxide is measured by a catheter positioned through the nostril in the hypopharynx. The comparison between the tracing obtained from lead 1 and lead 4 (O_2 Sat. and CO_2 Exp.) can easily distinguish "diaphragmatic" and "obstructive" apneas. (Lower) The same narcoleptic patient while asleep (stage 2 SWS early in the night). Example of typical "mixed apnea" with "diaphragmatic" apnea at the beginning and "obstructive" apnea which is seen when diaphragmatic moments resume. Note on the right of the figure that the pulmonary artery pressure begins to rise during the obstructive component of the apnea.

Another point that seems clear from our data is that the clinical complaint, which is usually only of a sleep disorder such as insomnia, hypersomnia with daytime sleep spells and dirunal somnolence, or narcolepsy with cataplexy, differs in relation with the type of sleep apneic episodes. That is, patients with predominant diaphragmatic apneas may complain of insomnia; those with predominant obstruction may complain of hypersomnia and diurnal somnolence, and the REM narcoleptic group seems to have nearly equal amounts of diaphragmatic and obstructive factors. On this basis, we disagree with Duron et al. (1972), who state that the peripheral factor may exist completely independent of the diaphragmatic component.

"Peripheral" or "Obstructive" Factors

When the sleep apneic condition is predominantly obstructive, the causative factor is often very obvious. Partial airway obstruction due to enlargement of tonsils and adenoids is a well recognized clinical entity in children. In some few cases, the chronic nasopharyngeal obstruction has lead to cardiomegaly and cor pulmonale. In addition, a typical alveolar hypoventilation syndrome manifested by CO_2 retention has developed (Menashe et al., 1965; Noonan, 1965; Luke et al., 1966; Levy et al., 1967).

Although Menashe et al. (1965) and Levy et al. (1967) did not study their patients during sleep, a sleep complaint was reported in several cases. Case 1 of Menashe et al., a 3 1/2-year-old girl, was hospitalized for "lethargy" and was sleeping "20 hours a day." Her sleep "was associated with cyanosis, diaphoresis, and stertorous breathing," and "the most striking findings were noted when the child was asleep. . .the abnormalities disappeared when she awakened." The same authors' Case 2, a 9-year-old boy, was hospitalized for "irresistible paroxysms of sleep which were associated with stertorous breathing and respiratory distress." His sleepiness had gradually increased for the past year to such an extent that during the month preceding his admission, "his normal activity was limited to a few morning hours. Throughout the day, he was handicapped by repeated desire for sleep." The child's nocturnal sleep was described as "very deep, with frequent enuresis, somnambulism and orthopnea."

The case of Levy et al., a 3-year-old boy, was hospitalized for "full-blown congestive cardiac failure with tachycardia." No definite etiologic diagnosis could be made to explain the congestive heart failure. However, "a striking pattern was appreciated: He was frequently semicomatose and during these spells. . .there was severe, noisy respiratory distress. He could be aroused from this with marked difficulty;" and "when not in this state (of sleep) he looked reasonably well." His parents confirmed that "he frequently slept like that at home."

Luke et al. (1966) reported 4 cases. These authors were primarily concerned with cardio-respiratory changes and did not give clinical histories that were sufficient to judge the degree of sleep disturbance except for their Case

2, a 3-year-old boy, who had "somnolence" before hospitalization: "Intermittent breathing and somnolence continued to such an extent that a central nervous system defect was suspected."

These 7 cases all demonstrated a narrowed nasopharnyx secondary to hypertrophied adenoids with a pulmonary hypertension and cardiac failure. They were specifically reported because of the rarity of such association, the importance of the hemodynamic changes, and the therapeutic effect of removal of the obstruction. In four of the seven children, a "hypersomnia syndrome" was mentioned in the clinical history; and in at least three, the authors realized that the respiratory abnormality was predominant or *only* present (1 case) during sleep. Finally, three of the children were described as "with mild obesity" (1 case) or as having recently gained weight (2 cases).

Akoun et al. (1971) and Duron et al. (1972) have dealt with a completely different population. Their patients had been classified as "Pickwickian" and were all adults (age range 43-54). They progressively developed a significant obesity and complained of marked daytime hypersomnolence. When their sleep was studied, all five patients presented an hypoxia-hypercapnia syndrome with obvious obstructive-type sleep apneic episodes. When checked for a possible cause, 3 patients had hypertrophied adenoids, and the others presented thyroid enlargement (intrathoracic goiter in one case).

In the adults, as in the children described earlier, an adenoidectomy (or the removal of the intrathoracic goiter in one adult) alleviated the diurnal somnolence. In children, this surgery also cured or ameliorated the cardiologic syndrome.

However, a few unsolved pathogenic problems are mentioned by several of the foregoing authors. Among the problems are those directly related to the symptomatology such as: Why is there sometimes an elevated left ventricular end diastolic pressure? Why could a continued moderate elevation in pulmonary artery pressure still be recorded several months after tonsillectomy and adenoidectomy (Case 1, Luke et al., 1966)? How can the secondary weight gain be explained (Menashe et al., 1965)?

For us, a major question is: Why do only a certain specific few children develop a cor pulmonale and cardiac failure, although many children are known to have hypertrophied tonsils and adenoids? Perhaps, as mentioned by Levy et al. (1967), this syndrome occurs more frequently than is supposed; but even if the incidence is underestimated, hypertrophied adenoids does not seem a sufficient explanation for the cardiac failure and the hypersomnolence. An analogous situation may pertain in the obesity-hypoventilation syndrome in both adults and children in which the same question arises since hypoventilation obviously does not develop in all obese persons.

Hypersomnia with obstructive sleep apneas has also been reported in connection with cranio-vertebral anomalies involving C_1 and C_2, and associating platybasia with basilar invagination (Krieger et al., 1969) and micrognathia (Valero and Alroy, 1975; Boonstra and Blokzi, 1970; Tammeling et al., 1972). However, the patients of Boonstra and Blokzi and Tammeling et al. did not present pure "obstructive" sleep apneas, but chiefly mixed apneic episodes in which " 'peripheral apnea' was nearly always preceded by 'central apnea'." None of these patients were obese, but all were hypersomniacs presenting sleep apneic episodes associated with very disturbed nocturnal sleep and an alveolar hypoventilation syndrome. Here, once again, Tammeling et al. (1972) asks the intriguing question, "why does hypersomnia not occur in every subject with micrognathia?"

In several of our cases at Stanford, the etiology of obstructive or peripheral sleep apnea is even more difficult to fully explain on the basis of a purely anatomical defect, such as enlarged adenoids or micrognathia. With Dr. F. Eldridge, we have diagnosed 10 patients complaining of hypersomnia with diurnal somnolence as sleep apnea cases. Four of these patients had a complete cardio-respiratory work-up during wakefulness and were also extensively studied during sleep. Cardiac catheterization was performed by floating a Swan-Ganz catheter into the pulmonary artery and a continuous recording of PAP was made over the next 14 to 18 hours which included substantial periods of both sleep and wakefulness. During sleep an ear oxymeter continuously measured the arterial oxygen saturation and arterial blood samples were drawn at strategic moments throughout the night for calibration of the oxymeter and independent validation. Peripheral air flow was analyzed by means of a buccal thermistor and a CO_2 pick-up catheter positioned in the nostril. A catheter tip transducer was positioned in the esophagus to measure intrathoracic pressure and diaphragmatic movements. Finally, EMG activity from cricopharyngeal and intercostal muscles was also recorded (Guilleminault et al., 1973b).

With these sophisticated measurements, we have identified mixed type sleep apneas with a predominant obstructive factor in all 4 cases. However, we have failed to demonstrate any obvious anatomical causes to explain such obstruction. For example, in the case of one patient, an 11-year-old boy, an adenoidectomy was performed in an attempt to relieve his hypersomniac condition; yet the diurnal somnolence remained unchanged after surgery. Other authors have reported similar cases (Schwartz and Escande, 1967; Gastaut et al., 1969; Coccagna et al., 1970a; Hishikawa et al., 1970; Tassinari et al., 1972).

It seems, then, that another factor—perhaps involving the central nervous system—may play a role in the obstruction of the upper airway during sleep. An abnormal collapse of the pharyngeal wall (Schwartz and Escande, 1967; Gastaut et al., 1969; Hishikawa et al., 1970; Tassinari et al., 1972) could be the key factor responsible for the apneic episodes. Our results would favor such an hypothesis.

The Pickwickian Syndrome Versus the Hypersomnia-Sleep Apnea Syndrome

As we have previously noted, the cardio-respiratory syndrome of obesity (Pickwickian Syndrome) was the first of the sleep apneic conditions to be described. Studies conducted since that time have suggested that the Pickwickian Syndrome should no longer be considered a discrete syndrome. A brief review of recent findings will explain the reasons for this new interpretation.

Gastaut et al. (1965; 1966) showed that, in a patient who presented the cardio-respiratory syndrome associated with obesity (Pickwickian Syndrome), 80% of the apneic episodes were of the obstructive type. Other investigators have also extensively studied the Pickwickian Syndrome and demonstrated its heterogeneity (Coccagna et al., 1968; Lugaresi et al., 1968a, c; Hishikawa et al., 1970; Kurtz et al., 1972; Tammeling et al., 1972; Tassinari et al., 1972). In other words, the following different clinical indications have all been called Pickwickian Syndrome: patients who present micrognathia, obesity with secondary cardiovascular changes, and hypersomnolence; children who present enlarged adenoids, obesity, secondary cardiovascular changes, and hypersomnolence; patients who present playtbasia with basilar invagination, obesity, secondary cardiovascular changes and hypersomnolence; and patients with hypersomnolence, obesity, without cardiovascular changes and with or without an abnormal CO_2 response curve. However, in all cases, sleep apneic episodes (of different types) with progressive development of an alveolar hypoventilation were observed. In 1969 (Lugaresi et al.) and 1970 (Coccagna et al.), the first cases of diurnal hypersomnolence with obstructive sleep apneas *without* obesity were reported. Coccagna et al. (1970b), in reviewing all their cases, showed that the semeiology and physiopathology of the sleep and respiratory disturbances were similar in the Pickwickian Syndrome, the hypersomnia syndrome with periodic apneas, and the "Ondine's Curse Syndrome" (first described by Severinghaus and Mitchell in 1962).

Ondine's Curse or primary alveolar hypoventilation is a very rare syndrome; since its first description, less than 40 patients have been reported. This syndrome involves an abnormality in the respiratory center in which the ventilatory response to inhaled CO_2 during the daytime is always perturbed. It appears that there is a failure of the automatic control of ventilation which is usually present, though not obvious, during the daytime, and which is predominant during sleep. Lugaresi et al. (1968b) found that 19 of the published cases of Ondine's Curse also presented a diurnal hypersomnolence with periodic sleep apneic episodes.

Coccagna et al. (1970b) have noted that, in these different syndromes, three major symptoms could always be found: 1) a diurnal hypersomnolence; 2) a respiratory abnormality during sleep; 3) an hypotonia of the muscle of the nasopharynx during sleep. In fact, all the disorders can be grouped under one generic term such as that proposed by Coccagna et al. (1970b), i.e., "hypersomnia-hypoventilation syndrome," or as we prefer to call it, "hypersomnia with periodic sleep apneas."

Thus, the notion of a Pickwickian Syndrome as a unique entity no longer exists. Similar types of apneic episodes can be recorded in both obese and nonobese patients (Tassinari et al., 1972; Kurtz et al., 1972). The significance of the alveolar hypoventilation syndrome also fluctuates from one patient to another with no obvious relationship to obesity nor to the degree of diurnal somnolence. Finally, when recorded, a number of so-called Pickwickian patients who have lost weight, continue to present marked abnormalities in their nocturnal sleep structure and in their respiratory patterns during sleep (Kurtz et al., 1972).

A Novel Approach to Sleep Apnea-Hypersomnia

A new concept of the hypersomnia-sleep apnea syndrome seems to appear. Diurnal hypersomnia with periodic sleep apneic episodes—whether completely discrete or associated with obesity, hypertrophied adenoids, mandibular malformation, laryngeal stenosis, etc.—always shows repetitive sleep apneas in which the obstructive type predominates (Lugaresi et al., 1972). However, the peripheral factor, no matter how obvious, is not sufficient by itself to induce the typical sleep apnea-hypersomnia syndrome. A central nervous system defect must be hypothesized to account for the fact that only a few obese patients, or a few patients with hypertrophied adenoids or micrognathia develop a hypersomnia and periodic sleep apnea syndrome.

Coccagna et al. (1970b) and Lugaresi et al. (1972a), as well as ourselves (Guilleminault et al., 1972c), have proposed the hypothesis that a defect in the reticular activating system may be responsible for both the periodic apneic episodes and the hypersomnia. In disagreeing, Gastaut et al. (1965) and Hishikawa et al. (1972) postulate that the primary problem is the respiration difficulty and that the hypersomnia arises as a direct result of the sleep apnea episodes. In other words, each time the patient needs to breathe during the night, he wakes up or presents an EEG arousal. He must then compensate during the day for the numerous "unconscious" arousals that occur during the night. Several factors make it difficult to accept this position. First, it is unclear that these unconscious arousals can lead to such marked increase in diurnal sleep as have been reported (Coccagna et al., 1970b; Lugaresi et al., 1972c) and that this profound hypersomnia is secondary *only* to a repetitive nocturnal insomnia. Secondly, certain patients, although they have a disturbed nocturnal sleep structure with little, if any, stage 3 or stage 4 sleep, may never achieve full arousals, but just pass to a lighter stage of sleep at the end of the apneic episode. It may be most logical to hypothesize that there is an interaction between a central factor and the repeated nocturnal sleep disturbance that leads to the hypersomnia in these patients. A final factor which should be considered in this regard is the role of carbon dioxide and oxygen fluctuations throughout the night.

The Role of Hypercapnia

Episodes of severe hypercapnia and hypoxemia are typical features of the sleep apnea-hypersomnia syndrome. Jung and Kuhlo (1965), Lugaresi et al. (1968c), and Brettoni et al. (1967, 1968) have affirmed that the problem of so called "carbonarcosis" should be considered.

The Role of CO_2 on the Length of the Apneic Episode

Jung and Kuhlo (1965) suggested that in the Pickwickian patient there is a low sensitivity to CO_2 stimulation. If this were true, one might find that longer periods of apnea would be required to reach levels of CO_2 sufficiently high to stimulate respiration in the Pickwickian as compared to the normal person. Drachmann and Gumnit (1962) have hypothesized a significant role for the hypoxemia in control of respiration, as have Semerano et al. (1972).

In our own experience, several patients with sleep apnea-hypersomnia appear to have an abnormal CO_2 response curve during the daytime without any other components of the Ondine's Curse Syndrome. However, we think that the combination of hypercapnia, hypoxia, and pH changes is a major influence on the respiration and that one cannot specifically implicate any one of these changes as being solely responsible for the length of the apneic episode. In fact, we also tend to think that the hypercapnia may play only a minor role, while the hypoxia and pH changes may be the primary factors. The studies of Robert et al. (1970) support such a hypothesis. These authors had a Pickwickian patient sleep in an atmosphere containing a mixture of CO_2 3% plus air during one night, and a mixture of oxygen 100% at 6 liters/minute plus air during another night. In this patient, the inhalation of an enriched CO_2 mixture did not increase the ventilatory frequency, nor did it change the number of apneic episodes during the night. On the other hand, hyperoxia led to a normalization of nocturnal sleep, with great reduction of nocturnal arousals, an increase in total stage 3 slow-wave sleep and REM sleep, and a significant reduction in the number of apneic episodes during sleep.

The Role of CO_2 on Hypersomnolence

Does a carbonarcosis develop and can the hypercapnia be partially responsible for the diurnal hypersomnolence? Lugaresi et al. (1972a) suggest that this factor should at least be considered. Bonvallet et al. (1955) have shown that the reticular activating system is extremely sensitive to CO_2, and that hypercapnia may very easily depress this structure. One could hypothesize that the pattern of recurrent respiratory pauses which leads to repetitive increases in CO_2 may decrease the sensitivity of some specific central nervous system structures that are normally involved in maintaining vigilance. However, we believe that even if this hypothesis is true, hypercapnia is not the only determining factor. It is likely that the hypercapnia, hypoxemia and pH oscillation all play a role in association, and it seems artificial to specifically dissociate the action of the CO_2 from the other major metabolic changes that occur simultaneously. For example, Wood et al. (1968) have shown that hypoxemia induces an abnormal increase in the cerebral content of gamma-aminobutyric-acid, an amino acid which supposedly has depressive effects on neural transmission and could also partially explain the hypersomnolence. Furthermore, as has been suggested by Semerano et al. (1972), hypoxia may also induce other important changes in the levels and metabolic turnover rates of the bioamines involved in the sleep-waking cycle which could also be considered as responsible for the hypersomnolent state. Thus, in our opinion, it is preferable to say that the major secondary metabolic changes play a role in hypersomnolence, and not that the CO_2 is entirely responsible.

Sleep Apnea-Hypersomnia and Secondary Cardiovascular Changes

One of the most striking findings in the past five years is the role that sleep apneas play in the development of right ventricle hypertrophy, high blood pressure, which supposes an involvement of the left ventricle, and complete cardiac failure. We wish to emphasize the fact that certain patients whose only complaint is of a sleep disorder, either hypersomnia, narcolepsy with cataplexy, or insomnia (Guilleminault et al, 1972c), may develop a severe cardiac condition due to the occult sleep apnea syndrome. A brief review of the cardiovascular changes that occur during sleep apnea is necessary to assess the consequences of the syndrome.

Coccagna et al. (1972), using continuous recording of pulmonary artery pressure (PAP) throughout the night in patients with sleep apnea-hypersomnia, have shown that a marked increase in PAP can be recorded in these patients during sleep. Since that study, these findings have been confirmed by several authors (Kuhlo and Doll, 1972; Lonsdorfer et al., 1972; Guilleminault et al., 1972c, 1973b). Alveolar hypoventilation is also a very well known cause of pulmonary hypertension and secondary development of cor pulmonale (Fishman, 1972; Fishman et al., 1966).

In every study of sleep apneic patients, continuous monitoring has shown extreme changes in PAP. Of particular interest is the finding that, even if the patient has respiratory movements between apneic episodes, the PAP does not always return to normal. Peak values of PAP are reached at the end of each apneic episode when the respiratory movements resume. Values as high as 100 mm Hg for the systolic PAP and 60 mm Hg for the diastolic PAP are not infrequent. The increase in PAP seems to be more pronounced in patients with a predominant obstructive apnea than in those with predominately diaphragmatic apneas. (Fig. 10)

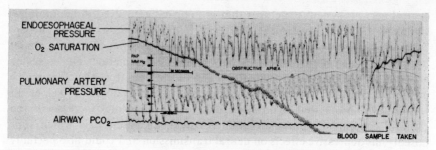

Fig. 10. Example of an obstructive apneic episode of 135 sec duration seen in a 46-year-old male who complained of hypersomnia while asleep (stage 2 NREM sleep) at 3:50 a.m. The pulmonary artery pressure progressively rises up to 90 mm Hg (diastolic) and 20 mm HG (systolic) at the end of the apneic period when respiration resumes through the upper airway (airway PCO_2). When the blood sample was drawn, the following values were obtained: pH = 7.28, $PaCO_2$ = 47 mm Hg, PaO_2 = 46 mm Hg, SaO_2 = 71.5%.

Coccagna et al. (1972) have shown a relationship between sleep stages and the values of PAP, with maximal levels recorded during REM sleep. Our studies of 10 patients at Stanford showed no significant relationships between sleep stages and PAP. Moreover, in those patients in whom a trend appeared, the relationship was in the direction of higher values of PAP occurring in stage 2 NREM sleep. However, these differences may be due to the different patient populations seen by each group. The Lugaresi and Coccagna group have seen much more marked obstructive sleep apneic episodes. In fact, the intrathoracic pressure in several of their patients rose as high as 100 cm H_2O, well above levels we have recorded in our own population of obstructive sleep apneic patients.

High blood pressure can also be noted in patients with sleep apnea-hypersomnia. Coccagna et al. (1972) continuously measured the arterial pressure of their patients during sleep. In these patients, the arterial pressure rose progressively in the successive NREM sleep stages and underwent an additional increase during REM sleep. Values as high as 210 mm Hg (systolic) and 110 mm Hg (diastolic) were frequently recorded. Furthermore, changes in heart rate paralleled those in the arterial pressure values.

To explain these changes, Coccagna et al. (1972) have evoked the role of the severe acidosis with hypoxia and hypercapnia which develop throughout the night. In our own experience, once again, only our patients with a predominant obstructive apnea presented high blood pressure. It is possible that the dramatic intrathoracic pressure increase observed during the obstructive phase of the apneic episode may be an important factor responsible for such blood pressure changes.

The Sleep Apnea-Insomnia Syndrome

Topics related to the complaint of insomnia will be covered elsewhere in this volume (see chapter by Kales et al.). However, as we indicated in the introduction, it may be inappropriate to always divide a consideration of sleep disorders along the lines of too much sleep (hypersomnia) versus too little (insomnia). An important case in point is the sleep apnea-insomnia syndrome.

In 1972, periodic breathing during sleep was discovered in patients complaining of insomnia (Guilleminault et al, 1972 b,c). In these patients, the prolonged apneas appeared to be predominantly of the diaphragmatic type (Guilleminault et al. 1973b, in press). At the present time, six patients with this syndrome have been identified within the population of insomniacs who have been referred to the Stanford Sleep Disorders Clinic. Needless to say, all insomniacs are now studied with respiratory measures in addition to the standard sleep parameters. The six patients represent about 10 percent of the total chronic insomniac population. While this is an extremely preliminary and potentially highly artifactual figure, it must nonetheless capture our attention because of the very large number of patients in the United States who complain of chronic insomnia. Again, as far as we can tell, this dramatic problem is completely unknown to the patient, who is only aware that his nocturnal sleep seems very disturbed and restless and that he is tired during the day.

Although the apnea in these insomniac patients is primarily or entirely diaphragmatic, in marked contrast to the predominantly obstructive apnea in hypersomniacs, it seems likely that the two disease processes are related in some way. This is primarily because there is a definite diaphragmatic component in the prolonged apneas of most hypersomniacs. Practical reasons would also favor considering these two entities in relation to each other; that is, they both require the same cardio-respiratory techniques for a thorough evaluation. Aside from obstructive versus diaphragmatic, major differences appear to exist in the objective total sleep time and in the sub-jective complaint. In general, the total sleep time is significantly less in the sleep apnea-insomniacs than in the sleep apnea-hypersomniacs. Although their sleep is also very disturbed, and although they may have a substantial number of arousals, the hypersomniacs tend to perceive their sleep as deep and uninterrupted. To some extent, the subjective differences may depend upon the fact that the sleep apnea-insomniacs are more likely to have full arousals following the apneas, while the hypersomniacs may have a shift to "lighter" stages of sleep.

The existence of the sleep apnea-insomnia syndrome has been confirmed in a preliminary report by Hauri (personal communication) who mentioned that he had identified sleep apnea in three patients complaining of insomnia.

The Relationship Between the Sleep Apnea Syndrome and Sudden Infant Death Syndrome [SIDS].

In 1967 a premature infant was recorded who presented prolonged apneic episodes during quiet (NREM) sleep (Guilleminault et al., 1973a). The infant seemed to breathe normally when awake. The longest apneic episode was 170 seconds with a severe bradycardia and marked cyanosis and seemed destined to terminate in death unless the infant was aroused. The infant subsequently died a few days later apparently during sleep. This case together with our studies of the sleep apnea syndrome in adults led us to elaborate an hypothesis, not only that SIDS might be the result of prolonged apneic episodes during sleep (NREM or possibly REM or both), but that the pervasive adult sleep apnea syndrome and SIDS might be manifestations of the same basic defect (Guilleminault et al. 1973a). A similar hypotheses is made by Weitzman and Graziani in chapter 7 of this volume. An implication is that the adult cases may have been "high risk" SIDS infants who survived. If so, a particularly intriguing question is why some and not others? One of the crucial issues would appear to be the effectiveness of the CNS processes that normally terminate sleep and facilitate respiration (arousal mechanisms). In this respect, it it noteworthy that all or nearly all of the adult cases are males.

Recently, we have been studying the relationship between apneic pauses and the different sleep stages in six prematures presenting apneic episodes and in two babies brought to the Stanford Hospital for a "stopped breathing" episode observed by the parents. Infants were monitored using standard sleep recording measures as well as thoracic and abdominal strain gauges and nostril and mouth thermistors. Our findings indicate that both diaphragmatic and obstructive apneic spells may exist in premature and young infants. From our very limited results, the prominence of the diaphragmatic apneas seems to be directly related to the number of months that the infant was prematurely born. An obstructive component was also seen in older infants (particularly in one infant studied after a "stopped breathing" episode).

Similar studies on infants have been conducted by Steinschneider (1972) and Deuel (1973). The former described prolonged apnea during sleep in five infants, two of whom subsequently died of SIDS. A more complete discussion of the relationship between sleep and SIDS can be found in this chapter 7 by Weitzman and Graziani.

TREATMENT OF DISORDERS OF "EXCESSIVE" SLEEP

Treatment of REM Narcolepsy

In terms of treating the characteristic diurnal sleep episodes and sleepiness of REM narcolepsy, one could very briefly summarize our view by the following conclusion: At the present time there is no good, i.e., effective and harmless, medication for daytime sleep attacks.

Amphetamines have long been considered the drugs of choice (Prinzmetal and Bloomberg, 1935; Yoss, 1969). However, the complications that can arise from chronic amphetamine use are numerous. As early as 1938, Young and Scoville reported the first case of amphetamine abuse in a narcoleptic patient. High blood pressure, addiction, depressive reactions, and amphetamine psychosis are not uncommon side effects seen with these medications. Nonetheless, amphetamines are widely prescribed for narcolepsy.

For example, in the inital screening of 50 REM narcoleptics (with cataplexy), we found that 31 patients were taking an average of 56 mg amphetamine each day (dose ranged from 10 to 300 mg). In six of the patients who were taking more than 100 mg amphetamine daily, the patients had raised the dose within the previous 3 years to cope with increasing frequency and severity of daytime sleep attacks. However, in no case had the larger amphetamine intake ameliorated the sleep attacks; on the contrary, all six patients showed a paradoxical increase of daytime sleepiness accompanying the greater amphetamine ingestion.

In these patients, a slow reduction of the daily amphetamine dose to 40 mg did not result in any increase in the symptomatology. In fact 3 of the patients reported an *improvement* in their condition with a reduction of daytime sleepiness (Guilleminault et al. in press). Furthermore, we have found that amphetamines, regardless of the dose level, are useless in controlling cataplexy, hypnagogic hallucinations or sleep paralysis except briefly in the initial treatment period.

In general, we tend to prescribe methylphenidate (Ritalin) to help daytime sleep attacks. Methylphenidate presents fewer side effects, particularly on blood pressure, and it also produces less tolerance and dependency than the amphetamines. However, this medication is not effective in controlling the auxiliary symptoms of narcolepsy and it may also induce psychiatric side effects in certain patients. One of our patients developed a paranoid psychosis with visual and auditory hallucinations while under 50 mg daily of methylphenidate. This psychotic behavior stopped within 36 hours after withdrawal of the drug.

Tricyclic antidepressants have been reported to be effective in narcoleptics with cataplexy by Akimoto et al. (1960), Hishikawa et al. (1966), Passouant et al. (1970; 1972), Roth et al. (1971), and ourselves (Guilleminault et al., submitted). The efficacy of this medication seems to be more evident on the so-called auxiliary symptoms (cataplexy, sleep paralysis, and hypnagogic hallucinations) than on the daytime sleep attacks. We have obtained satisfactory results on the auxiliary symptoms with imipramine and desmethylimipramine in 90 percent of our patients during the first year of treatment. However, the medications resulted in no improvement of the daytime sleepiness, and 4 patients presented an "escape" from control of cataplexy after six months.

Dunleavy et al. (1972) have shown that a certain number of tricyclic antidepressant drugs induce a complete suppression of REM sleep in normal controls, but that the duration of action and the suppressive effect of the medication is variable from one tricyclic antidepressant to another. These findings appear to be confirmed by the therapeutic effect of these drugs on cataplexy. The most effective compound for the treatment of the auxiliary symptoms of narcolepsy with cataplexy seems to be chlorimipramine, followed by imipramine and desmethylimipramine. Thus, the efficacy of these agents seems to be directly related to their REM suppressive properties. Trimipramine and iprindole, which do not suppress REM sleep in normal controls, appear to be useless in controlling the auxiliary symptoms of narcolepsy.

Wyatt et al. (1971) treated seven intractable narcoleptic patients with the monoamine oxidase inhibitor (MAOI) phenelzine. Striking reductions in the amount of cataplectic attacks, sleep paralysis, and hypnagogic hallucinations were noted. Daytime sleep attacks and daytime drowsiness were also reduced. However, in several of the patients, the narcoleptic symptoms periodically seemed to recur. Phenelzine almost completely suppressed REM sleep for periods of more than a year. However, MAOIs are drugs with considerable toxicity (Jarvik, 1965). In addition to being potentially lethal when taken in combination with tyramine-containing foods, they have numerous troubling side effects. Wyatt et al. (1971) reported orthostatic hypotension, edema, and impaired sexual function. When the drug was suddenly discontinued in two cases, they also reported a complete nocturnal insomnia with continuous frightening visual hallucinations when in darkness. Fisher et al. (1972) report a very similar case. The conclusion of Wyatt et al. (1971) was: "We do not recommend their (MAOI drugs) use except under the most careful scrutiny and in patients with disabling and otherwise intractable symptoms."

Because a neurotransmitter defect is suspected in narcolepsy, several investigators (Gunne et al, 1972; Saletu et al., 1971; Guilleminault et al., 1972a) have tried l-DOPA or DOPA-like medications such as amantadine (Guilleminault et al, 1972a) to control daytime sleep attacks. We are currently continuing such investigations. The following results have been reported to date (Guilleminault et al, 1972a). Amantadine has shown no positive effects on the symptoms of narcolepsy. Peripheral DOPA decarboxylase inhibitor, which supposedly would increase the amount of "central" l-DOPA, dopamine, and hopefully noradrenaline (a neurotransmitter involved in alertness) did not present any statistical changes in the daytime sleepiness of six patients. Finally, in spite of the fact that l-DOPA appeared to be effective in several patients (Guilleminault et al, 1972a), we have not used it too freely because of the psychiatric side effects induced in most of the patients.

Treatment of SWS Hypersomnia, Sleep Drunkenness, and "Maintenance of Vigilance" Syndromes

At the present time there are no known specific treatments for SWS hypersomnia, sleep drunkenness, or the "maintenance of vigilance" syndromes. As was apparent in our earlier discussion of these syndromes, there is an urgent need for further investigation of the pathogenesis of these illnesses before an effective treatment can be considered.

Treatment of Sleep Apnea Syndromes

The urgent need to deal with the severe cardiovascular changes which may develop secondarily in the sleep apnea syndromes has stimulated extensive therapeutic trials on sleep apnea-hypersomnia patients in Europe.

In patients with predominantly obstructive apnea, Kuhlo et al. (1969) were the first to propose and to perform a chronic tracheostomy. Since that time, Lugaresi, Coccagna et al. (1970, 1972, 1973), Boonstra and Blokzi (1970), Tammeling et al. (1972), and Walsh et al. (1972) have reported the following beneficial effects of such surgery:

Effect on Sleep

All authors agree that the diurnal somnolence disappeared on the day of the operation or very shortly thereafter. The nocturnal sleep became more restful immediately.

Effect on Arterial Pressure [Coccagna et al., 1972]

After the tracheostomy, the arterial pressure level in sleep and wakefulness was consonant with that observed in a normal control group.

Effect on Pulmonary Artery Pressure
[Coccagna et al., 1972; Tammeling et al., 1972]

Subsequent to tracheostomy, the pulmonary artery pressure during sleep tended to normalize. In other words, when the patients were asleep, the pulmonary artery pressure showed only a slight increase and not the high elevations that had been present before the operation.

Effect on Respiration

In most cases, a tendency to breathe periodically and to have true diaphragmatic apneas in all stages of sleep persisted. However, the apneic episodes were much shorter than before the tracheostomy, and produced few of the pathological changes that accompanied the preoperative sleep apneas. If the tracheostomy was closed, an immediate reappearance of the full symptomatology was observed (Coccagna et al., 1972).

In conclusion, when obstructive sleep apnea-hypersomnia syndrome is diagnosed, tracheostomy appears to be a very effective treatment. But it must be emphasized that the tracheostomy is a life-long condition that many patients find difficult to accept. However, at this time, chronic tracheostomy is the only treatment that we are able to propose for obstructive sleep apnea-hypersomnia.

As was mentioned previously, we have never seen a *purely* diaphragmatic sleep apnea-hypersomnia patient, but we have observed several cases of diaphragmatic sleep apnea-insomnia, and of mixed-type sleep apnea-narcolepsy. In one of these patients we have tried chlorimipramine as it had been reported effective in one patient by Kumashiro et al. (1971). The patient reported a great improvement of his sleep complaint and polygraphic recording confirmed a significant reduction in the number of apneic episodes during nocturnal sleep. However, the symptomatology was not completely cured, and more trials must be conducted before this medication can be proved effective.

CONCLUSION

"Hypersomnias" are a group of complaints that have been poorly understood by physicians for years. Even in the case of REM narcolepsy where a history of cataplectic attacks is extremely characteristic, patients are often told somewhat preemptively that they are "lazy" or "just need more sleep." In the first 35 REM narcoleptics that were seen in the Stanford Sleep Disorders Clinic, (circa 1971-72), the mean interval between the onset of symptoms and the establishment of a definitive diagnosis was 15 years! There is also a general attitude that, aside from some very obvious primary pathology such as encephalitis, brain tumor, etc., sleepiness or daytime sleep is not exactly a legitimate medical problem. In spite of their problem, many patients believe that sleep is "good" and "healthful" and that you cannot get too much of a good thing. This is particularly true if this attitude is reinforced by a similar attitude on the part of the physician to whom the patient timidly presents his complaint.

In our own geographic area, we have made strenuous efforts to acquaint community physicians with the material we have presented in this review. This may be partly responsible for the fact that 45 percent of our referrals are patients who complain of "excessive" sleep. This is almost exactly the same as the number of referrals of chronic insomniacs (48%). At any rate, both because of the fact that there are probably many more "hypersomniacs" than most people realize and because many of them have serious sleep related pathology, we must consider the disorders of excessive sleep as a significant public health problem.

Another point which we have demonstrated in this presentation is that the word "hypersomnia" or the term "excessive sleep," which we use to classify these sleep disorders, is often a misnomer when applied to specific cases. This is particularly true in REM narcolepsy where the complaint is of "inappropriate" or "irresistible" sleep episodes which, although they unquestionably interfere with the patients' daily life, do not represent an "excessive" amount of sleep.

It is commonly suggested that although a hypersomniac may not actually sleep an extraordinary amount, he is sleepy during the day because he really needs much more sleep at night. His employment situation, family demands, and other environmental constraints do not allow him to obtain the needed amount. This suggestion is readily refuted by our studies of the "non-maintenance of vigilance syndrome". As we mentioned earlier, four patients were allowed to sleep *ad libitum* during a 48 hour polygraphic recording session. These patients never slept more than 8 hours per 24 hour period. Rechtschaffen and Roth (1969) also recorded total sleep time in several non-narcoleptic patients who complained of hypersomnia (they did not rule out sleep apnea) and found unremarkable amounts (mean around 8 hours).

Of course, we can no longer consider hypersomniacs as a homogeneous group even from the standpoint of sleep parameters. Whether or not there is excessive sleep in some cases will depend upon the specific pathology. However, in the final analysis, our knowledge of these syndromes is still very limited. In fact, there is one group of patients about whom we know virtually nothing and therefore did not even mention them in this presentation. We hide our ignorance of this condition behind the label "idiopathic hypersomnia".

We have attempted to present basic frameworks within which to consider the disorders, but we have not dealt with some of the more complex problems that arise. For example, in the past 12 months, we have diagnosed the sleep apnea syndrome in 8 patients who complained of sleep attacks, cataplexy, hypnagogic hallucinations, and sleep paralysis and who presented a sleep onset REM period when recorded (Guilleminault et al., 1972c, 1973b). Sieker et al. (1960) and Kurtz et al. (1971) had previously reported the association of narcolepsy with cataplexy and the Pickwickian Syndrome. We have also found the sleep apnea syndrome in 6 patients complaining of insomnia (Guilleminault et al., 1973c). What do these findings imply about the etiology, pathophysiology, prevalence, etc., of the sleep apnea syndrome? Do we now begin to refute traditional popular and medical belief and say that sleep is bad? In other words, in terms of the potential prevalence of the sleep apneas, we may wonder if natural sleep actually undermines or impairs the respiratory functions in everyone with only certain individuals developing an overt pathology.

The answers to these and many other questions must await the results of much needed investigation into the disorders of excessive sleep. There is a need for more descriptive data, for the creation of animal models, for the study of etiology, genetic components, and prevalence of these illnesses. And, finally, there is an urgent need to develop safe and effective treatments to offer these patients. At the present time, several centers located in Europe, North America, and Japan are working on the problem areas. But the field is still in its infancy and the answers will not be achieved overnight.

The work of Dr. Dement and Dr. Guilleminault is supported by National Institutes of Neurological Diseases and Stroke Grant NS 10727 and Research Scientist Development Award MH 05804. The cardio-respiratory studies of sleep apnea were conducted in collaboration with Dr. Frederic L. Eldridge whose research is supported by Public Health Services Grant NS 09390.

The authors wish to thank members of the Stanford University Sleep Disorders Clinic, Dr. Vincent P. Zarcone, Dr. Richard A. Wilson, and Dr. Seymour Kessler, who have participated in the experiments reported in this paper; they wish to thank Mary Carskadon and Lynn Hassler for their assistance in editing the manuscript.

REFERENCES

Akimoto, H., Honda, Y. and Takahashi, Y. Pharmacotherapy in narcolepsy. *Dis. Nerv. Syst. 21*, 704-706 (1960).

Akoun, G., Schwartz, B., Farge, B., Engle, M., Vannier, R. and Brocard, H. Syndrome Pickwickien, bronchite chronique et hypertrophie amygdalienne. *J. Franc Med. Chir. Theoret. 25*, 555-568 (1971).

Aserinsky, E. Periodic respiratory pattern occurring in conjunction with eye movements during sleep. *Science 150*, 763-766 (1965).

Aserinsky, E. Physiological activity associated with segments of the rapid eye movement period. in, *Sleep and Altered States of Consciousness,*E. Evarts, S. Kety, and H. Williams, Eds., Williams and Wilkins, Baltimore, 1967, pp. 335-350.

Berti-Ceroni, G., Coccagna, G., Gambi, D. and Lugaresi, E. Considerazioni clinico paligrafiche sulla narcolessia esseuziole "a sonno lento". *Sist. Nerv. 19*, 81-89 (1967a).

Berti-Ceroni, G., Coccagna, G. and Lugaresi, E. L'organizzazione ipnica nitermerale nei narcolettiai. *Riv. Pat. Nerv. Ment. 88*, 343-354 (1967b).

Berti-Ceroni, G., Pazzaglia, P., Mantovani, M. et al. The effects of total sleep deprivation in narcoleptics. *Electroencephal. Clin. Neurophysiol. 30*, 373 (1971).

Birchfield, R., Sieker, H. and Heyman, A. Alterations in blood gases during natural sleep and narcolepsy: A correlation with electroencephalographic stages of sleep. *Neurology 8*, 107-112 (1958).

Bonvalet, M., Hugelin, A. and Dell, P. Sensibilite comparee du systeme reticule activateur ascendant et du centre respiratoireaux gaz du sang et l'adrenaline. *J. Physiol.* (Paris) *47*, 651-654 (1955).

Boonstra, S. and Blokzi, J. Genesis and dramatic cure in two patients suffering from severe diurnal hypersomnia. *Electroencephal. Clin. Neurophysiol 28*, 423-430 (1970).

Bowling, G. and Richards, N. Diagnosis of the narcolepsy syndrome. *Cleveland Clin. Quart. 28*, 38-45 (1961).

Brettoni, B., Baccini, A., Paci, P. and Parenti, R. La syndrome di Pickwick (contributo Casistico) *Giorn. Pneumol. 11*, 555-569 (1967).

Brettoni, B., Palatresi, R., Paci, P. and Parenti, R. L'acidosi respiratoria degli obesi. *Mal. Tor. Cardiovasc. 4*, 37-51 (1968).

Bristow, J. Honour, A., Pickering, T. and Sleight, P. Cardiovascular and respiratory changes during sleep in normal and hypertensive subjects. *Cardiovasc. Res. 3*, 476-485 (1969).

Bruhova, S. and Roth, B. Heredo familial aspects of narcolepsy and hypersomnia. *Arch. Suisse. Neurol. Neurochir. Psychiat. 110*, 45-54 (1972).

Bulow, K. Respiration and wakefulness in man. *Acta Physiol. Scand. 59* (suppl.) 209 (1963).

Bulow, K. and Ingvar, D. Respiration and state of wakefulness in normals studied by spyrography, capnography and EEG. *Acta Physiol. Scand. 51*, 230-238 (1961).

Burwell, C., Robin, E., Whaley, R., and Bikelman, A. Extreme obesity associated with alveolar hypoventilation: A Pickwickian syndrome. *Amer. J. Med. 21*, 811-818 (1956).

Cadilhac, J.,Tomka, R. et Passouant, P. Les hypersomnies paroxystiques essentielles (Interet de la telemetrie). *Rev. EEG Neurophysiol. [Paris] 1 [3],* 309-313 (1971).

Coccagna, G., Petrella, A., Berti-Ceroni, G., Lugaresi, E. and Pazzaglia, P. Polygraphic contribution to hypersomnia and respiratory troubles in Pickwickian Syndrome. in, *The Abnormalities of Sleep in Man,* H. Gastaut, E. Lugaresi, G. Berti-Ceroni, and G. Coccagna, Eds. Gaggi, Bologna, Italy, 1968, pp. 215-221.

Coccagna, G., Lugaresi, E. and Mantovani, M. Le ipersonnie con respirazione periodica. *Proc. Conf. Soc. Ital. EEG Neurofisiol.* (Rimini) 1970a, pp. 255-264.

Coccagna, G., Mantovani, M., Berti-Ceroni, G., Pazzaglia, P., Petrella, A. and Lugaresi, E. Sindromi ipersonniche-ipoventilatore. *Min. Med. 61*, 1073-1084 (1970b).

Coccagna, G., Mantovani, M., Brignami, F., Manzini, A., and Lugaresi, E. Arterial pressure changes during spontaneous sleep in man. *Electroenceph. Clin. Neurophysiol. 31*, 277-281 (1971).

Coccagna, G., Mantovani, M., Brignami, F., Parchi, C. and Lugaresi, E. Continuous recording of the pulmonary and systemic arterial pressure during sleep in syndromes of hypersomnia with periodic breathing. *Bull. Physiopathol. Resp. [Nancy] 8*, 1159-1172 (1972).

Coccagna, G., Mantovani, M., Brignami, F., Parchi, C. and Lugaresi, E. Tracheostomy in hypersomnia with periodic breathing. *Bull. Physiopathol. Resp. [Nancy] 8*, 1217-1227(1972).

Cohn, L. and Cruvant, M. Relation of narcolepsy to epilepsy. *Arch. Neurol. Psych. [Chicago] 51*: 163-170, 1944.

Daly, D., and Yoss, R. A family with narcolepsy. *Mayo Clin.Proc. 34*, 313-320 (1959).

Daniels, L. Narcolepsy. *Medicine 13*, 1-122 (1934).

Dement, W. Eye movements during sleep. in, *The Oculomotor System,* M. Bender, Ed., Hoeber Medical Division, Harper and Row, New York, 1964, pp. 366-416.

Dement, W., Rechtschaffen, A. and Gulevich, G. A polygraphic study of the narcoleptic sleep attack. *Electroenceph. Clin. Neurophysiol. 17*, 608-609 (1964).

Dement, W., Rechtschaffen, A. and Gulevich, G. The nature of the narcoleptic sleep attack. *Neurology 16*, 18-33 (1966).

Dement, W. and Rechtschaffen, A. Narcolepsy: polygraphic aspects, experimental and theoretical concepts. in, *The Abnormalities of Sleep in Man,* H. Gastaut et al., Eds. Gaggi, Bologna, Italy, 1968, pp. 147-164.

Dement, W.,Zarcone, V., Varner, V., Hoddes, E., Nassau, S., Jacobs, B., Brown, J., McDonald, A., Horan, K., Glass, R., Gonzales, P., Friedman, E. and Phillips, R. The prevalence of narcolepsy. *Sleep Res. 1*, 148 (1972).

Dement, W., Carskadon, M. and Ley, R. The prevalence of narcolepsy II. *Sleep Res.*, 1973 (in press).

Dement, W., Guilleminault, C., and Mitler, M. Cataplectic attack: Polygraphic recording in man and experimental induction in cat. *Neurology 23*, 403-404 (1973a).

Dement, W., Guilleminault, C., Mitler, M., Wilson, R. and Zarcone, V. Disorders of "excessive" sleep. in,*Proceedings of the First Canadian Meeting on Sleep.* McClure, Ed.,1973b, pp. 23-40.

Deuel, R. Polygraphic monitoring of apneic spells. *Arch. Neurol. 28*, 71-76 (1973).

Drachman, D. and Gumnit, R. Periodic alteration of consciousness in the "Pickwickian" syndrome. *Arch. Neurol. 6*, 471-477 (1962).

Dunleavy, D., Brezinova, V., Oswald, I., Maclean, A. and Tinker, M. Changes during weeks in effects of tricyclic drugs on the human sleeping brain. *Brit. J. Psychiat. 120*, 663-672 (1972).

Duron, B. La fonction respiratoire pendant le sommeil physiologique. *Bull. Physiopathol. Resp. [Nancy] 8*, 1277-1288 (1972).

Duron, B., Tassinari, C. and Gastaut, H. Analyse spirographique et electromyographique de la respiration au cours du sommeil controle par l'EEG chez l'homme normal. *Rev. Neurol. 115*, 562-574 (1966).

Fisher, C., Byrne, J., Edwards, A., Kahn, E. A psychophysiological study of nightmares. *J. Amer. Psychoanal. Assoc. 18*, 747-782 (1970).

Fisher, C., Kahn, E., Edwards, A. and Davis, D. Total suppression of REM sleep with Nardil in a patient with intractable narcolepsy. *Sleep Res. 1*, 159 (1972).

Fishman, A. The syndrome of chronic alveolar hypoventilation. *Bull. Physiopathol. Resp.* [*Nancy*] *8*, 971-980 (1972)

Fishman, A., Goldring, R. and Turino, G. General alveolar hypoventilation: A syndrome of respiratory and cardiac failure in patients with normal lungs. *Quart. J. Med. 35*, 261-274 (1966).

Fujiki, A. and Kaneko, Z. Electroenephalographic study in narcolepsy especially concerning the symptoms of cataplexy, sleep paralysis and hypnagogic hallucination. *Proc. Jap. EEG Soc.*, 52-55 (1963).

Gastaut, H., Tassinari, C. and Duron, B. Etude polygraphique des manifestation épisodiques (hypniques et respiratoires) diurnes et nocturnes du syndrome de Pickwick. *Rev. Neurol. 112*, 573-579 (1965).

Gastaut, H., Duron, B., Papy, J., Tassinari, C. and Waltregny, A. Etude polygraphique comparative du cycle nychtemerique chez les narcoleptiques, les pickwickiens, les obeses et les insuffisants respiratoires. *Rev. Neurol. 115*, 456-462 (1966).

Gastaut, H., Duron, B., Tassinari, C., Lyagoubi, S. and Saier, J. Mechanism of the respiratory pauses accompanying slumber in the Pickwickian syndrome. *Act. Nerv. Super. 11*, 209-215 (1969).

Gelineau, J. De la narcolepsie. *Gaz. d. hop.* [*Paris*] *53*, 626-628 (1880).

Goode, G. Sleep paralysis. *Arch. Neurol. 6*, 228-234 (1962).

Grandjean, T. Une microtechnique du catheterisme cardiaque droit praticable au lit du malade sans controle radioscopique. *Cardiologia* [*Basel*] *51*, 184-192 (1967).

Guilleminault, C., Castaigne, P. and Cathala, H. Observation on the effectiveness of amantadine, L-dopa, L-dopa plus dopa decarboxylase inhibitor, and dopa decarboxylase inhibitor in the treatment of narcolepsy. *Sleep Res. 1*, 150 (1972a).

Guilleminault, C., Dement, W., Wilson, R. and Zarcone, V. Respiration problems and sleep disorders. *Sleep Res. 1*, 151 (1972b).

Guilleminault, C., Eldridge, F. and Dement, W. Narcolepsy, insomnia and sleep apneas. *Bull. Physiopathol. Resp.* [*Nancy*] *8*, 1127-1138 (1972c).

Guilleminault, C., Dement, W. and Monod, N. Nouvelle hypothese a propos du syndrome "mort subite du nourrisson": Apnees au cours du sommeil. *Nouv. Pres. Med.*, May (1973a).

Guilleminault, C., Eldridge, F. and Dement, W. Sleep apnea: A syndrome associated with several sleep disorders. *Neurology 23*, 389-390 (1973b).

Guilleminault, C., Eldridge, F. and Dement, W. Sleep apnea—a unique syndrome with important cardio-respiratory changes. *Sleep Res.* (1973c, in press).

Guilleminault, C., Phillips, R. and Dement, W. A new approach utilizing EEG spectral analysis and vigilance tests to study "idiopathic hypersomnia". *Proc. of Marseille 8th International Congress of EEG and Clinical Neurophysiol.*, 1973d, (in press).

Guilleminault, C., Raynal, D., Wilson, R. and Dement, W. Continuous polygraphic recording in narcoleptic patients. *Sleep Res.* (1973e, in press).

Guilleminault, C., Smythe, H. and Dement, W. Cataplexy, H reflex and therapeutic trial. *Sleep Res.* (1973f, in press).

Guilleminault, C., Eldridge, F. and Dement, W. Insomnia with sleep apnea: Preliminary report of a new syndrome. *Science* (in press).

Guilleminault, C., Carskadon, M. and Dement, W. On the treatment of REM narcolepsy. *Arch. Neurol.* (in press).

Gunne, L. Lidvall, H. and Widen, L. Preliminary clinical trial with L-Dopa in narcolepsy. *Psychopharmacology, 19,* 204 (1971)

Hishikawa, Y., Tabushi, K., Ugyama, M., Hariguchi, S., Fujiki, A. and Kaneko, Z. Electroencephalographic study in narcolepsy especially concerning the symptoms of cataplexy, sleep paralysis and hypnagogic hallucination. *Proc. Jap. EEG Soc.,* 52-55 (1963).

Hishikawa, Y. and Keneko, A. Electroencephalographic study on narcolepsy. *Electroenceph. Clin. Neurophysiol. 18*; 249-259 (1965).

Hishikawa, Y., Ida, H., Nakai, K. and Kaneko, Z. Treatment of narcolepsy with imipramine (Tofranil) and desmethylimipramine (Pertofran). *J. Neurol. Sci. 3*; 453-461 (1966).

Hishikawa, Y., Nanno, H. Tachibana, M. et al. The nature of sleep attack and other symptoms of narcolepsy. *Electroenceph. Clin. Neurophysiol. 24*; 1-10 (1968).

Hishikawa, Y., Furuya, E., Wakamatsu, H. and Yamamoto, J. A polygraphic study of hypersomnia with periodic breathing and primary alveolar hypoventilation. *Bull. Physiopathol. Resp. [Nancy] 8*; 1139-1151 (1972).

Hodes, R. and Dement, W. Depression of electrically induced reflexes ("H-reflexes") in man during low voltage EEG "sleep". *Electroenceph. Clin. Neurophysiol. 17*; 617-629 (1964).

Imlah, N. Narcolepsy in identical twins. *J. Neurol. Neurosurg. Psychiatry 24*; 158-160 (1961).

Ingvar, D. and Bulow, K. Respiratory regulation in sleep in· *Regulation of Respiration Ann. N.Y. Acad. Sci. 109*; 870-879 (1963).

Jarvik, M. Drug used in the treatment of psychiatric disorders. in; *The Pharmacological basis of Therapeutics* 3rd ed., L. Goodman, and A. Gilman, eds. Macmillan, New York, 1965, pp. 159-214.

Jones, B., Bobillier, P. and Jouvet, M. Effets de la destruction des neurones contenant des catecholamines du mesencephale sur le cycle veille—sommeil du chat. *C. R. Soc. Biol. [Paris] 163*; 176-180 (1969).

Jones, H. and Oswald, I. Two cases of healthy insomnia. *Electroenceph. Clin. Neurophysiol. 24*; 378-380 (1968).

Jouvet, M. The role of monoamines and acetylcholine-containing neurons in the regulation of the sleep-waking cycle. *Ergeb Physiol. 64*; 166-307 (1972).

Jouvet, M. and Pujol, I. Etude neurophysiologique et biochimique. *Rev. Neurol. [Paris] 127;* 115-138 (1972).

Jung, R. and Kuhlo, W. Neurophysiological studies of abnormal night sleep and the Pickwickian syndrome. in; *Sleep Mechanism.,* K. Akert, C. Bally, and J. Schade, eds., Elsevier, Amsterdam, 1965, pp. 140-159.

Kerr, W. and Lagen, J. The postural syndrome to obesity leading to postural emphysema and cardio-respiratory failure. *Ann. Int. Med. 10*; 569-578 (1936).

Kessler, S., Guilleminault, C. and Dement, W. A genetic study on REM narcolepsy. *Sleep Res.* (1973, in press).

Khatri, I. and Freis, E. Hemodynamic changes during sleep. *J. Appl. Physiol. 22;* 867-873 (1967).

Krieger, A., Rosomoff, H., Kuperman, A. and Zingesser, L. Occult respiratory dysfunction in a craniovertebral anomaly. *J. Neurosurg. 31*; 15-20 (1969).

Krabbe, E. and Magnussen, G. Familial narcolepsy. *Nord. Med. (Hospitalstid) 15*; 2519-2526 (1942).

Kuhlo, W. Sleep attack with apneas. in *The Abnormalities of Sleep in Man.* H. Gastaut, I. Lugaresi, G. Berti-Ceroni, and G. Coccagna, eds., Gaggi, Bologna, Italy, 1968, pp. 205-207.

Kuhlo, W., Doll, E. and Franc, M. Exfolgreiche behandlung eines Pickwick syndrome durch eine dauertracheal kanule. *Dtsch. Med. Wochenschr. 94*; 1286-1290 (1969).

Kuhlo, W. and Doll, E. Pulmonary hypertension and the effect of tracheotomy in a case of Pickwickian syndrome. *Bull. Physiopathol. Resp. [Nancy] 8*; 1205-1216, (1972).

Kumashiro, H., Sato, M., Hirata, J., Baba, O. and Otsuki, S. Sleep apnea and sleep regulating mechanism. *Folia Psychiat. Neurol. Jap. 25*; 41-49 (1971).

Kurtz, D., Bapst-Reiter, J., Fletto, R., Micheletti, G., Meunier-Carus, J., Lonsdorfer, J. and Lampert-Benignus, E. Les formes de transition du syndrome Pickwickien. *Bull. Physiopathol. Resp.* [*Nancy*] *8*; 1115-1125 (1972).

Kurtz, D., Meunier-Carus, J., Bapst-Reiter, J., Lonsdorfer, J., Micheletti, G., Benignus, E. and Rohmer, F. Problemes nosologiques poses par certaines formes d'hypersomnie. *Rev. EEG Neurophysiol. 1*; 227-230 (1971).

Levin, M. Aggression, guilt and cataplexy. *Amer. J. Psychiat. 116*; 133-136 (1959).

Levy, A., Tabakin, B., Hanson, J. and Narkewicz, R. Hypertrophied adenoids causing pulmonary hypertension and severe congestive heart failure. *New Eng. J. Med. 277*; 506-511 (1967).

Lonsdorfer, J., Meunier-Carus, J., Lampert-Benignus, E., Kurtz, O., Bapst-Reiter, J., Fletto, R. and Micheletti, G. Aspects hemodynamiques et respiratoires du syndrome Pickwikien. *Bull. Physiopathol. Resp.* [*Nancy*] *8*; 1181-1192 (1972).

Lugaresi, E., Coccagna, G., Berti-Ceroni, G. Syndrome de Pickwick et syndrome d'hypoventilation alveolaire primaire. *Acta Neurol. Belg. 68*; 15-25 (1968a).

Lugaresi, E., Coccagna, G., Berti-Ceroni, G., Petrella, A. and Mantovani, M. La "maledizione di Ondine" il disturbo del respiro e del sonno nell' ipoventilazione alveolare primaria. *Sist. Nerv. 20*; 27-37 (1968b).

Lugaresi, E., Coccagna, G., Patrella, A., Berti-Ceroni, G. and Pazzaglia, P. Il disturbo del sonno e del respito nella sindrome pickwickiana. *Sist. Nerv. 20*; 38-50 (1968c).

Lugaresi, E., Coccagna, G., Mantovani, M. and Brignami, F. Effets de la tracheotomie dans les hypersomnies avec respiration periodique. *Rev. Neurol.* [*Paris*] *123*; 267-268 (1970).

Lugaresi, E., Coccagna, G., Mantovani, M., Cirignotta, F., Ambrosetto, G. and Baturic, P. Hypersomnia with periodic breathing—periodic apneas and alveolar hypoventilation during sleep. *Bull. Physiopathol. Resp.* [*Nancy*] *8*; 1103-1113 (1972a).

Lugaresi, E., Coccagna, G., Mantovani, M. and Lebrun, R. Some periodic phenomena arising during drowsiness and sleep in man. *Electroenceph. Clin. Neurophysiol. 32*; 701-705 (1972b).

Lugaresi, E., Coccagna, G. and Mantovani, M. Effects of tracheotomy in two cases of hypersomnia with periodic breathing. *J. Neurol. Neurosurg. Psychiat. 36*; 15-26 (1973).

Luke, M., Mehrizi, A., Folger, G., Jr. and Rowe, R. Chronic nasopharyngeal obstruction as cause of cardiomegaly, cor pulmonale, and pulmonary edema. *Pediatrics 37*; 762-768 (1966).

Menashe, V., Farrehi, C. and Miller, M. Hypoventilation and cor pulmonale due to chronic upper airway obstruction. *J. Pediat. 67*; 198-203 (1965).

Mouret, J., Renaud, B., Quenin, P., Michel, D. and Schott, B. Monoamines et regulation de la vigilance. Apport et interpretation biochimique des donnees polygraphiques. in, *Les Mediateurs Chimiques*, P. Girard and R. Couteaux eds., Masson, Paris, 1972, pp. 139-155.

Nan'no, H., Hishikawa, Y., Koida, H. et al. A neurophysiological study of sleep paralysis in narcoleptic patients. *Electroenceph. Clin. Neurophysiol. 28*; 328-390 (1970).

Noonan, J. Reversible cor pulmonale due to hypertrophied tonsils and adenoids: Studies in two cases. *Circulation 32* (sup.), 2-164 (1965).

Passouant, P., Cadilhac, J. and Baldy-Moulinier, M. Physiopathologie des hypersomnies. *Rev. Neurol. 116*; 585-629 (1967).

Passouant, P., Schwab, R., Cadilhac, J. and Baldy-Moulinier, M. Narcolepsi- cataplexie. *Rev. Neurol. 111*; 415-426 (1964).

Passouant, P., Popoviciu, L., Velok, G. et Baldy-Moulinier, M. Etude polygraphique des narcolepsies au cours du nycthemere. *Rev. Neurol. 118*; 431-441 (1968).

Passouant, P., Halberg, F., Genicot, R., Popoviciu, L. et Baldy-Moulinier, M. La periodicite des acces narcoleptiques et le rythme ultradien du sommeil rapide. *Rev. Neurol. 121*; 155-164 (1969).

Passouant, P., Baldy-Moulinier, M. et Aussilloux (Ch.) Etat de mal cataplectique au cours d'une maladie de Gelineau; influence de la clomipramine. *Rev. Neurol. 123*; 56-60 (1970).

Passouant, P., Cadilhac, J. and Ribstein, M. Les privatious de sommeil avec mouvements oculaires par les antidepresseurs. *Rev. Neurol. 127;* 173-192 (1972).

Petit, J. and Milic-Emili, G. Measurement of endoaesophageal pressure. *J. Appl. Physiol. 13;* 481-485 (1958).

Petitjean, F. and Jouvet, M. Hypersomnie et augmentation de l'acide 5-hydroxy indolacetique cerebral par lesion isthmique chez le chat. *C. R. Soc. Biol. (Paris) 164;* 2288-2293 (1970).

Phillips, R., Guilleminault, C. and Dement, W. A study on hypersomnia. *Sleep Res.* (1973, in press).

Pivik, T. and Dement, W. Phasic changes in muscular and reflex activity during non-REM sleep. *Exper Neurol. 27;* 115-124 (1970).

Prinzmetal, M. and Bloomberg, W. The use of benzedrine for the treatment of narcolepsy. *Amer. Med. Acad. 105;* 2051-2054 (1935).

Rechtschaffen, A., Wolpert, E., Dement, W., Mitchell, S. and Fisher, C. Nocturnal sleep of narcoleptics. *Electroenceph. Clin. Neurophysiol. 15;* 599-609 (1963).

Rechtschaffen, A. and Dement, W. Studies on the relation of narcolepsy, cataplexy, and sleep with low voltage random EEG activity. in; S. Kety, E. Evarts, and H. Williams, Eds.; *Sleep and Altered States of Consciousness,* Williams and Wilkins, Baltimore, 1967, pp. 488-505.

Rechtschaffen, A. and Dement, W. Narcolepsy and hypersomnia. in; *Sleep—Physiology and Pathology.* (A Symposium), A. Kales, Ed.; J. B. Lippincott, Philadelphia, 1969, pp. 119-130.

Rechtschaffen, A. and Roth, B. Nocturnal sleep of hypersomniac. *Act. Nerv. Super. 11,* 229-233 (1969).

Rechtschaffen, A., Molinari, S., Watson, R. and Wincor, M. Extra-ocular potentials: A possible indicator of PGO activity in the human. *Psychophysiology 7,* 336 (1971).

Richardson, D., Honour, A., Fenton, G., Stott, F. and Pickering, G. Variation in arterial pressure throughout the day and night. *Clin. Sci. 26,* 445-460 (1964).

Robert, M., Probst, H., Krassoievitch, M. and Tissot, R. Les pauses respiratoires survenant au cours du sommeil chez le patient avec syndrome de Pickwick. *Praxis 59,* 1767-1776 (1970).

Robin, E., Whaley, R., Crump, C. and Travis, D. Alveolar gas tension, pulmonary ventilation and blood pH during physiologic sleep in normal subjects. *J. Clin. Invest. 37,* 981-989 (1958).

Roth, B. *Narkolepsie a hypersomnie s Hlediska Fysiologie Spanku.* Statni Zdravotnicke Nakladetelstvi, Prague, 1957, p. 331.

Roth, N. Problems in narcolepsy. *Bull. Menninger Clin. 10,* 160-170 (1946).

Roth, B., Bruhova, S. and Lehovsky, M. REM sleep and NREM sleep in narcolepsy and hypersomnia. *Electroenceph. Clin. Neurophysiol. 26,* 176-182 (1969).

Roth, B., Faber, J., Nevsimalova, S. and Tosovsky, J. The influence of imipramine, dexphenmetrazine and amphetaminsulphate upon the clinical and polygraphic picture of narcolepsy-cataplexy. *Arch. Suisse. Neurol. Neurochir. Psychiat. 108* (2), 251-260 (1971).

Roth, B., Nevsimalova, S. and Rechtschaffen, A. Hypersomnia with "sleep drunkenness". *Arch. Gen. Psychiat. 26,* 456-462 (1972).

Saletu, B., Itil, T. and Keskiner, A. Prediction of drug treatment effective in narcolepsy based on digital computer analyzed EEG. *Clin. Electroenceph. 2,* 154-167 (1971).

Schwartz, B. and Escande, J. Etude cinematographique de la respiration hypnique Pickwickienne. *Rev. Neurol. 116,* 667-678 (1967).

Scollo-Lavizzari, G. A note on cataplexy with simultaneous EEG recordings. *Eur. Neurol. 4,* 57-63 (1970).

Semerano, A., Bevilacqua, M., Battistin, L. Blood gas analysis and polygraphic observations in the Pickwickian syndrome. *Bull. Physiopathol. Resp. (Nancy) 8,* 1193-1201 (1972).

Serejski, M. and Frumkin, I. Narkolepsie und epilepsie. *Ztschr. Ges. Neurol. Psychiat. 123,* 233-250 (1930).

Severinghaus, J., Mitchell, R. Ondine's curse: Failure of respiratory center automatically while awake. *Clin. Res. 10,* 122 (1962).

Sieker, H.O., Heyman, A., Birchfield, R.I. The effects of natural sleep and hypersomnolent states on respiratory function. *Ann. Intern. Med. 52,* 500-516 (1960).

Smirne, S., Castellotti, V., and Graziani, G. Aspetti patogenetici in un caso di respirazione periodica e ipersonnia. *Riv. Neurol. 41,* 342-349 (1971).

Snyder, F., Hobson, J., and Goldfrank, F. Blood pressure changes during human sleep. *Science* *142*, 1313-1314 (1963).

Snyder, F., Hobson, J., and Goldfrank, F. Changes in respiration, heart rate and systolic blood pressure in human sleep. *J. Appl. Physiol. 19* 417-422 (1964).

Sours, J.A. Narcolepsy and other disturbances in the sleep-waking rhythm: A study of 115 cases with review of the literature. *J. Nerv. Ment. Dis. 137*, 525-542 (1963).

Steinschneider, A. Prolonged apnea and the sudden infant death syndrome: Clinical and laboratory observations. *Pediatrics 50*, 646-654, (1972).

Suzuki, J. Narcoleptic syndrome and paradoxical sleep. *Folia Psychiat. Neurol. Jap. 20*, 123-149 (1966).

Takahashi, Y. and Jimbo, M. Polygraphic study of narcoleptic syndrome with special reference to hypnagogic hallucinations and cataplexy. *Folia Psychiat. Neurol. Jap. Suppl. 7*, 343-347 (1963).

Tammeling, G.J., Blokzi, E.J., Boonstra, S., and Sluiter, H.J. Micrognathia, hypersomnia and periodic breathing. *Bull. Physiopathol. Resp. (Nancy) 8*, 1229-1238 (1972).

Tassinari, C.A., Dalla Bernardina, B., Cirignotta, F., and Ambrosetto, G. Apnoeic periods and the respiratory related arousal patterns during sleep in the Pickwickian syndrome: A polygraphic study. *Bull. Physiopathol. Resp. (Nancy) 8*, 1087-1102 (1972).

Valero, A. and Alroy, G. Hypoventilation in acquired micrognathia. *Arch. Int. Med. 115:* 307-310, (1965).

Vizioli, R. Les bases neurophysiologiques de la cataplexie. *Electroenceph. Clin. Neurophysiol. 16*, 191-193 (1964).

Vogel, G. Studies in psychophysiology of dreams III. The dream of narcolepsy. *Arch. Gen. Psychiat. 3*, 421-428 (1960).

Wadd, W. Cursory remarks on corpulence. Royal College of Surgeons, London, 1810.

Walsh, R.E., Michaelson, E.D., Harkleroad, L.E., Zighelboim, A., and Sackner, M.A. Upper airway obstruction in obese patients with sleep disturbance and somnolence. *Ann. Intern. Med. 76*, 185-192 (1972).

Westphal, C. Eigenthumliche mit einschlafen verbundene anfälle. *Arch. F. Psychiat. 7*, 631-635 (1877).

Wilson, R., Raynal, D., Guilleminault, C., Zarcone, V., and Dement, W. REM sleep latencies in daytime sleep recordings of narcoleptics. *Sleep Res.* (1973, in press).

Wilson, S.A.K. Epileptic variant. *J. Neurol. Psychopath. 8*, 223-240 (1928).

Wood, J.D., Watson, J., and Drucker, A.J. The effect of hypoxia on brain gamma amino butyric acid levels. *J. Neurochem. 15*, 603-608 (1968).

Wyatt, R., Fram, D., Buchbinder, R., and Snyder, F. Treatment of intractable narcolepsy with a monoamine oxidase inhibitor. *New Eng. J. Med. 285*, 987-991 (1971).

Yoss, R.E. Treatment of narcolepsy. *Mod. Treat. 6*, 1263-1274 (1969).

Yoss, R.E. The inheritance of diurnal sleepiness as measured by pupillography. *Mayo Clin. Proc. 45*, 426-437 (1970).

Yoss, R.E. and Daly, D. Narcolepsy. *Med. Clin. North Am. 44*, 953-968 (1960).

Yoss, R.E. and Daly, D. Treatment of narcolepsy with Ritalin. *Neurology 9*, 171-173 (1959).

Yoss, R.E. and Daly, D. On the treatment of narcolepsy. *Med. Clin. North Am. 52*, 781-787 (1968).

Young, D. and Scoville, W.B. Paranoid psychosis in narcolepsy and possible danger of benzedrine treatment. *Med. Clin. North Am. 22*, 637-646 (1938).

Zarcone, V. Narcolepsy: A review of the syndrome. *New Eng. J. Med. 288*, 1156-1166 (1973).

Advances in Sleep Research, Vol. 1
© 1974, Spectrum Publications, Inc.

CHAPTER 9

Role of the Sleep Research and Treatment Facility: Diagnosis, Treatment and Education

ANTHONY KALES
EDWARD O. BIXLER
JOYCE D. KALES

Understandably, the early years of the modern sleep research era, which followed the discovery of REMs, were devoted primarily to the investigation and definition of normal sleep (Aserinsky and Kleitman, 1953, 1955; Dement and Kleitman, 1957a,b; Agnew et al., 1967; Feinberg et al., 1967; Kales et al., 1967a,b). But as the field expanded with each normative discovery, clinicians began to realize the potential value of evaluating, in the sleep laboratory, those conditions in which sleep was abnormal, i.e., disrupted and/or altered. Consequently, the number and scope of studies relating to clinically pertinent aspects of sleep have greatly increased in recent years.

One approach to clinically oriented sleep research has involved only the use of sleep laboratory studies. A more recent trend, however, is the development of specialized "sleep centers" which utilize clinical studies both in the sleep laboratory and in an outpatient clinical setting. There are now several such centers in the country.

This multi-faceted approach to the evaluation and treatment of sleep disorders originated with the pioneering efforts of the Sleep Research and Treatment Facility, founded at UCLA in 1963 and presently based at the Hershey Medical Center of Pennsylvania State University. The Sleep Research and Treatment Facility includes, in addition to a Sleep Laboratory and a Sleep Disorders Clinic, extensive Educational Programs, designed to educate and assist the general physician in the management of patients with sleep disorders.

With the development of sleep centers, there has arisen a controversy as to who should treat the majority of sleep disorder patients—the primary physician or the "sleep specialist" (Dement and Guilleminault, 1973; Kales, 1973a). Because of the magnitude and variety of sleep problems seen in medical practice, and the importance of treating the "whole patient", our philosophy is that the primary physician is best able to treat these patients and the role of the sleep specialist should be to assist the primary physician.

By developing and disseminating new methods for recognizing and treating sleep disorders, we feel we can significantly help the physician to manage these patients more effectively in his everyday clinical practice. Thus, our educational programs, directed toward physician consultation, constitute an extremely important and unique facet of our total program.

Fig. 1 illustrates the functional scope of the Sleep Research and Treatment Facility and how these programs ultimately assist the general physician with the diagnosis and treatment of sleep disorder patients. In the Sleep Laboratory, sleep disorders and other conditions with disturbed sleep are evaluated in depth. Then, in the Sleep Disorders Clinic, these findings are applied in a variety of studies to the evaluation and treatment of a larger number of patients. Finally, our Educational Programs extend these findings to physicians, government agencies, and private industry.

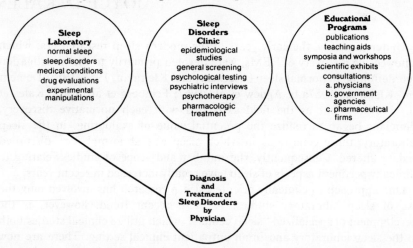

Fig. 1 Illustration of how our Sleep Research and Treatment Facility, through its Sleep Laboratory, Sleep Disorders Clinic and Educational Programs, has provided the physician with information which better enables him to diagnose and treat sleep disorders.

Tables I and II describe the range of studies that we have conducted in the Sleep Laboratory and Sleep Disorders Clinic that relate to the evaluation and treatment of disturbed sleep. In all of these studies, where appropriate, the skills of the adult and child psychiatrist, neurologist, pediatrician, endocrinologist, urologist, and internist as well as the clinical psychologist and clinical pharmacologist, are utilized on both a staff and consultative basis. Table I lists a variety of studies related to normal sleep as well as a number of investigations of sleep disorders and other clinical conditions associated with disturbed sleep. These include studies of sleepwalking, night terrors, insomnia, bed-wetting, and clinical conditions such as duodenal ulcer, hypothyroidism, child and adult asthma, and Parkinson's disease (Armstrong et al., 1965; Oswald and Priest, 1965; Kales et al., 1966a,b, 1967a; Monroe, 1967; Kales et al, 1968a; Kales and Jacobson, 1969; Kales et al., 1969b,

TABLE I

Evaluation of Disturbed Sleep;
Electrophysiological and Clinical Studies

NORMAL	Baseline Sleep
	    children
	    young adults
	    elderly
	
	Dream Recall
	    children
	    young adults
	    elderly
	
	Laboratory Adaptive and Readaptation
	
	Physiology
	    muscle tonus
	    neuroendocrine
	    phasic phenomena

EXPERIMENTAL
 	
MANIPULATIONS
	REM Deprivation
	    normal adults
	    autistic children
	
	Sleep Deprivation

ABNORMAL	General Patient Evaluation
	    epidemiology
	    psychiatric interview
	    psychological testing
	
	Sleep Disorders
	    sleep walking
	    pavor nocturnus
	    nocturnal "seizures"
	    sleep apnea
	    insomnia
	    enuresis
	    narcolepsy
	    hypersomnia
	
	Medical Conditions
	    duodenal ulcer
	    hypothyroid
	    child & adult asthma
	    Parkinson disease
	    coronary artery disease
	    ophthalmic patients

1970a-d; Kales and Cary, 1971; Kales and Kales, 1971; Kales et al., 1971a--, 1972, 1973; Kales and Kales, in press; Kales et al., in press). Table II pertains to studies relevant to the pharmacological and psychological treatment of disturbed sleep. Of particular importance here are the short and long term studies of hypnotic drug effectiveness and investigations of drug-withdrawal insomnia and hypnotic drug dependence.

TABLE II

Treatment of Disturbed Sleep;
Electrophysiological, Psychological, and Pharmacological Studies

	Hypnotic Drug Effectiveness

	Short-term administration
	  normal subjects
	  insomniac patients

	Intermediate Administration
	  normal subjects
	  insomniac patients

HYPNOTIC DRUG THERAPY	Long-term administration insomniac patients
	Chronic use insomniac patients
	Sleep Stage Alterations Short, intermediate, long-term and chronic use

	Drug Withdrawal Insomnia
	  Hypnotic drug withdrawal
	  Gradual vs. abrupt withdrawal
	  Dilantin & drug withdrawal

	DOPA administration
	  normal subjects
	  Parkinson patients

	Hallucinogenic drug administration
	  normal adults
	  autistic children

OTHER DRUG
THERAPY
	Antidepressant administration
	  insomnia
	  enuresis
	  nocturnal seizures
	  sleep apnea

	Stage 4 suppression
	  sleepwalking
	  night terrors

	Psychotherapy
	  insomnia
	  hypersomnia
	  enuresis
	  adult somnambulism

OTHER
THERAPY
	Electrotherapy (electrosleep)
	  normal
	  insomniac
	  hypertensive

	Environmental manipulation fluidized bed

SLEEP LABORATORY AND SLEEP DISORDERS CLINIC STUDIES

In this section, we will discuss the findings from our combined sleep laboratory and sleep disorders clinic studies of insomnia, somnambulism, night terrors, and enuresis as well as related studies by other sleep investigators, and our recommendations for the management and treatment of these disorders. Later we will discuss the need for, and our implementation of, educational programs directed toward extending these findings.

Insomnia

Certainly, if one considers the very transient, situational disturbance, insomnia is indeed ubiquitous. Of all sleep disturbances, insomnia is the one most frequently treated by the general physician (Kales and Cary, 1971). Insomnia may consist of difficulty in falling asleep, difficulty in staying asleep, too early final awakening, or a combination of these (Fig. 2).

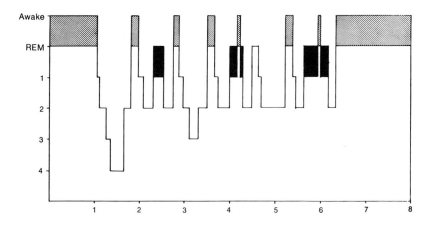

Fig. 2 Sleep patterns in insomnia. Depicted are a composite of three different types of insomnia: difficulty falling asleep, difficulty staying asleep, difficulty staying asleep (with frequent awakenings), and early final awakening. Insomnia may consist of one, or a combination, of these difficulties.

What Medical or Psychological Conditions Have Been Found to be Associated with the Symptom of Insomnia?

Insomnia is often a symptom associated with medical disorders, including any condition where pain and physical discomfort are significant symptoms. Where insomnia is associated with medical conditions, both physical and emotional factors must be considered, since it can be assumed that there is always an emotional response to a disease process, varying only in degree.

However, through psychological testing and interviews, we have found an extraordinarily high percentage of psychological disturbances in insomniac patients (Kales and Cary, 1971; Kales et al., 1972; Kales and Kales, 1973). Over 85% of the insomniac patients we tested had one or more major MMPI scales in the pathological range. The scales for depression, sociopathy, obsessive-compulsive features, and schizophrenic trends were most frequently elevated. In a previous study, Monroe found that "poor" sleepers had significant psychological disturbances compared to "good" sleepers, as demonstrated by the MMPI (Monroe, 1967). From their MMPI data, the poor sleepers appeared to be more anxious and depressed and had more peculiarities of thought but surprisingly they did not demonstrate more hypochondriasis than good sleepers.

Of course, insomnia may also occur independent of any medical or psychiatric disorder, secondary to a stressful situation such as a death in one's family or financial problems. In these cases, the insomnia is usually transient.

What Are the Physiological Characteristics of the Sleep of Insomniacs?

Monroe compared physiological parameters of good and poor sleepers and found that the two groups differed significantly in this respect (Monroe, 1967). Poor sleepers had more body movements as well as increased heart rate, peripheral vasoconstriction, and slightly elevated rectal temperature when compared to good sleepers, both during sleep and during the 30 minutes just prior to sleep. These findings indicate a higher level of "physiological arousal" for poor sleepers during sleep.

What Information Have All-Night Sleep Laboratory Studies
Yielded in Regard to the Effectiveness of Hypnotic Drugs?

Many hypnotic drugs are purported to be effective in single clinical doses, yet many insomnia patients complain of persistent and severe sleeplessness despite chronic use of multiple doses of these drugs. This unfortunate but common situation raises the question of whether many hypnotic drugs are actually effective in inducing and maintaining sleep, especially under conditions of prolonged use. The staff of our Sleep Research and Treatment

TABLE III
22 Night Protocol Design
and Reasons for Design

Night	P	D	Lab	Home	Reason
1	X		X		Adaptation to environment
2 to 4	X		X		Baseline measurements
5 to 7		X	X		Initial and short-term drug effects
8 to 15		X		X	Evaluation in home surroundings
16		X	X		Readaptation to laboratory
17 & 18		X	X		Long-term (2 wks) drug effectiveness
19 to 22	X		X		Evaluation of withdrawal effects

Facility, since 1966, has been extensively involved in the evaluation of hypnotic agents (Kales et al., 1970b,d), particularly in regard to their effectiveness with long-term use. The results of these studies, utilizing insomniac subjects, have led to the conclusion that many commercially available hypnotic drugs are not effective with prolonged used, in either inducing or maintaining sleep (Kales et al, 1970b, 1973).

We evaluated individually the following drugs and dosages, using our standard 22-night protocol (Table III): chloral hydrate (Noctec) 1000mg; flurazepam (Dalmane) 30 mg; glutethimide (Doriden) 500 mg; methaqualone (Sopor) 150 and 300 mg; and secobarbital (Seconal) 100 mg. We found that all of the drugs were initially moderately to markedly effective in inducing or maintaining sleep, or both (Table IV). However, we found that at the end of the two-week period of drug administration, significant tolerance had developed with all of these drugs except flurazepam. These favorable findings for flurazepam effectiveness were corroborated in a subsequent 17-night investigation (Table V) (Kales et al., 1971b).

In another study, we evaluated the sleep of ten insomniac patients all of whom had been chronically taking hypnotic drugs, mostly in multiple doses, over prolonged periods of time (Kales et al., in press). Their sleep was monitored in the laboratory while they continued to take their medication in the usual manner and dosage. The drugs evaluated included glutethimide, pentobarbital, secobarbital, a combination of amobarbital and secobarbital, and chloral hydrate. When the sleep of these patients chronically using hypnotic drugs was compared to that of age-matched insomniac controls who were not taking sleep medication, it became clear that the chronic drug patients had as great or greater difficulty in falling asleep, staying asleep, or both, as the nondrug controls (Fig. 3).

How Does the Treatment of Insomnia Vary,
According to Different Etiological Factors?

In cases of mild insomnia or insomnia secondary to situational disturbances, pharmacological therapy alone is most sufficient. In medical conditions, in addition to treating the primary disease process, pharmacological treatment is often indicated (Kales and Cary, 1971; Kales and Kales, 1973). Despite the fact that insomniacs are frequently disturbed, they are rarely referred for psychiatric treatment and rarely seek it themselves. They tend to reject the possiblity of pathology and focus instead on somatic aspects of their problem. The prognosis for this group would be greatly improved if they were more often referred for psychiatric treatment despite their rejection of psychological factors. In severe or chronic cases, where psychological disturbances are significant, best results are obtained with a combination of psychotherapy and pharmacological treatment (Kales and Cary, 1971; Kales and Kales, in press). We recommend flurazepam for the pharmacological treatment of insomnia. This recommendation is based on our sleep

TABLE IV
Drug Effectiveness
A Comparison of Five Hypnotic Agents:
22 Night Schedule

Glutethimide (500 mg)

	Nights*	Sleep Latency (minutes)	Wake Time (minutes)	Number of Wakes	Total Sleep %
Baseline	2-4	76.2	13.7	6.8	82.7
Drug	5-7	38.0	19.7	10.9	88.7
Drug	17-18	90.2	16.4	6.6	79.1
Withdrawal	19-22	62.9	23.3	6.5	83.1

Secobarbital (100 mg)

	Nights*	Sleep Latency (minutes)	Wake Time (minutes)	Number of Wakes	Total Sleep %
Baseline	2-4	29.3	57.7	11.6	81.9
Drug	5-7	17.6	20.7	8.4	92.0
Drug	17-18	30.0	47.0	6.6	84.0
Withdrawal	19-22	19.8	63.8	10.1	82.6

Flurazepam (30 mg)

	Nights*	Sleep Latency (minutes)	Wake Time (minutes)	Number of Wakes	Total Sleep %
Baseline	2-4	35.8	14.3	4.1	90.0
Drug	5-7	13.9	5.0	2.7	96.4
Drug	17-18	21.2	3.8	2.3	94.7
Withdrawal	19-22	25.4	10.4	3.2	92.2

*Night 16 allowed for re-adaptation to the laboratory.

TABLE IV (continued)

Chloral Hydrate (1000 mg)

	Nights*	Sleep Latency (minutes)	Wake Time (minutes)	Number of Wakes	Total Sleep %
Baseline	2-4	52.5	21.4	9.2	85.6
Drug	5-7	31.3	23.6	9.1	89.3
Drug	17-18	43.7	11.7	5.2	89.1
Withdrawal	19-22	61.2	8.8	5.7	86.2

Methaqualone (300 mg)

	Nights*	Sleep Latency (minutes)	Wake Time (minutes)	Number of Wakes	Total Sleep %
Baseline	2-4	39.9	76.2	10.8	75.8
Drug	5-7	26.1	47.5	5.2	84.7
Drug	17-18	27.8	80.5	7.5	77.4
Withdrawal	19-22	27.3	136.9	11.6	65.3

laboratory findings of its effectiveness in inducing and maintaining sleep (Kales et al., 1970a, 1971b). Since flurazepam has been shown to be more effective on the second and subsequent nights of administration, patients should be advised that they may not notice marked improvement on the first night.

Drug Withdrawal Insomnia

What Sleep Stage Alterations Occur with Hypnotic Drug Use and Withdrawal?

Sleep laboratory studies have demonstrated that hypnotic drugs produce a variety of sleep stage alterations, and that these alterations frequently are dose-related (Oswald and Thacore, 1963; Oswald and Priest, 1965; Kales et al, 1967a,b, 1969b). Table VI summarizes the results for a number of different hypnotic drug evaluations in which each drug was assessed over an 8-consecutive-night schedule. The first 2 nights were for adaptation to the laboratory, the third for obtaining base-line measurements; 3 drug nights for measuring initial and short-term effects of the drugs, and 2 placebo

TABLE V
Effects of Placebo and Flurazepam
on Sleep Induction and Maintenance

Group	Nights	Condition	Sleep Latency (minutes)	Wake Time after Sleep Onset (minutes)	Total Wake Time (minutes)	No. of Wakes
A	2-4	O	29.9	35.2	65.1	12.7
	5-9	D	13.1	11.2	24.3	5.7
	10-14	P	18.7	31.5	50.2	10.8
	15-17	O	26.2	38.1	64.3	11.4
B	2-4	O	63.4	40.2	103.6	8.0
	5-9	P	69.3	38.3	107.6	6.3
	10-14	D	27.0	15.6	42.6	4.5
	15-17	O	32.2	24.9	57.1	5.8
C	2-4	O	46.9	21.3	68.2	7.8
	5-9	P	42.7	31.6	74.3	8.5
	10-14	P	37.7	33.2	70.9	8.9
	15-17	O	41.0	23.8	64.8	6.7

O=No medication administered; P=placebo administration; D=active drug (flurazepam 30 mg) administration.

nights for measuring the effects of withdrawal, if any. In group A are drugs producing significant changes in REM sleep with drug administration and withdrawal; in group B are those that do not produce significant changes under similar conditions. In general, REM sleep suppression with drug administration was followed by increases in REM sleep above base-line after drug withdrawal. Also, REM sleep suppression was usually accompanied by a delay in the onset of the first REM period of the night and by decreased REM time in the first two-thirds of the night. It was also noted with pentobarbital that a rebound in REM sleep occurred in the last third of a drug night as the duration of action of the drug was exceeded. We also observed that with most drugs the degree of REM suppression had lessened by the last drug night (N 6), although generally still remaining below baseline levels.

In the same short-term drug studies (Kales et al, 1969b), we found that the benzodiazepine drugs, expecially flurazepam and diazepam and pentobarbital and glutethimide produced significant decreases in stage 4 sleep. The decreases in stage 4 sleep with flurazepam and diazepam are progressive and marked and carry over into the withdrawal period.

In patients who had been taking hypnotic drugs for several years, in single or multiple doses (glutethimide, pentobarbital, secobarbital) we found a significant decrease in REM sleep compared to insomniac controls who were not taking any medication (Kales et al., in press). There was also a suggestion of a decrease in stage 3 sleep in the patients chronically using barbiturate drugs (Fig. 3).

We have also studied patients who have been "addicted" to massive doses of hypnotic drugs, after taking them on a chronic basis (Kales et al., 1968b), 1969a). Two of these patients, one taking 1000 mg of pentobarbital and the other 1200 mg of a mixture of amobarbital and secobarbital (Tuinal) daily,

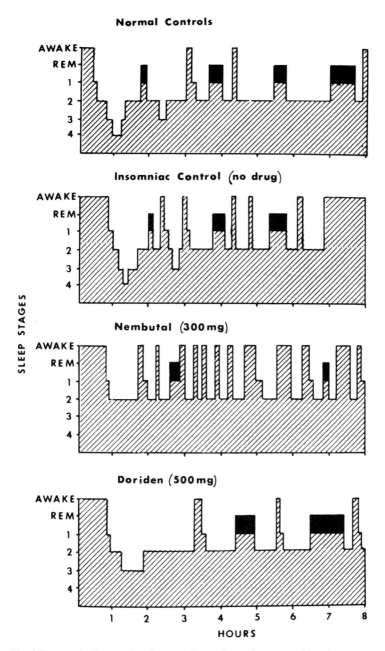

Fig. 3 Sleep cycle of normal subjects and insomniac patients not taking drugs are compared with two patients chronically taking hypnotic medication. The patients chronically taking medication experienced marked insomnia as illustrated by the long sleep latency and multiple awakenings. In addition, marked sleep stage alterations are demonstrated with chronic drug use.

TABLE VI
Stage REM Alterations Following Drug Administration and Withdrawal. Eight Night Studies

Group* and drugs	% Stage REM on study nights (Ni)						% Change from baseline night	
	Baseline Ni 3	Ni 4	Drug Ni 5	Ni 6	Withdrawal Ni 7	Ni 8	1st drug night	1st withdrawal night
Group A								
Glutethimide (DORIDEN), 500 mg (N = 5)	27.0	14.3	16.2	18.0	31.4	30.7	−47.0	+16.3
Methyprylon (NOLUDAR), 300 mg (N = 7)	25.3	18.4	18.9	25.3	31.5	31.6	−27.3	+24.5
Secobarbital (SECONAL), 100 mg (N = 2)	20.2	15.3	19.8	19.0	21.1	21.2	−24.5	+ 4.5
Methaqualone (QUAALUDE), 300 mg (N = 5)	23.4	18.8	23.4	21.6	27.6	22.4	−19.7	+17.9
Pentobarbital (NEMBUTAL), 100 mg (N = 4)	21.7	18.3	21.1	20.9	26.4	25.6	−15.7	+21.7
Diphenhydramine (BENADRYL), 50 mg (N = 2)	20.8	17.6	15.6	15.2	26.7	20.1	−15.4	+28.4
Promethazine (PHENERGAN), 25 mg (N = 4)	18.3	18.5	23.0	17.3	33.3	26.2	+ 1.1	+82.0
Group B								
Chloral hydrate (NOCTEC), 1000 mg (N = 5)	23.0	21.7	23.7	22.4	23.3	24.8	− 5.7	+ 1.3
Diazepam (VALIUM), 10 mg (N = 3)	20.1	19.2	20.1	18.8	20.1	20.7	− 4.5	0
Flurazepam (DALMANE), 30 mg (N = 8)	22.5	21.5	18.0	19.1	21.9	22.3	− 4.0	− 2.7
Chloral hydrate (NOCTEC), 500 mg (N = 10)	21.4	21.3	23.0	21.4	18.5	23.5	− 0.5	−13.6
Chlordiazepoxide (LIBRIUM), 50 mg (N = 4)	22.6	23.3	18.6	21.9	21.3	22.7	+ 3.1	− 4.9
Methaqualone (QUAALUDE), 150 mg (N = 5)	21.2	21.9	22.9	24.2	24.6	23.1	+ 3.3	+16.0

* Group A = drugs producing marked alterations with drug administration and withdrawal; Group B = drugs producing no change or minimal change with drug administration and withdrawal; N = number of subjects.

were monitored before, during, and after gradual withdrawal of these drugs. Both patients showed a marked decrease in REM sleep, as well as in stage 3 and 4, at the start of the study that were accompanied by a marked increase in stage 2 sleep.

As the drugs were gradually withdrawn over a prolonged period, there were marked immediate increases in REM sleep above base-line levels accompanied by occasional nightmares. REM percentages reached levels of 35 to 40 per cent as compared to 10 to 15 percent when the patients were using the drugs. In contrast, stages 3 and 4 sleep returned very gradually to base-line values and did not rebound above these levels (Fig. 4).

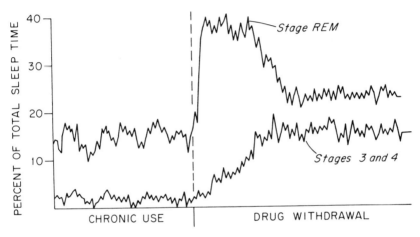

Fig. 4 Sleep patterns during chronic drug use and following drug withdrawal. With many hypnotic drugs chronic use, especially in multiple doses, produces a suppression of both REM and stages 3 and 4 sleep. When the drugs are withdrawn abruptly, there is often marked insomnia. When the subjects do fall asleep, there is a marked increase in REM sleep associated with an increase in the frequency and intensity of dreaming. Nightmares may even occur. These disturbances of sleep result in even further insomnia.

What Is the Clinical Significance of Drug-Induced Sleep Stage Alteration?

While considerable information has been amassed in sleep research regarding the physiology of sleep stages, we do not at this time know the specific significance of any sleep stage, nor can we draw any conclusions regarding the necessity of a given sleep stage. For example, patients have been totally deprived of stage 4 sleep and of REM sleep for prolonged periods, without any apparent adverse effects (Wyatt et al, 1969; Kales et al., 1970b; Kales and Scharf, 1973).

The only sleep stage alterations that we have noted to have clinical significance, are those occurring with abrupt hypnotic drug withdrawal. Abrupt withdrawal may result in disturbed sleep, more frequent and intense dreams, and occasionally nightmares, when the drug has been used regularly in multiple doses for a protracted period of time (Oswald and Thacore, 1963;

Oswald and Priest, 1965; Kales et al., 1969b; Kales and Kales, 1971). All of these changes contribute to a condition we call "Drug Withdrawal Insomnia", which results from both psychological factors and physiological changes involved in drug withdrawal and is an important factor in the development of "Hypnotic Drug Dependence" (Kales et al., 1969b; Kales and Kales, 1971; Kales et al., in press). When a patient abruptly withdraws from the regular and prolonged use of multiple doses of a hypnotic, he frequently first experiences marked insomnia, i.e., difficulty in falling asleep. This insomnia may be due to both psychological apprehension over his ability to get along without the drug as well as an abstinence syndrome manifested by jitteriness and nervousness. In addition, once the patient falls asleep, his sleep is frequently fragmented and disrupted. Sleep research has helped to explain this aspect of drug withdrawal insomnia. If the hypnotic, which is abruptly withdrawn, is a REM suppressant, there is a marked increase or rebound in REM sleep associated with an increased intensity and frequency of dreaming (Fig. 4). At times even nightmares occur (Oswald and Thacore, 1963; Oswald and Priest, 1965; Kales et al., 1969b). These altered sleep and dream patterns disturb sleep and contribute additionally to the "Drug Withdrawal Insomnia." It should be emphasized that altered sleep patterns and "Drug Withdrawal Insomnia" can occur not only when a drug is intentionally withdrawn, but also on an actual drug night when the patient sleeps past the duration of pharmacological action of the drug.

Based on Sleep Research Findings, How Can
Drug Withdrawal Insomnia and Hypnotic Drug Dependence
be Prevented or Minimized?

In those situations where the drug does indeed appear to be ineffective with prolonged use and withdrawal is desirable, we have made the following specific recommendations in order to minimize sleep stage alterations and Drug Withdrawal Insomnia (Kales et al., 1969b; Kales and Kales, 1971; Kales et al., in press): 1) withdraw the hypnotic drug very gradually at the rate of one therapeutic dose every 5 or 6 days; 2) inform the patient that severe changes may occur, including increased dreaming, vivid dreams, and even nightmares and that these are reflections of transient physiological changes; 3) where total withdrawal of the drug is difficult, replace the drug with a hypnotic which has been demonstrated in the sleep laboratory to be effective in inducing and maintaining sleep, without a loss of effectiveness developing in a short period of time.

Sleepwalking

Somnabulism, or sleepwalking, has been extensively investigated in the sleep laboratory, utilizing both child and adult somnambulists (Gastaut and Broughton, 1965; Kales et al., 1966a; Broughton, 1968; Kales and Jacobson, 1969). The results of these studies refute some popular beliefs concerning sleepwalking episodes.

What Is the Relationship Between Sleepwalking and Sleep Stages?

Despite the popular notion that sleepwalking is the acting out of a dream, sleep laboratory studies of somnambulists, involving primarily children, have shown that sleepwalking incidents occur exclusively out of NREM sleep especially stages 3 and 4 sleep (fig. 5) (Gastaut and Broughton, 1965; Kales et al., 1966a; Broughton, 1968; Kales and Jacobson, 1969). Sleepwalking episodes in the laboratory lasted from 30 seconds to several minutes and the sleepwalker was totally amnesic for the event upon awakening. Investigators were able to induce these episodes by lifting the subjects onto their feet during NREM sleep. All incidents, whether spontaneous or induced, characteristically began with a paroxysmal burst of high voltage, slow EEG activity (Fig. 6) (Gastaut and Broughton, 1965; Kales et al., 1966a; Kales and Jacobson, 1969).

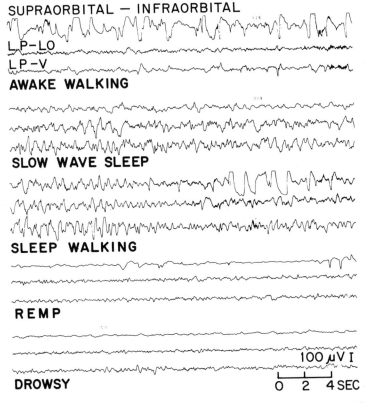

Fig. 5 Relationship of sleepwalking to sleep stage. Illustrated are tracings from a child somnambulist while awake and also during various stages of sleep. Note the similarity between the tracings of stages 3 and 4 sleep and the recordings at the onset of the sleepwalking episode.

*What Behavior Was Observed During Sleepwalking Episodes
in the Sleep Laboratory?*

During the laboratory incidents, the sleepwalkers appeared to be somewhat aware of but indifferent to their environment. Their eyes were open and expressions blank, creating a dazed appearance (Gastaut and Broughton, 1965; Kales et al., 1966a; Kales and Jacobson, 1969). Less often, a fearful expression was seen. The movements were somewhat rigid and not uncommonly repetitive and purposeless, such as rubbing a blanket or a door. Activity ranged from sitting up to slowly walking aimlessly about the laboratory, to pulling at the electrodes and cables, and rarely more violent activity such as running, jumping, and appearing to be searching for something. Contrary to popular belief, the sleepwalkers, at all times, functioned at a very low level of awareness and critical skill.

Somniloquy was common; if spoken to, the subjects answered monosyllabically as if annoyed or preoccupied. At no time did the somnambulists initiate conversation or contact with the personnel. Most often the subjects returned to bed spontaneously; however, if they did not, they usually could be led there easily. There was complete amnesia for the incidents when they awakened in the morning. The subjects were also amnesic if they awakened spontaneously during an incident, as well as being markedly disoriented. Dream recall in the morning was infrequent; however, when recall did occur, the manifest content did not resemble the activity during the somnambulistic incidents of the previous night.

*Are There any Specific Psychological Factors
Associated with Sleepwalking?*

Psychiatric disturbances were not found to be primary in the child somnambulists studied in the sleep laboratory (Kales et al., 1966b). Our psychological testing did not demonstrate any consistent psychopathology in these children. Further, our follow-up studies demonstrated that most of the child somnambulists had "outgrown" the disorder after several years, suggesting a delayed CNS maturation in these children (Broughton, 1969). In adult somnambulists, psychological disturbances are frequent. Sours evaluated adult male somnambulists with psychological tests and consistently found moderate to severe psychopathology (Sours et al., 1963).

*What Treatment Recommendations Are Suggested Regarding
the Management of Sleepwalking?*

Since most child somnambulists "outgrow" their sleepwalking episodes and since, as previously mentioned, the sleepwalker's critical skill is minimal and he is relatively unaware of his surroundings, we feel that the most important consideration is to protect the somnambulist from injury to himself (Kales and Kales, 1971). Prophylactic measures such as locking doors and windows, removing potentially dangerous objects and having him sleep on the first floor if possible, are essential to the safety of the sleepwalker.

When the sleepwalking is frequent and severe as well as when the child does not outgrow the disorder, the use of stage 4 suppressant drugs is under investigation. As mentioned, we have found that a number of drugs, primarily the benzodiazepines, such as diazepam and flurazepam, very effectively suppress stages 3 and 4 sleep (Kales and Scharf, 1973) (TableVII). However, use of these drugs with somnambulists in our laboratory has not resulted in a clear-cut decrease in the incidence of sleepwalking episodes.

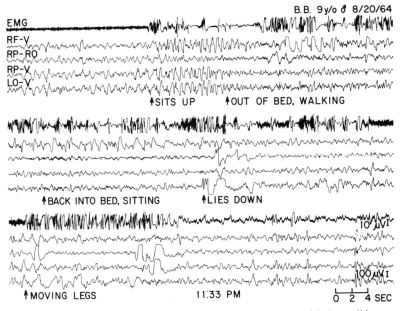

Fig. 6 A typical sleep EEG recording of a child somnambulistic episode. All sleepwalking occurs exclusively out of NREM sleep, especially stages 3 and 4. All incidents whether spontaneous or induced, characteristically began with a paroxysmal burst of high voltage, slow wave EEG activity.

Night Terrors

The night terror is the most dramatic of sleep disorders. The attack is characteristically heralded by a blood-chilling scream, and at the conclusion of the episode the individual is confused, disoriented, and often amnesic regarding the attack (Gastaut and Broughton, 1965; Broughton, 1969).

How Does a Night Terror Differ from a Nightmare?

Gastaut and Broughton (1969) found that night terrors, which are characterized by profound clinical and autonomic changes, occur out of stages 3 and 4 sleep, while the more frequent and common nightmare, or frightening dream, occurs out of REM sleep. In the night terror, the child (or adult) suddenly, out of "deep" sleep, sits up with a piercing scream. Motor activity is intense with occasional sleepwalking, the child is confused and incoherent, and heart and respiratory rate are profoundly elevated. Subjectively there are feelings of intense anxiety and respiratory oppression, and a sensation of doom, while content recalled is usually limited to a single frightening image. In the REM nightmare, or frightening dream, autonomic

TABLE VII

Benzodiazepines: Effects on Sleep Stages

Drug	Dose (mg)	REM Sleep		Stage 4 sleep	
		Drug administration	Drug withdrawal	Drug administration	Drug withdrawal
Flurazepam	30	slight decrease, moderate decrease in eye movement, density	return to baseline, no REM rebound, no decrease	marked decrease	decrease maintained over several drug withdrawal periods. No rebound. Some return toward baseline
	15	slight increase	movement not studied return to baseline. No REM rebound	No rebound not studied	moderate return toward baseline
	60	clear-cut decrease	movement in eye movement return to baseline. No REM rebound	moderate decrease	could not be evaluated—only 1 drug night in protocol
Diazepam	5–10	no change	no change	progressive decrease	marked decrease maintained over several drug withdrawal periods. No rebound
Chlordiazepoxide	50	slight decrease	return to baseline. No REM rebound	moderate decrease	some return toward baseline
RO 5-4200	2	moderate decrease	return to baseline. No REM rebound	marked decrease	moderate return toward baseline
	1	no change	no change	no change	subjects had essentially no stage 4 sleep; thus could not evaluate
	0.25	no change	no change	slight decrease	returns essentially to baseline levels

changes, if present, are slight, the individual is more easily aroused and content recalled is more lengthy and developed.

How Can Night Terrors Best Be Managed?

As with child somnambulists, follow-up studies have shown that most children with night terrors outgrow this disorder eventually, again suggesting a delayed CNS maturation which manifests in impaired arousal during sleep. Broughton (1969) has classified both sleepwalking and night terrors as "arousal disorders".

Psychological disturbance is frequent in adults with night terrors. Gastaut and Broughton have reported that daytime anxiety, while rare in children with night terrors is common in adults with this disorder. Therefore, psychological evaluations and treatment are often indicated in the adult patients.

Pharmacologic management of this disorder is under investigation. Fisher has applied our findings with drugs that suppress stages 3 and 4 to patients afflicted with night terrors, since night terrors occur exclusively out of stages 3 and 4 sleep (Fisher et al., 1971). He has found a significant decrease in both the amount of stage 4 sleep and in the frequency of these attacks following the administration of diazepam.

Enuresis

Enuresis which is by far the most frequent and distressing of the childhood sleep disorders, is often complicated and magnified by a lack of accurate information and a resultant lack of proper handling on the part of the parents and physicians.

Is Enuresis Primarily a Psychological or Physiological Disorder?

The precise etiology of enuresis is difficult to determine. The physician must first establish whether the enuresis has continued since infancy (primary enuresis) or whether the child was dry for a period of time but has since relapsed (secondary enuresis) (Fraser, 1972). Secondary enuresis is often due to psychological factors with the child relapsing only occasionally because of organic factors such as polyuria with diabetes or infection or other uropathology.

Sleep laboratory evaluations of children with enuresis have in great part contradicted the popular misconception that bedwetting represents hostile or dependent feelings on the part of the child. Further, enuretic episodes are uncommon when the child is in bed and awake, and usually occur during NREM sleep, especially in the first third of the night when stages 3 and 4 predominate. Studies of enuretic children have shown that if subjects were left wet following an enuretic episode and awakened during subsequent REM periods their recall contained fragments of being wet. This partially explains the misconception of a one-to-one relationship between enuresis and dreaming, i.e., when a child has an enuretic episode out of NREM sleep but is not changed, he may subsequently incorporate the wetness into a REM period dream and in the morning actually believe that the enuresis occurred while he was dreaming (Gastaut and Broughton, 1965; Broughton, 1969).

*What Precautions Are Indicated in the Evaluation
and Treatment of Enuresis?*

Unless there is a specific indication of possible uropathology, young children should not be considered for urological procedures as the psychological effects may be quite detrimental. In the case of primary enuresis, the probability of a "maturational lag" should be considered, especially if there is both a strong family history of bedwetting and a history of other family members outgrowing the disorder in a reasonable period of time.

In clinical and sleep laboratory studies, imipramine HCL (Tofranil) has been found to be effective in decreasing enuretic frequency, especially if dosage is properly adjusted. The length of these studies was usually for periods of only one to three months (Bindelglas et al., 1968). Whether the drug is effective with prolonged use and, if so, whether such potent pharmacological treatment should be used chronically in young children needs to be evaluated. In our sleep laboratory evaluation of Tofranil in enuretic children, we found the drug to be quite effective in reducing enuretic frequency, but this reduction was unrelated to any sleep stage alterations observed (Kales et al., 1971c). Tofranil produced a marked REM suppression with a marked REM rebound with withdrawal. Stage 4 sleep was unchanged across both conditions.

*How Can Parents Minimize Their Child's Anxiety
Concerning his Bedwetting?*

Parents of enuretic children are invariably deeply concerned but they should be educated to recognize the consequences of overreacting. Frequently, this exaggerated response is in large part a result of the parents themselves having had a history of enuresis; the child's enuresis in effect revives their own previous feelings of anxiety and guilt. They should be informed that with patience and understanding, children generally outgrow this disorder. This is extremely important in preventing the superimposition of severe guilt and anxiety on the enuresis problem through parental mishandling of the bedwetting incidents (Kales and Kales, 1971).

EDUCATIONAL PROGRAMS

As we stressed earlier in this chapter, an extensive and comprehensive education and consultation program is essential to the function of our Sleep Research and Treatment Facility.

In order to make safe, effective treatment of sleep problems a reality for the general population, the findings of the sleep laboratory studies and clinical evaluations must be communicated to physicians, government agencies such as the FDA, and pharmaceutical firms (Fig. 7). The following is a discussion of our efforts to extend our knowledge to these groups.

Physician-Patient

We are hopeful that as physicians become more knowledgeable in the findings of modern sleep research, especially sleep laboratory-clinical studies, they will approach nocturnal disturbances with the same diligence and confidence that they direct to daytime disorders. Not only will the patients be directly benefitted initially, but an indirect benefit will also result as the physician obtains additional clinical information on these disorders, which in turn can be shared with the sleep laboratory-clinician.

One of our major educative efforts was directed toward preparing a scientific exhibit, "Sleep Research in Modern Medicine", which described normal sleep and dream patterns and in addition, findings from the sleep laboratory which related to the evaluation and treatment of disturbed sleep (Kales, 1970). A second scientific exhibit, "The Evaluation and Treatment of Insomnia", deals in depth with this sleep disorder (Kales, 1971). Our third such exhibit, "The Evaluation and Treatment of Sleep Disorders by the General Physician", covers the general field of sleep disturbances with recommendations for treatment of these disorders (Kales, 1973). These three exhibits have been shown at ten national medical and scientific conventions. The exhibits include: movies describing the Sleep Laboratory, normal sleep patterns, and sleep disorders. In addition, educational reprints describing the evaluation and treatment of sleep disorders are distributed.

Food and Drug Administration

A number of basic principles have evolved that are important to the methodology of all drug evaluation studies both clinical and sleep laboratory (Kales and Kales, 1970). These include:

1) allowing for adaptation and readaptation to the sleep laboratory or hospital environment

2) the use of consecutive nights from condition to condition

3) within a given protocol, a second drug can be evaluated only after an adequate withdrawal period has been allowed following administration of the first drug

4) evaluating long-term as well as short-term efficacy, since our studies showed that within a 2-week period, decreased effectiveness had developed for most of the drugs studied.

5) evaluating the withdrawal period. We have demonstrated that significant carry-over occurs with some drugs for sleep induction and maintenance, and as originally pointed out by Oswald and his associates, REM rebound accompanied by increases in dream frequency and intensity often occurs during this period (Oswald and Priest, 1965).

All of these principles are incorporated in our 22-night protocol which is the primary design that we utilize for evaluating short-term and long-term (2 weeks) efficacy as well as sleep stage effects.

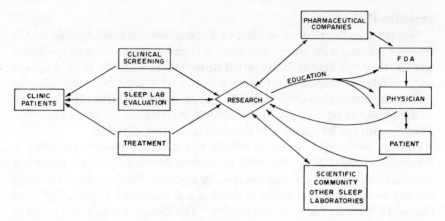

Fig. 7 Multidimensional approach of the Sleep Research and Treatment Facility. Useful and educational information is made available to the general physician, government agencies, and pharmaceutical firms which results in improved diagnosis and treatment of the sleep disorder patient.

The proposed FDA "Guidelines for the Evaluation of New Hypnotic Drugs" contain specific requirements for sleep laboratory evaluations of new hypnotic drugs, based on these methodological recommendations (Kales and Lasagna, 1971).

Since we found that most hypnotic drugs produce decreased efficacy at the end of a 2-week drug-administration period, we are strongly recommending that all hypnotic drugs be evaluated in sleep laboratory studies, including drug-administration periods of 2 weeks to 2 months. Although hypnotic drugs may be prescribed for only brief periods of time, they are often prescribed and used for chronic periods extending for many years. If they are going to be used in this fashion, it is obvious that their efficacy must be proven in an objective manner over such intervals of time.

Pharmaceutical Firms

Until recently, advertisements in medical journals for hypnotic drugs provided the physician with practically no specific information on the effectiveness of the drug or the length of the effectiveness. In these advertisements, references listed are frequently not published articles, but rather information listed as "on file" with the pharmaceutical firm. Generally, the advertisements contain broad unscientific statements to the effect that the specific drug produces "peaceful, sound and uninterrupted sleep". Another typical practice is to advertise the superiority of a drug based on the presence or absence of drug-induced sleep stage alterations. As we do not know the significance of sleep stages or of their suppression, this type of advertising is inaccurate and misleading.

However, some of the recent advertisements have been most informative and scientific and detail the effectiveness of the drug as demonstrated in both sleep laboratory and traditional clinical studies.

We consider the continued effectiveness and safety of a hypnotic drug to be the primary factors in recommending its use. However, there have been very few studies in which the effectiveness of a hypnotic drug has been evaluated beyond several consecutive nights to one week of drug administration. Therefore, with regard to both our concern for properly evaluating the effectiveness of hypnotic drugs, as well as accurately promoting them, we have recommended the following (Kales et al., in press):

1) All hypnotic drugs should be evaluated in traditional and sleep laboratory studies in which the drug is administered for at least two consecutive weeks and in some cases for one month or longer. These recommendations, as mentioned, are now included in the proposed FDA Guidelines for Evaluating Hypnotic Drugs.

2) If a drug is shown to lose its effectiveness within two weeks or a month of consecutive use, then this should be clearly indicated in the package insert and advertising for the drug. If a drug's effectiveness has not been established in such an objective and rigorous manner, then physicians should be aware of this, and of the distinct possibility that the drug may be effective for only a brief period of time.

3) Since we do not know the specific significance of any sleep stage, pharmaceutical firms should not attempt to advertise the superiority of their drug on the basis of the presence or absence of drug-induced sleep stage alterations as this would be incorrect and misleading to the physician.

In this chapter, we have described the role of the Sleep Research and Treatment Facility in the evaluation and treatment of sleep disorders. In our model, the sleep laboratory-clinician serves primarily as a consultant to the primary physician, providing him through Educative Programs, with the latest findings from the Sleep Laboratory and Sleep Disorders Clinic. The sleep laboratory-clinician also serves as a backup resource for evaluating and treating the more complex sleep problems.

REFERENCES

Agnew, H.W., Webb, W.B. and Williams, R.L. Sleep patterns in late middle age males: An EEG study. *Electroenceph, Clin. Neurophysiol.* 23:168-171 (1967)

Aserinsky, E. and Kleitman, N. Regularly occurring periods of eye motility and concomitant phenomena during sleep. *Science 118*:273-224(1953).

Aserinsky, E. and Kleitman, N. Two types of ocular motility occurring in sleep. *J. Appl. Physiol.* 8:1-10(1955).

Armstrong, R.H., Burnap, D., Jacobson, A., Kales, A. Ward, S. and Golden, J.S. Dreams and gastric secretions in duodenal ulcer patients. *New Physician 14*:241-243(1965).

Bindelglas, P.M., Dee, G.H. and Enos, F.A. Medical and psychological factors in enuretic children treated with imipramine hydrocholoride. *Amer. J. Psychiat. 124(8)*:125-130(1968).

Broughton, R.J. Sleep disorders. Disorders of arousal? *Science. 159*:1070-1078(1968).

Dement, W. C. and Kleitman, N. Cyclic variations in EEG during sleep and their relation to eye movements, body motility and dreaming. *Electroenceph. Clin. Neurophysiol.9*:673-690(1957).

Dement, W.C. and Kleitman, N. The Relation of eye movements during sleep to dream activity: An objective method for the study of dreaming. *J. Exper. Psychol.* *53*:339-346(1957).

Dement, W. and Guilleminault, C. A 'position' paper on sleep disorders. presented at the Annual Meeting of the Assoc. Psychophysiological Study of Sleep, San Diego, 1973.

Feinberg, I., Koresko, R.L. and Heller, N. EEG sleep patterns as a function of normal and pathological aging in man. *J. Psychiat. Res.* *5*:107-144(1967).

Fisher, C., Kahn, E., Edwards, A. and Davis, D. Effects of Valium on NREM night terrors. *Psychophysiology* *9(1)*:91(1971).

Fraser, M.S. Nocturnal enuresis. *Practitioner* *208*:203-211 (1972).

Gastaut, H. and Broughton, R.A. A clinical and polygraphic study of episodic phenomena during sleep. in, *Recent Advances Biological Psychiatry*. Vol. 1. J. Wortis, Ed., Plenum Press, New York, 1965, pp197-221.

Kales, A. Sleep research in modern medicine. Reprint from Scientific Exhibit shown at the annual meetings of Amer. Medical Assoc., Amer. Pharmaceutical Assoc., Amer. Psychiatric Assoc., Amer. Acad. of General Practice, Aerospace Medical Association, and American Neurological Assoc., 1970.

Kales, A. Evaluation and treatment of insomnia: A. Introduction to sleep research in modern medicine and B. Sleep laboratory and clinical studies. Reprint from Scientific Exhibit shown at the Amer. Medical Assoc. annual convention, New Orleans, La., November 28-December 1, 1971.

Kales, A. Discussion of a 'position' paper on sleep disorders by W. Dement. Presented at the Annual Meeting of the Assoc. Psychophysiological Study of Sleep, San Diego, 1973.

Kales, A. The Evaluation and treatment of sleep disorders by the general physician. Reprint from Scientific Exhibit shown at the Amer. Psychiatric Assoc. annual convention, Honolulu, Hawaii, 1973.

Kales, A., Jacobson, A., Paulson, M.J., Kales, J.D., and Walter, R.D. Somnambulism: Psychophysiological correlates I. All-night EEG studies. *Arch. Gen. Psychiat.* *14*:586-594(1966a).

Kales, A. Paulson, M.J., Jacobson, A. and Kales, J.D. Somnombulism: Psychophysiological correlates II. Psychiatric interviews, psychological testing and discussion. *Arch. Gen. Psychiat.* *14*:595-604(1966b).

Kales, A., Heuser, G., Jacobson, A., Kales, J.D., Hanley, J., Zweizig, J.R. and Paulson, M.J. All night sleep studies in hypothyroid patients, before and after treatment. *J. Clin. Endocrinol. Metabol.* *27*:1593-1599 (1967a).

Kales, A., Jacobson, A., Kales, J.D., Kun, T., and Weissbuch, R. All-night EEG sleep measurements in young adults. *Psychol. Sci.* *7*:67-68(1967b).

Kales, A., Wilson, T. Kales, J.D., Jacobson, A., Paulson, M.J., Kollar, E., and Walter, R.D. Measurements of all-night sleep in normal elderly persons: Effects of aging. *J. Amer. Ger. Soc.* *15*; 405-414(1967c).

Kales, A., Beall, G.N., Bajor, G.F., Jacobson, A. and Kales, J.D., Sleep studies in asthmatic adults: Relationship of attacks to sleep stage and time of night. *J. Allergy* *41*:164-173(1968a).

Kales, A., Malmstrom, E.J., Rickeles, W.H., Hanley, J., Tan, T.L., Stadel, B., and Hoedemaker, F.S. Sleep patterns of a pentobarbital addict: Before and after withdrawal. *Psychophysiol.* *5*:208(1968b).

Kales, A., Adams, G., Hanley, J., Preston, T., and Rickles, W. Sleep patterns during withdrawal of Tuinal: Effects of Dilantin administration. *Psychophysiology* *6*:262(1969a).

Kales, A. and Jacobson, A. Clinical and electrophysiological studies of somnambulism. in, *Abnormalities of Sleep in Man* (XVth Europ. Meeting on Electroenceph., Bologna, Italy), M. Critchley and H. Gasataut, Eds., 1969, pp. 296-302.

Kales, A., Malmstrom, E.J., Scharf, M.B. and Rubin, R.T. Sleep disturbances following sedative use and withdrawal. in, *Sleep: Physiology and Pathology*, A. Kales, Ed., Philadelphia, J.B. Lippincott, 1969b, pp. 331-343.

Kales, A., Allen, W.C. Jr., Scharf, M.B. and Kales, J.D. Hypnotic drugs and their effectiveness: All-night EEG studies of insomniac subjects. *Arch. Gen. Psychiat. 23*:226-232(1970a).

Kales, A. and Kales, J.D. Sleep laboratory evaluation of psychoactive drugs. *Pharmacol. Physicians 4*:1-6(1970).

Kales, A., Kales, J.D., Scharf, M.B. and Tan, T.L. Hypnotics and altered sleep and dream patterns: II. All-night EEG studies of chloral hydrate, flurazepam and methaqualone. *Arch. Gen. Psychiat. 23*:219-225(1970b).

Kales, A., Kales, J.D., Sly, R.M., Scharf, M.B., Tan, T.L. and Preston, T.A. Sleep patterns of asthmatic children: All night EEG studies. *Allergy 46*:300-308(1970c).

Kales, A., Preston, T., Tan, T.L. and Allen, W.C. Jr. Hypnotics and altered sleep and dream patterns: I. All-night EEG studies of glutethimide, methyprylon and pentobarbital. *Arch. Gen. Psychiat. 23*:211-218(1970d).

Kales, A. Ansel, R.D., Markham, C.H., Scharf, M.B. and Tan, T.L. Sleep in patients with Parkinson's Disease and normal subjects prior to and following levodopa adminstration. *Clin. Pharmacol. Therap. 12*:397-406(1971a).

Kales, A. and Cary, G. Insomnia, evaluation and treatment. in, *Psychiatry, 1971, Medical World News*(Suppl.), E. Robins, Ed., 1971, pp. 55-56.

Kales, A. and Kales, J.D. Evaluation, diagnosis and treatment of clinical conditions related to sleep. *JAMA 123*:229-2235(1971).

Kales, J.D., Kales, A., Bixler, E.O. and Slye, E.S. Effects of placebo and flurazepam on sleep patterns in insomniac subjects. *Clin. Pharmacol. Therap. 12*:691-697(1971b).

Kales, A. and Lasagna, L. (Consultants) Food and drug administration guidelines for the evaluation of new hypnotic drugs. Prepared by a joint committee of the Pharmaceutical Manufacturers Assoc. and the Food and Drug Administration, 1971.

Kales, A., Scharf, M.B., Tan, T.L., Zweizig, J.R., and Alexander, P. Sleep laboratory and clinical studies of the effects of Tofranil, Valium and placebo on sleep stages and enuresis. *Psychophysiology 7*:348(1971c).

Kales, A., Caldwell, A., Goring, P. and Healey, S. Psychological evaluation and treatment studies of insomniac subjects. *Psychophysiology 9*:91 (1972).

Kales, A., Bixler, E.O., Scharf, M.B., and Kales J. Sleep laboratory effectiveness studies of secobarbital and methaqualone. Presented to the 74th Annual Meeting of the Amer. Soc Clinical Pharmacology and Therapeutics, New Orleans, 1973.

Kales, A. and Scharf, M.B., Sleep laboratory and clinical studies of the effects of benzodiazepines on sleep: flurazepam, diazepam, chlordiazepoxide and RO5-4200. in, *The Benzodiazepines,* S. Garattini, E. Mussini, and L.O. Randall, Eds., Raven Press, New York, 1973, pp. 577-598.

Kales, A., Bixler, E.O., Tan T.L., Scharf, M.B., and Kales, J.D. Chronic hypnotic use: Ineffectiveness, drug withdrawal insomnia, and drug dependency. (in press).

Kales, A., Kales, J.D. "Recent Advances in the Diagnoses and Treatment of Sleep Disorders." in, *The Relevance of Sleep Research to Clinical Practice* (American College of Psychiatry) G. Usdin, Ed., Brunner/Mazel Inc. N.Y., 1973, pp. 61-94.

Monroe, L.J. Psychological and physiological differences between good and poor sleepers. *J. Abnorm. Psychol. 72*:255(1967).

Oswald, I., and Thacore, V.R. Amphetamine and phenmetrazine addiction: Physiological abnormalities in the abstinence syndrome. *Brit. Med. J. 2*:427(1963).

Oswald, I and Priest, R.G. Five weeks to escape the sleeping pill habit. *Brit Med. J. 2*:1093-1099(1965).

Sours, J.A., Frumkin, P. and Indermill, R. Somnambulism. *Arch. Gen. Psychiat. 9*:112-125(1963).

Wyatt, R., Kupfer, D.J., Scott, J., Robinson, D.S. and Snyder, F. Longitudinal studies of the effects of monoamine oxidase inhibitors on sleep in man. *Psycholopharmacologia (Berlin) 15*:236-244(1969).

Index